日英対訳
Japanese & English

リンパ浮腫の
外科的治療

東京大学 名誉教授
広島大学病院国際リンパ浮腫治療センター 特任教授

編集　光嶋　勲

Professor Emeritus of the University of Tokyo

*Professor and Chief of the International Center
for Lymphedema , Hiroshima University Hospital*

Edited by **Isao Koshima**

Surgical
Treatments
for
Lymphedema

ぱーそん書房

●執筆者一覧

●編集

光嶋　　勲（東京大学 名誉教授、広島大学病院国際リンパ浮腫治療センター 特任教授）

●執筆者（執筆順）

辛川　　領（東京大学医学部形成外科・美容外科）

伊藤　太智（東京大学医学部形成外科・美容外科）

水田　栄樹（国立がん研究センター東病院形成外科）

森下　悠也（東京大学医学部形成外科・美容外科）

森脇　裕太（東京大学医学部形成外科・美容外科）

光嶋　　勲（東京大学 名誉教授、広島大学病院国際リンパ浮腫治療センター 特任教授）

小谷　正彦（熊本大学 名誉教授、京都医療技術短期大学 名誉教授）

飯田　拓也（東京大学医学部形成外科・美容外科 准教授）

播摩　光宣（東京大学医学部形成外科・美容外科）

関　　征央（聖マリアンナ医科大学形成外科）

山下　修二（東京大学医学部形成外科・美容外科 特任講師）

加藤　　基（埼玉県立小児医療センター形成外科・リンパ外来）

山本　　匠（国立国際医療研究センター形成外科 診療科長）

山本　奈奈（東京都立墨東病院形成外科）

林　　明辰（地方独立行政法人総合病院国保旭中央病院形成外科 医長）

三浦　真弘（大分大学医学部医学系研究科生体構造医学講座 講師）

濱田　裕一（日本赤十字社福岡赤十字病院形成外科）

平島　正則（神戸大学大学院医学研究科生理学・細胞生物学講座血管生物学分野 准教授）

原　　尚子（埼玉県済生会川口総合病院リンパ外科・再建外科 医長）

三原　　誠（埼玉県済生会川口総合病院リンパ外科・再建外科 主任医長）

林　　伸子（地方独立行政法人総合病院国保旭中央病院形成外科）

大島　　梓（国立がん研究センター東病院形成外科）

成島　三長（三重大学医学部形成外科 教授）

戸所　　健（高島平中央総合病院 総合医局長・形成外科）

田代　絢亮（国立がん研究センター中央病院形成外科・東京大学医学部形成外科・美容外科）

江﨑　太一（東京女子医科大学医学部解剖学・発生生物学講座 教授・講座主任）

吉田　周平（広島大学国際リンパ浮腫治療センター）

●List of Authors

●Editor

Isao Koshima (Professor Emeritus, the University of Tokyo/Professor and Chief, the International Center for Lymphedema, Hiroshima University Hospital)

●Authors (order of writing)

Ryo Karakawa (Department of Plastic, Reconstructive and Aesthetic Surgery, Faculty of Medicine, the University of Tokyo)

Taichi Ito (Department of Plastic, Reconstructive and Aesthetic Surgery, Faculty of Medicine, the University of Tokyo)

Haruki Mizuta (Department of Plastic Surgery, National Cancer Center Hospital East)

Yuya Morishita (Department of Plastic, Reconstructive and Aesthetic Surgery, Faculty of Medicine, the University of Tokyo)

Yuta Moriwaki (Department of Plastic, Reconstructive and Aesthetic Surgery, Faculty of Medicine, the University of Tokyo)

Isao Koshima (Professor Emeritus, the University of Tokyo/Professor and Chief, the International Center for Lymphedema, Hiroshima University Hospital)

Masahiko Kotani (Professor Emeritus, University of Kumamoto and Kyoto College of Medical Science)

Takuya Iida (Associate Professor, Department of Plastic, Reconstructive and Aesthetic Surgery, Faculty of Medicine, the University of Tokyo)

Mitsunobu Harima (Department of Plastic, Reconstructive and Aesthetic Surgery, Faculty of Medicine, the University of Tokyo)

Yukio Seki (Department of Plastic and Reconstructive Surgery, St. Marianna University School of Medicine)

Shuji Yamashita (Assistant Professor, Department of Plastic, Reconstructive and Aesthetic Surgery, Faculty of Medicine, the University of Tokyo)

Motoi Kato (Department of Plastic Surgery/Lymph Clinic, Saitama Children's Medical Center)

Takumi Yamamoto (Chief, Department of Plastic and Reconstructive Surgery, National Center for Global Health and Medicine)

Nana Yamamoto (Department of Plastic Surgery, Tokyo Metropolitan Bokutoh Hospital)

Akitatsu Hayashi (Assistant Chief, Department of Plastic and Reconstructive Surgery, Asahi General Hospital)

Masahiro Miura (Senior Lecturer, Department of Human Anatomy, Faculty of Medicine, Oita University)

Yuichi Hamada (Department of Plastic Surgery, Japanese Red Cross Fukuoka Hospital)

Masanori Hirashima (Associate Professor, Division of Vascular Biology, Kobe University Graduate School of Medicine)

Hisako Hara (Medical Director, Department of Lymphatic and Reconstructive Surgery, Saiseikai Kawaguchi General Hospital)

Makoto Mihara (Chief Medical Director, Department of Lymphatic and Reconstructive Surgery, Saiseikai Kawaguchi General Hospital)

Nobuko Hayashi (Department of Plastic and Reconstructive Surgery, Asahi General Hospital)

Azusa Oshima (Department of Plastic Surgery, National Cancer Center Hospital East)

Mitsunaga Narushima (Professor, Department of Plastic Surgery, Faculty of Medicine, Mie University)

Takeshi Todokoro (General Director, Department of Plastic Surgery, Takashimadaira Chuo General Hospital)

Kensuke Tashiro (Department of Plastic Surgery, National Cancer Center Hospital/Department of Plastic, Reconstructive and Aesthetic Surgery, Faculty of Medicine, the University of Tokyo)

Taichi Ezaki (Professor and Chief, Department of Anatomy and Developmental Biology, Faculty of Medicine, Tokyo Women's Medical University)

Shuhei Yoshida (The International Center for Lymphedema, Hiroshima University Hospital)

序　文

　この度「リンパ浮腫の外科的治療」が出版されることになった。本書は 2011 年に出版した「よくわかるリンパ浮腫のすべて」（永井書店刊）の姉妹編でもあるが、この書籍は極めて好評で、特に海外のリンパ浮腫を専門とする外科医から英語訳の要望が多く出ていた。そこで今回は、日本語に加えて英語翻訳を行い、われわれのもとで研修を行った海外の多くの外科医にその滞在中に快く英文添削を行って頂いた。日英表記されたこの書籍が今後、医療のみならず日本の保守的出版業界に革命を起こしてくれることを期待している。また、リンパ浮腫治療にかかわる世界中の多くの専門家にとっても、本書が最新のバイブルとなることを願っている。

　全国のリンパ浮腫患者は、2009 年の時点で 10 万人とも 15 万人ともいわれている。海外も含めると、膨大な患者が理学療法さえも受けられず苦悩している。リンパ浮腫の治療は、圧迫療法を中心とした理学療法が行われ外科治療は否定され続けてきた。連日のスリーブ・ストッキングの着用は浮腫の増悪予防には必須であるが、患者たちにとっては身体的にも精神的にも大きな負担である。このため患者は浮腫と同時に理学療法からの解放を外科療法に求め続けてきたが、外科医はその期待に100％応ずることはできなかった。

　近年、基礎分野でのリンパ管の機能に関する研究やリンパ系の解剖、リンパ管の新生や再生など分子細胞生物学の研究が急速に進んできた。これらの基礎を基盤として、本邦において 1990 年以後、臨床の分野で超微小血管吻合手技（スーパーマイクロサージャリー）を用いた低侵襲のリンパ管細静脈吻合術（LVA）が開発された。その後、この術式による著効例が報告され、血管柄付きリンパ管・リンパ節移植など新たな術式も急速に開発されつつある。さらに、2007 年以後、われわれのグループによって ICG 蛍光リンパ管造影法が導入され、手術が容易となり残っているリンパ管機能が推測でき、stage 0 の浮腫の診断や浮腫予防までもが可能となってきた。これらの術式・診断法は本邦から発信され、2000 年以降、海外のライブ手術でその術式を供覧したことで外科的治療法は世界各国に広まった。この発達の背景には、リンパ学の基礎と臨床の両分野における舟岡（京大）や山田（名大）など本邦の先駆者たちの激動の時代下での独自の努力がその礎にあったことを忘れてはならない。

　本書はリンパ系の仕組み、浮腫の分類、症状、検査・診断、そして過去と最新の外科治療までをわかりやすく簡潔にまとめた。中でも ICG 蛍光造影を用いたリンパ管の還流機能評価、超微小外科手技を用いたこれまでの外科的治療の変遷にまで踏み込んでリンパ管について詳細に解説した書籍は、海外を含めて類をみないであろう。

　リンパ浮腫の外科的治療に携わる基礎と臨床のそれぞれの専門分野の集大成がここに完成したことは大きな喜びである。本書は、今後各分野の専門家が手を取り合ってリンパ浮腫という難治疾患に対する新たな治療法を開発する礎になるであろう。

編者は本書の完成と同時に、13年間にわたりリンパ浮腫の外科治療の開発を行ってきた東京大学を定年退職することになったが、この間、約300名の外国人留学者や邦人約150名の熱い心をもったリンパ浮腫の専門家を目指す若手医師とともに術式の進化に邁進してきた。本書はこれまで得られた知見のまとめとして完成させたものである。幸いにも、本年4月から新しい職場である広島大学付属病院に国際リンパ浮腫治療センターの開設とともに、さらなる内外の専門家の育成や術式の進化を行う機会を得ることができた。今後は広島の地において新しいリンパ学の創設と海外への発信を行いたいと考えている。

　最後になったが、本書の刊行にあたり、東大時代に私の秘書を長く勤めてくれた山崎連子さんには大変お世話になった。ここに記して謝意を表したい。また、本書の完成は、姉妹本に引き続き永井書店から独立されたぱーそん書房の山本美惠子さんの情熱によるものである。忙殺される編者を絶えず激励して頂いた彼女の貢献に深く感謝したい。

―第8回世界リンパ浮腫外科治療シンポジウム招待講演（2017.3.16 バルセロナ・サンパウ病院）の帰路、機内にて―

編者　光嶋　勲

Preface

This textbook is the renewal of primary publication on lymphedema published in 2011. It was Japanese edition and very popular, but many foreigners were eager to be edited in English. Therefore, this time, we translated English in addition to Japanese, and many overseas surgeons who conducted training under us got pleasantly corrected English sentences during their stay. With their great contribution, the second version is published in both Japanese and English styles. This bilingual trial is very rare in Japanese publishers, so I strongly expect this would be a revolution in conservative culture of Japanese publications. Also, I expect this would be new bible for specialists in all over the world.

Now many patients are suffered lymphedema, at 2009, lymphedema patients throughout our country are said to be 150,000 or 100,000 people, but almost all of them are left without any treatments. Even if they treated with physio and compression therapy, many especially in hot area feel discomfort for daily compression to prevent progression of edema. Although wearing sleeve stockings every day is indispensable for prevention of exacerbation of edema, it is a heavy burden both physically and mentally for patients. For this reason, the patient has been requesting surgical therapy to open up from physiotherapy at the same time as edema, but the surgeon could not respond to that expectation 100%. After 1990, surgeries for lymphedema were started but until 1990, those were denied and physiotherapy used be mainly employed.

Recently, based on the basic knowledges on lymphatic systems, which have been rapidly well known, low invasive new lymphaticovenular anastomosis using supermicrosurgery was established by the editor after 1990. This techniques and related surgical methods such as vascularized lymphatic channel transfers have been also developed for lymphatic diseases including lethal lymphedema. In 2007, ICG fluorography was also reported by our group to detect the channels and evaluate remaining lymph-drainage functions. These techniques and knowledges were rapidly popularized in the world after demonstrating in live surgeries in many foreign countries. In the background of these clinical advancements, we should remember the preliminary works by Japanese specialists including Prof. Funaoka in University of Kyoto, and Dr. Yamada in University of Nagoya.

In this text book, it was summarized on anatomy of lymphatic systems, classification, symptoms, examinations and diagnosis, past and present update history on surgery for lymphedema. Among them, the detailed evaluation of lymphatic vessel reflux function using ICG fluorescence imaging has the originality. Also, this book describes detailed stepping into the transition of conventional surgical treatments and ultra-microsurgical techniques which is not regarded as books in other countries.

Combination of basic and clinical knowledge is very important for advanced treatments for lymphedema. I believe this textbook would be a keystone to open new strategies in future.

At the end of March in this year, the editor retired the University of Tokyo, where I proceeded to establish new concepts and surgical treatments for lymphatic diseases. During the last 13 years, 300 foreign and 150 Japanese doctors are worked together. The editor has now established and proposed new surgical treatments in the International Center of Lymphedema in the University of Hiroshima.

Finally, I would like to thank for two women. Mrs Renko Yamasaki, my secretary in the University of Tokyo, took care many foreign visitors and gave us great effort to complete this book. Also, Ms Mieko Yamamoto, who used to be a member of Nagai Publisher and now become owner of Person Publish Company, dedicated to publish this text book as well as the first version from Nagai Publisher. She always encouraged the editor to complete the publication. I sincerely thank for their great contribution.

—Described in the flight back to Tokyo after the invited key note lecture (March 16, 2017), The eighth Annual International Symposium of Lymphedema in SanPau Hospital in Baecelona—

Editor *Isao KOSHIMA*

■目　次

1. 歴史─リンパ浮腫の外科療法

──────────────（辛川　領、伊藤太智、水田栄樹、森下悠也、森脇裕太、光嶋　勲）**1**

 Ⅰ.リンパ研究と外科治療の歴史 ······································· 1
 Ⅱ.リンパシンチグラム法 ··· 5
 Ⅲ.リンパ浮腫外科治療法の歴史 ····································· 6
 Ⅳ.リンパ管吻合術 ··· 12
 Ⅴ.合併外科治療：予防的リンパ管細静脈吻合術 ················· 21

●Important Reference
 【リンパ節郭清後のリンパ節の再生とリンパ道の回復について】──（小谷正彦）**25**
  1. リンパ節の再生…25
  2. リンパ道の回復…26

2. 解　剖 ──────────────────────── 27

1 頭頸部領域におけるリンパ解剖 ─────────────（飯田拓也）27
 Ⅰ.頭部のリンパ節 ··· 27
 Ⅱ.顔面、頭部のリンパ流 ··· 28
 Ⅲ.頸部のリンパ節 ··· 29
 Ⅳ.MSKCC(Memorial Sloan-Kettering Cancer Center)分類 ········· 31
 Ⅴ.頭頸部のリンパに関する臨床との関係 ························· 32

2 四肢のリンパ管解剖 ───────────────────（播摩光宣）34
 Ⅰ.四肢リンパ管のミクロ解剖 ······································· 34
 Ⅱ.上肢リンパ管のマクロ解剖 ······································· 36
 Ⅲ.下肢リンパ管のマクロ解剖 ······································· 38

3. 分　類 ──────────────────────── 41

1 リンパ浮腫の分類 ──────────────────── (関　征央) 41
 Ⅰ.特発性リンパ浮腫 ··· 41
 Ⅱ.続発性リンパ浮腫 ··· 44

i

2 リンパ浮腫症候群 ———————————————（山下修二）**47**
Ⅰ. ターナー症候群 ······························· 47
Ⅱ. ヌーナン症候群 ······························· 48
Ⅲ. ミルロイ病 ································· 49
Ⅳ. Milroy-like lymphedema ······················ 50
Ⅴ. MCLMR 症候群 ···························· 50
Ⅵ. Lymphedema distichiasis syndrome ················· 51
Ⅶ. メージュ病 ································· 51
Ⅷ. Hennekam 症候群 ·························· 51
Ⅸ. WILD 症候群 ····························· 52

4. 病態・重症度評価 ———————————————— 54

1 リンパ浮腫の病態 ——————————————（加藤　基）**54**
Ⅰ. むくみとリンパ ······························ 54
Ⅱ. リンパ浮腫の種類 ····························· 56
Ⅲ. リンパ浮腫の病態 ····························· 59
Ⅳ. リンパ浮腫の進行・ステージ分類 ··················· 61

2 リンパ管変性・硬化 ———————（山本　匠、山本奈奈、林　明辰）**64**
Ⅰ. リンパ流閉塞によるリンパ循環の変化 ················· 64
Ⅱ. リンパ浮腫の進行とリンパ管変性・硬化 ················ 65
Ⅲ. ICG リンパ管造影所見によるリンパ管硬化の評価 ··········· 67

3 ICG リンパ管造影による病態生理的重症度評価 ————（山本　匠）**70**
Ⅰ. リンパ循環動態の変化と身体所見による評価 ·············· 70
Ⅱ. ダイナミック ICG リンパ管造影によるリンパ循環動態の評価 ····· 71
Ⅲ. ICG リンパ管造影所見と DB stage ·················· 74
Ⅳ. 原発性リンパ浮腫の評価と ICG 分類 ················· 81

●Important Reference
【四肢リンパ浮腫患者の走査電子顕微鏡所見—リンパ管静脈吻合術で観察される
皮下組織の微細構造的特徴】————————————（三浦真弘、濱田裕一）**86**
　　1. LVA にて術中観察される皮下組織内の構造的特徴（電顕所見）···88
　　2. まとめ···101

●Important Reference
【遺伝子変異マウスの胎児浮腫とリンパ管形成異常】——————（平島正則）**103**
　　1. 胎児浮腫···103

2. リンパ管の発生…104

3. リンパ管形成異常をきたす遺伝子変異…107

5. 術前評価 ——————————————— 112

1 CT・MRI ————————————————（原　尚子）112
Ⅰ. CT ……………………………………………………………… 112
Ⅱ. MRI ……………………………………………………………… 114

2 リンパシンチグラフィ・SPECT-CT ——————（原　尚子、三原　誠）119
Ⅰ. リンパシンチグラフィ ……………………………………………… 119
Ⅱ. SPECT-CT ……………………………………………………… 126
Ⅲ. 種々の画像診断の比較 …………………………………………… 127

3 エコーによるリンパ管の同定とリンパ浮腫の評価
——————————————————（林　明辰、林　伸子）129
Ⅰ. エコーによるリンパ管の同定と手術への応用 ……………………… 130
Ⅱ. Real-time Elastography を用いたリンパ浮腫の評価 ……………… 132

4 ICG リンパ管造影を用いた術前評価 ——————（山本　匠）135
Ⅰ. ICG リンパ管造影所見の評価 …………………………………… 135
Ⅱ. 造影所見による術中所見予測 …………………………………… 137
Ⅲ. 術前評価における Linear パターンの意義 ……………………… 139
Ⅳ. ICG リンパ管造影所見に基づいた手術戦略 …………………… 140
Ⅴ. DB stage に応じた治療戦略 …………………………………… 142

5 早期診断 ————————————————————（大島　梓）148
Ⅰ. 早期診断 ………………………………………………………… 148
Ⅱ. 予測・予防 ……………………………………………………… 153

6. 治療方針・適応 ——————————————— 156

1 二次性リンパ浮腫の治療方針 ——（山本　匠、山本奈奈、林　明辰、成島三長）156
Ⅰ. 二次性リンパ浮腫の病態 ………………………………………… 156
Ⅱ. 二次性リンパ浮腫の診断と重症度評価 ………………………… 157
Ⅲ. 二次性リンパ浮腫の治療戦略 …………………………………… 159
Ⅳ. 不顕性リンパ浮腫の概念と予防的治療 ………………………… 163

2 原発性リンパ浮腫の治療方針 ——（山本　匠、山本奈奈、林　明辰、成島三長）167
Ⅰ. 原発性リンパ浮腫の病態 ………………………………………… 167

Ⅱ. 原発性リンパ浮腫の診断と ICG リンパ管造影分類 ················· 168
　Ⅲ. 原発性リンパ浮腫の治療戦略 ············· 169

3　骨盤リンパ嚢胞の治療 ─────────── （戸所　健）**172**
　Ⅰ. 骨盤リンパ嚢胞とは ················· 172
　Ⅱ. 随伴症状 ················· 173
　Ⅲ. 既存の治療法について ················· 174
　Ⅳ. LVA の適応について ················· 175
　Ⅴ. 治療プロトコール ················· 175
　Ⅵ. 症例・結果 ················· 177

7. 外科治療 ───────────────── 180

1　リンパ管細静脈吻合術（LVA） ─────── （林　明辰）**180**
　Ⅰ. 術前評価・適応 ················· 181
　Ⅱ. 必要な器具・技術 ················· 184
　Ⅲ. 手術手技 ················· 186
　Ⅳ. 吻合方法 ················· 189
　Ⅴ. 周術期管理 ················· 192
　Ⅵ. 術後評価 ················· 193
　Ⅶ. 症例 ················· 197

2　リンパ脂肪弁によるリンパ管移植法 ──── （田代絢亮、光嶋　勲）**201**
　Ⅰ. 手術法 ················· 202
　Ⅱ. 症例提示 ················· 204
　Ⅲ. 考察 ················· 208

3　リンパ節移植 ───────────── （原　尚子）**211**
　Ⅰ. 総論 ················· 211
　Ⅱ. リンパ節移植の適応 ················· 215
　Ⅲ. Reverse lymphatic mapping ················· 216
　Ⅳ. 乳房再建とリンパ節移植 ················· 216
　Ⅴ. リンパ節移植の応用 ················· 217

●Important Reference
【リンパ学に残された不思議―リンパ系と脂肪とのかかわり―】 ──── （江﨑太一）**219**
　　1. リンパ組織と脂肪組織は共に細網組織を基本構築としている…220
　　2. 油でリンパ管腫が誘導される…221
　　3. リンパ組織は加齢とともに脂肪化（加齢退縮）をきたす…222

4. リンパ組織はステロイドホルモンの影響を受けやすい…223

　　5. 慢性リンパ浮腫や自己免疫病は女性に多い…224

4 Brorson 法 ——————————————————————（原　尚子）**229**
Ⅰ. 手術手技………………………………………………………… 230
Ⅱ. 術後の圧迫療法………………………………………………… 230
Ⅲ. 合併症…………………………………………………………… 231
Ⅳ. 長期経過………………………………………………………… 231
Ⅴ. 脂肪吸引術後の患肢の血流…………………………………… 231
Ⅵ. 脂肪吸引術とリンパ管機能…………………………………… 232
Ⅶ. 考察……………………………………………………………… 232

5 合併外科治療 ——————————————————————（吉田周平）**235**
Ⅰ. 術前評価・適応………………………………………………… 236
Ⅱ. 手術手技………………………………………………………… 236
Ⅲ. 周術期評価・管理……………………………………………… 241
Ⅳ. 術後評価………………………………………………………… 241

6 症例提示 ————（辛川　領、伊藤太智、水田栄樹、森下悠也、森脇裕太、光嶋　勲）**243**
Ⅰ. リンパ管細静脈吻合術………………………………………… 243
Ⅱ. 顕微鏡下リンパ管細静脈吻合術……………………………… 244
Ⅲ. 症例……………………………………………………………… 249
Ⅳ. 外科療法と圧迫療法の併用…………………………………… 258
Ⅴ. 両側性下肢リンパ浮腫の頻度と予防………………………… 264
Ⅵ. 予防的吻合術の必要性………………………………………… 265
Ⅶ. 陰部リンパ浮腫（瘻）………………………………………… 265

7 その他の外科治療および有用なテクニック ———————————— 268
a. IVaS 法を用いた LVA ————————————————（成島三長）**268**
Ⅰ. IVaS 法とは…………………………………………………… 269
Ⅱ. IVaS 法の実際………………………………………………… 269
Ⅲ. さまざまな吻合法……………………………………………… 272

b. LVA 小技集 ————————————————————（山本　匠）**278**
Ⅰ. 術野の展開……………………………………………………… 278
Ⅱ. 脈管の準備……………………………………………………… 280
Ⅲ. 吻合……………………………………………………………… 283

c. The Superior-Edge-of-the-Knee Incision method
—Effective LVA for lower extremity lymphedema— ——— (関　征央) **289**
Ⅰ. SEKI 法に必要な基本吻合技術 ……………………………………… 291
Ⅱ. SEKI 法の手術方法 ……………………………………………… 292
Ⅲ. SEKI 法の治療効果とメカニズム …………………………………… 295

8. 今後の展望 ——（辛川　領、伊藤太智、水田栄樹、森下悠也、森脇裕太、光嶋　勲）**299**
Ⅰ. 世界におけるリンパ浮腫外科治療の現況 ………………………………… 299
Ⅱ. リンパ浮腫外科治療の世界のパイオニアたち ………………………… 301
Ⅲ. 今後の治療戦略：より効果的な外科的治療法の必要性 ………………… 305
Ⅳ. 今後の治療の進め方：チーム医療を含めて ………………………… 306

■ CONTENTS

1. History of surgical treatment for lymphedema
—— (Ryo Karakawa, Taichi Ito, Haruki Mizuta, Yuya Morishita, Yuta Moriwaki, Isao Koshima) **1**

●Important Reference
【Regeneration of lymph nodes and recovery of the lymphatic tract after lymph node dissection】 ——————————— (Masahiko Kotani/Ryo Karakawa) **25**

2. Anatomy ———————————————————————— 27
1　Lymphatic anatomy in head and neck region ————— (Takuya Iida) 27
2　Anatomy of the lymphatic vessels in the limbs —— (Mitsunobu Harima) 34

3. Classification ——————————————————————— 41
1　Classification of lymphedema ———————————— (Yukio Seki) 41
2　Lymphedema syndrome ———————————— (Shuji Yamashita) 47

4. Assessment of clinical condition and severity ————— 54
1　Pathophysiology of lymphedema ————————— (Motoi Kato) 54

CONTENTS

2 Lymphatic vessels' degeneration and sclerosis
——————————— (Takumi Yamamoto, Nana Yamamoto, Akitatsu Hayashi) **64**

3 Pathophysiological severity staging using dynamic ICG lymphography
——————————————————————— (Takumi Yamamoto) **70**

●Important Reference
〔Scanning electron microscopy findings in patients with lower-and upper-extremity lymphedema : fine-structure characteristics of subcutaneous tissues observed during lymphaticovenous anastomosis〕
——————————————————— (Masahiro Miura, Yuichi Hamada) **86**

●Important Reference
〔Embryonic edema and defective lymphatic vascular development in gene mutant mice〕 ——————————————— (Masanori Hirashima) **103**

5. Preoperative evaluation —————————————————— 112

1 CT・MRI ———————————————————— (Hisako Hara) **112**

2 Lymphoscintigraphy and SPECT-CT ——— (Hisako Hara, Makoto Mihara) **119**

3 Identification of the lymphatic vessels and evaluation of lymphedema using ultrasound ——— (Akitatsu Hayashi, Nobuko Hayashi) **129**

4 Preoperative evaluation using ICG lymphography
——————————————————————— (Takumi Yamamoto) **135**

5 Early diagnosis ————————————————— (Azusa Oshima) **148**

6. Treatment plan and indication —————————————— 156

1 Management of secondary lymphedema
——— (Takumi Yamamoto, Nana Yamamoto, Akitatsu Hayashi, Mitsunaga Narushima) **156**

2 Management of primary lymphedema
——— (Takumi Yamamoto, Nana Yamamoto, Akitatsu Hayashi, Mitsunaga Narushima) **167**

3 Treatment of pelvic lymphocele ——————————— (Takeshi Todokoro) **172**

7. Surgical treatment ———————————————————— 180

1 Lymphaticovenular anastomosis(LVA) ——————— (Akitatsu Hayashi) **180**

2 Lymphadiposal flaps for severe leg edema functional reconstruction for lymph drainage system
——————————————— (Kensuke Tashiro, Isao Koshima/Shuhei Yoshida) **201**

3 Lymph node transfer ———————————————— (Hisako Hara) **211**

●Important Reference
〔The mysteries in lymphology—Relationships between the lymphatic system and the fat—〕 ————————————————————— (Taichi Ezaki) **219**

vii

4 Brorson's method ——————————————— (Hisako Hara) **229**

5 Treatment of surgery for a complication ———————— (Shuhei Yoshida) **235**

6 Case presentation
 – (Ryo Karakawa, Taichi Ito, Haruki Mizuta, Yuya Morishita, Yuta Moriwaki, Isao Koshima) **243**

7 Other surgical treatment and valuable technique ——————— **268**
 a. IVaS (intravascular stenting) method for LVA - (Mitsunaga Narushima) **268**
 b. Little tricks for LVA ————————————— (Takumi Yamamoto) **278**
 c. The Superior-Edge-of-the-Knee Incision method
 —Effective LVA for lower extremity lymphedema— ———————— (Yukio Seki) **289**

8. Future prospects
 – (Ryo Karakawa, Taichi Ito, Haruki Mizuta, Yuya Morishita, Yuta Moriwaki, Isao Koshima) **299**

■ English Check (Alphabetical order)

Chih-Sheng, Lai (Division of Plastic and Reconstructive Surgery, Taichung Veterans General Hospital, Taiwan)

Dalia Tobbia (Division of Plastic, Reconstructive and Microsurgery, Plastische Chirurgie am Klosterstern Medical Center, Germany)

Jan Bumbera (Hospital Košice-Šaca, Slovakia)

Jeff Chang (Division of Plastic Surgery, Stanford Hospital, USA)

Jin Wang (Department of Breast Surgery, Beijing Renhe Hospital of Peking University, China)

Karan Shetty (Dr. Tulip's Obesity & Diabetes Surgery Centre, India)

Sanket Shetty (Bhagwati Hospital, India)

CHAPTER **1**

History of surgical treatment for lymphedema

歴史—リンパ浮腫の外科療法

■ I ■ リンパ研究と外科治療の歴史

　1622年、Aselliusは、イヌにミルクを飲ませた後に開腹したところ、腸間膜に白く染まっている部位があることを報告し、それを乳び管と命名した。これが初めてのリンパ管の発見であった。1650年、Paquetは動物で胸管を発見している。1692年、Anton Nuckはリンパ管の描出に水銀が非常に有効であることを発見した。水銀を皮下に注入すると、微小な管腔臓器が描出される。それ以後、ヒト死体におけるリンパ系組織の解明が進んだ。Cruckshank（1786）やPaolo Mascagni（1787）、Sappey（1874）やほかの多くの開拓者たちが水銀を使用して、詳細なリンパ系の解剖を明らかにした。1874年、Sappeyは正確な全身のリンパ系を詳細で美しい解剖図で示した。しかし、水銀は毒性があるため使用が禁じられ、同様の実験は行えなくなった。さらに、水銀は室温で揮発するために、死体解剖時にも使用できなくなった。1896年、Gerotaは水銀の代用品としてテレビン油より精製されるプルシャンブルーを発見した。プルシャンブルーを使用することで、肉眼的にも顕微鏡下にもはっきりと脈管構造を認識できるようになった。1909年、Bartelsはこの手法で非常に優れたリンパ系解剖の教科書をつくった。この物質では、注入した部分の近傍までしか染色されなかったため、彼らの研究は、小児や胎児のみにとどまり短い距離のリンパ系の描出に非常に優れた功績を残した。しかしこの方法では、成人における染色は不可能で、体表面上の限られた部位のリンパ管においては有用でも、全体のリンパ系を観察することはできなかった。このような理由で、リンパ系の解明には、放射線学的な解析は行われず、一部の体表面上リンパ管の理解にのみ終わっていた。

　20世紀に入り、臨床の分野でリンパ系の解析が大いに進んだ。HudackとMcMasterは水溶性の染色液であるパテントブルーを皮下に注入すると、徐々に皮下のリンパ管に広がり、染色されることを発見した。同様の手法を利用して、1952年にKinmonthによってリンパ管造影検査が確立された。Kinmonthの手法は、リンパ管を描出するために四肢末梢皮下に染色液を注射し、リンパ管を染色したところで、局麻下に発見したリンパ管に水溶性の造影剤を注入する手技であった。この方法によって、リンパ管を放射線学的に描出することが初めて可能になった。しかしこの方法には、注入後の2時間は体動してはいけないこと、1回の検査で1つのリンパ管しか検査できないという2つの欠点があったことから、リンパ管造影は徐々に行われなくなり、代わりに悪性腫瘍のリンパ節転移の検索にはCTが用いられるようになってきた[1]。

　本邦においては1774年に、杉田玄白、前野良沢によって『解体新書』が完成し胸管の記載がみられる。京都大学解剖学初代教授の足立文太郎は、ヒトの動静脈の解剖研究とともにリンパ管の研究に情熱を傾けた。足立の後を継いだ京大解剖学の舟岡省吾教授は、Kinmonthよりも早く、世界で初めてリンパ管造影を行いドイツ語論文として発表している（1930）。彼の研究はヨード製剤

を家ウサギの顎下リンパ節、膝窩リンパ節に注入して、輸出リンパ管を造影した後、首や膝の屈伸運動を行わせることによりリンパの流れが受動的に促進されること、造影剤を精巣に注入して胸管を造影し、呼吸運動によって流れが変化することを観察している（**Fig. 1-1**）[2)3)]。当時は日本から海外に向けた外国語論文が出ることは極めて稀であった。光嶋がハーバード大学医学部留学中に過去の再建外科分野の歴史を勉強中に、舟岡先生の鮮明なリンパ管造影結果の示された論文を発見したときは大変感激した。京都大学で舟岡先生の著書を探すのは難しいようであるが、ハーバード大学の地下書庫では現在でも閲覧できる。また、舟岡は日本で初めてリンパ液の化学的組成の研究に取り組んだようである。

1928 年、Milroy は、先天性家族性リンパ浮腫の症例を最初に報告している。1953 年頃より、リンパ管シンチグラフィが行われるようになった。これはラジオアイソトープを腫瘍周囲に注入し、その放射活性をリンパ系に沿って追うものである。悪性黒色腫や乳癌において、センチネルリンパ節検査が必須のものとなっている。これはパテントブルーとラジオアイソトープを使って、腫瘍の広がりを確認し、リンパ節郭清部位を決定する方法である。1967 年に Spalteholtz & Spanner は、リンパ管の分布に関する詳細な解剖図譜を発表している[1)]。

これまでの各種リンパ管造影による解剖学的検索結果の致命的な欠点は、集合リンパ管同士の交通枝が確認されていないことである。手術中のリンパ管の観察で、集合リンパ管には至るところに多数の交通枝が存在することが最近わかった。筆者が推測するには、これまでのリンパ管造影法では、弁があるためリンパ管は順向性にしか造影されないためであろう。また、末梢は太く、中枢側は細いといわれるが、これはアーチファクトで実際の像とは異なるものと思われる。

最近のリンパ管観察法に関して、2005 年に Suami（須網）& Taylor らは、ヒト成人屍体におけるリンパ系の新しい描出技法を開発した。これにより、過酸化水素より発生する酸素の泡は、リンパ管を描出するのに非常に適した薬剤であることが証明された。過酸化水素を使用することで、微小血管とリンパ管をはっきりと区別することができるようになった。混合造影剤を注入することで、X 線上でも肉眼的に見るのと同じくらいはっきりとリンパ管を確認できるようになった。須網は、この手法を用いて上肢と胸部の詳細なリンパ管の分布を報告した[4)−7)]。さらに、最近では、大橋ら（信州大学）は、実験でリンパ管の収縮機序に関して詳細な研究を行っている。また、佐藤（東京医科歯科大学解剖学名誉教授）は、主に骨盤腔・胸郭腔内や縦隔部のリンパ管の詳細な解剖を明らかにした。

I. The history of lymph research and surgical treatment

In 1622, Asellius observed that dog's mesenteric lymphatics were stained white after he fed the dog some milk, so he named them lymphatic vessels. This was the first discovery of lymphatic vessel. In 1650, Paquet delineated thoracic duct in animals. In 1692, Anton Nuck found that mercury was very effective on detection of lymphatics because it could figure out small organs after being injected within subcutaneous tissue. Thereafter, the elucidation of lymphatic system in cadavers was improved. Cruckshank (1786), Paolo Mascagni (1787), Sappey (1874) and many other pioneers reported detailed anatomy of lymphatic system by using mercury. In 1874, Sappey used detailed and beautiful anatomical drawings to show correct whole body lymphatic system. However, mercury was prohibited because of its toxicity so that the same experiments could not be carried on. In addition, since mercury evaporated at room temperature, it was banned to be used at cadaver dissection. In 1896, Gerota found Prussian Blue, which was refined from turpentine, as a substitute for mercury. By using Prussian Blue, vasculature was clearly identified from macroscopy and microscopy. In

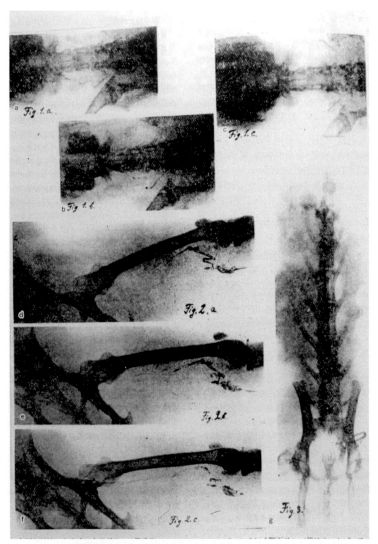

Fig. 1-1. 舟岡省吾による世界初のリンパ管造影(京都大学, 1930年)
First report on lymphangiography by Prof. Funaoka (Kyoto University, in 1930)
(Funaoka S: Untersuchungen uber die physiologie der lymphbewegung. Heft 1. Die rontgenographie des lymphgefasses. 京都帝国大学解剖学第3講座論文集, 1930による)

1909, Bartels published a very good textbook about lymphatic system anatomy by using this method. However, this substance only stained the tissue nearby the injected part. Therefore, their research made great achievements at depiction of short distance lymphatic system, but it was only limited to children and fetuses. This method was impossible in adults staining. Even though it was useful for lymphatic vessels of limited part of body surface, it could not be used to observe the entire lymphatic system. For this reason, elucidation of lymphatic system, for which radiological analysis was not performed, only ended on lymphatic vessels of a portion of body surface.

In the 20th century, analysis of lymphatic system in clinical field was greatly advanced. Hudack and McMaster found the gradual staining of human lymphatic vessels after subcutaneous injection of patent blue, a kind of water-soluble dye. With this technique, in 1952, Kinmonth established clinical lymphangiography.

Kinmonth's approach, in order to identify lymphatics, is a technique to inject water-soluble dye into peripheral limbs subcutaneously and to visualize lymphatic vessels at stained place under local anesthesia. By this way, it became possible to show lymphatic vessels radiologically for the first time. However, this method has two disadvantages : the patients could not move in 2 hours after the injection and only one lymphatic vessel can be detected by a single examination. For these reasons, lymphangiography was gradually replaced by CT detection for lymph node metastasis of malignant tumors[1].

In Japan, in 1774, Genpaku Sugita and Ryotaku Maeno completed a new anatomy text book and described thoracic duct in it. Buntaro Adachi, the first professor of anatomy in Kyoto University, started research on lymphatic system as well as anatomy of human vascular system. In 1930, Professor Seigo Funaoka of anatomy in Kyoto University, who is successor of Adachi and earlier than Kinmonth, published the first report on lymphangiography in the world in German (in 1996 the author found this book in underground book holder in Conway Library of Harvard Medical School, Boston). He injected Iodine into submandibular and popliteal lymph nodes of rabbit and found that lymphatic flow could be passively promoted by bending and stretching rabbit's neck and knees. He also reported lymphangiography of thoracic duct after Iodine injection into testis and observed that lymphatic flow could be changed by respiration movement (**Fig. 1-1**)[2)3)]. Around that time, it was extremely rare that original researches in Japan were published in Western countries. When the author was studying the history of reconstructive surgery in Harvard Medical School, he was very impressed by Funaoka's thesis about lymphangiography result. Now it is difficult to find this book including his work in Japan, but easy in underground library of Harvard Medical School. In addition, Funaoka seems to be the first scholar who was dedicated to the study of chemical composition of lymph fluid in Japan.

In 1928, Milroy first reported cases of congenital hereditary lymphedema. Since 1953, scintigraphy of lymphatic system was available. This technique is to inject radioisotope around the tumor, then the radioactivity is tracked through the lymphatic system. For malignant melanoma or breast cancer, the sentinel lymph nodes must be examined. This method uses patent blue and radioisotopes to confirm the spread of the tumor and determine the region of lymphadenectomy. In 1967, Spalteholtz and Spanner published a detailed anatomy atlas about the distribution of the lymphatic vessels[1].

So far, the fatal defect of the anatomical examination results from various lymphangiographies is its incapability of confirming the cross branches of collecting lymphatic vessels. In the observation of the lymphatic vessels during the operation, it is found recently that there are multiple communicating branches among the collecting lymphatic vessels. The author speculates that the lymphangiography method is just able to provide anterograde angiography along the lymphatic vessels due to the existence of the valves. Also, the opinion that the proximal ducts are smaller while the distal ducts are bigger seems different from our actual images during human surgeries. The size is almost the same in each level of extremities, but smaller in lateral thoracic region.

Regarding the recent study on anatomy of lymphatics, in 2005, Suami, Taylor and other colleagues developed a new radiographic cadaver injection technique for investigating the lymphatic system. This technique proves that oxygen bubbles generated from hydrogen peroxide are very suitable substance for drawing lymphatic vessels. By using hydrogen peroxide, it has become possible to clearly distinguish lymphatic vessels from arteries and veins. After the injection of the mixed contrast agents, the lymphatic vessels can be clearly macroscopically visualized as same as that obtained by the X-ray observation. Suami mapped detailed anatomy of lymphatic vessels in upper arms and chest regions[4)-7)]. In addition, Ohashi (Physiology Department of Sinshu University, Japan) recently conducted a detailed research on the contraction mechanism of lymphatic vessels. Furthermore, Sato (Emeritus professor, Anatomy Department of Tokyo Medical and Dental University) revealed the detailed lymphatic system of the pelvic cavity, thoracic cavity and the mediastinum.

1. 歴史―リンパ浮腫の外科療法

Ⅱ　リンパシンチグラム法

　前川ら（横浜市立大学形成外科）は、リンパ浮腫に対するリンパ管静脈吻合術を行っており、シンチグラムでリンパ浮腫例を分類した。その結果、それぞれのパターンで吻合術の効果が異なることを報告している。

1．ICG 造影法の確立

　緒方（東京大学形成外科）らは、インドシアニングリーン（ICG）と赤外線カメラによるリンパ管造影法を用いてリンパ浮腫例のリンパ管の検索を行い、還流機能が障害され、ICG のうっ滞がみられることを報告した[8]。さらに、山本（東大形成）らは、症例によってパターンが異なり手術後の予後を推定できる可能性を述べている。2010 年、大島（東大形成）らは、子宮癌切除後早期 Stage 0 においても既に ICG 造影で下肢のリンパ液のうっ滞が起こる例が多いことを発見し、これらの患者は吻合術の適応とすべきであること、また、この吻合術によって浮腫が予防できる可能性があることを報告している。ICG 造影法の導入によって、これまで不可能であった四肢のリンパ還流機能が容易に観察可能となり、浮腫例の平滑筋機能が、この造影法で評価でき始め、Stage 0 のリンパ浮腫の診断が可能となった。今後のリンパ浮腫の治療法の開発にとって極めて画期的な検査法といえるであろう。

2．術前のリンパ流の観察法：ICG と赤外線照射によるリンパ管還流能の評価と同定

　色素（メチレンブルー、インドシアニンブルーなど）の皮下注によるリンパ管の識別法は、われわれの経験では正常なリンパ管では有効である。しかし、リンパ浮腫例のリンパ管は染色性が低く無効なことが多い。これは患肢のリンパ管が既に還流機能を失っているためと思われる。

　ICG を足背真皮内に注射後 20 分程度で赤外線を照射すると、リンパ液が蛍光を発しながらリンパ管の近位側に向かって流れ、その走行がみられる。正常者に比べるとリンパ管が早期にみられるのは下腿中央部程度までであり、大腿部の発現は少ない。また鼠径部まで染まるにはかなり時間が経過してからで、リンパ浮腫例ではリンパ液の還流がかなり障害されているのがわかる。リンパ浮腫となる症例のリンパ系の還流障害はかなり早期（Stage 0）から進行している。現在あるリンパ還流機能の評価法として最も正確なものであり、本法は現在世界中に広まりつつある。現在、リンパ浮腫例の手術適応、予後や進行度の判定に必須の検査法となった。リンパ浮腫の専門家は、本法に精通する必要がある。

Ⅱ. Lymphoscintigraphy

Maekawa et al. (Department of Reconstructive Surgery, Yokohama City University) performed a lymphovenous anastomosis for lymphedema, and classified the lymphedema by scintigraphy. The report showed the different results in the effects of different anastomosis patterns.

　1. **Establishment of indocyanine green (ICG) fluorescence lymphography**：Ogata et al. (Department of Reconstructive Surgery, University of Tokyo) indicated that the lymphatic dysfunction and ICG stasis could be checked during lymphatic examination for lymphedema by lymphography using indocyanine green

5

(ICG) and near-infrared fluorescence imaging[8]. In addition, Yamamoto et al.(Department of Reconstructive Surgery, University of Tokyo) discovered several patterns of ICG images and mentioned the possibility to predict the prognosis after surgeries. In 2010, by ICG imaging, Oshima et al.(Department of Reconstructive Surgery, The University of Tokyo) confirmed the lymph stasis of lower extremities of a number of early stage (stage 0) lymphedema cases after resection of uterine cancer, and these cases were suitable for lymphaticovenular anastomosis. Moreover, they mentioned the possibility to prevent lymphedema by lymphaticovenular anastomosis. ICG fluorography makes the lymphatic flow of extremities observable. The diagnosis of lymphedema at Stage 0 becomes possible by evaluation of the function of smooth muscle cells with ICG fluorography. It is an innovative method for the development of lymphedema therapy.

2. Preoperative observation method of lymphatic flow-evaluation and identification of lymphatic flow by indocyanine green (ICG) and infrared irradiation : In our experience, the identification of lymphatic vessels by subcutaneous injection of dye(methylene blue, indocyanine blue, etc.) is effective in normal functional lymphatic vessels. But it is often invalid for the lymphatic vessels of lymphedema patients because of the poor staining in most cases. This seems to be due to the loss of lymphatic drainage of the affected limb.

When irradiate with infrared ray about 20 minutes after injection of ICG into the intradermal layer of dorsal aspect of the foot, fluorescence of the dye traveling in the lymphatics towards the proximal side is observed. Compared to normal persons, lymphatic vessels of lymphedema patients at an early stage can be seen up to central part of lower leg but the expression at the thigh is rare. In addition, the staining at the groin will be observed after a period of time, which means that lymphatic drainage function is impaired in lymphedema patients. The drainage disorder of lymphatic system is progressing from early stage (stage 0). This technology is the most accurate method for assessing the function of lymphatic circulation, which is becoming widely used in the world. Currently, ICG lymphography has become an essential examination for evaluation of surgical indication, prognosis and progress of lymphedema. The experts of lymphedema should be familiar with this method.

Ⅲ リンパ浮腫外科治療法の歴史

　現在行われているリンパ浮腫の外科的治療法には、リンパ管静脈吻合術、リンパ管吻合術、リンパ節入り大網移植、リンパ節移植、血管柄付きリンパ節移植、脂肪吸引法などがある。保存的治療法としては、複合的理学療法(Földi 法)が有名である[9][10]。これらの方法は、圧迫、マッサージ、弾性ストッキングなどによる複合的リンパ管還流療法であるが根治は難しく、あくまでも補助療法である。リンパ浮腫の手術的治療法としては、これまでに下記のものが報告されてきた(現在使われていない術式も含む)。

1. リンパ管新生法(絹糸埋没法) (lymphangioplasty : Handrey's silk thread method, 1908)

　絹糸を皮下に留置し、リンパ管新生を促進する方法である。異物感染の問題があり、効果は期待できない。現在ではまったく行われない。

2．ドレナージ術

ドレナージ・チューブを皮下に留置し持続吸引を行う単純皮下ドレナージ法とナイロン・ネット埋没法などがある。これらの方法は重症の浮腫を一過性に軽減させるには有用かも知れないが、ドレナージ・チューブやネットの逆行性感染の問題があり、長期間の改善には不適で、現在ではまったく行われない。

3．皮膚切除・植皮術 (Charles法, 1912[11]、Kondoleon法, 1912[12]、Sistrunk法, 1918[13]、Homan法, 1936)

減量のために患肢の皮膚を含めて軟部組織を切除縫縮する (Kondoleon法)[12]。切除後植皮で被覆する (Charles法)(**Fig. 1-2**)[11]。下肢の内側と外側を2期に分けて切除する方法 (Homan法) などがある。病的組織を広範囲に切除するため術直後では有効であるが、長期では浮腫が増悪し、縫合線の肥厚性瘢痕化など整容的に問題が多い。

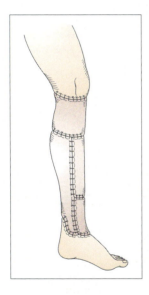

Fig. 1-2. 外科的治療法の歴史：皮膚切除・植皮術 (Charles法, 1912)
History of surgical treatment for lymphedema：Skin resection and skin graft (Charles method in 1912)
皮膚を含めて軟部組織を切除縫縮する (Kondoleon法)。切除後植皮で被覆する (Charles法)。下肢の内側と外側を2期に分けて切除する方法 (Homan法) などがある。
Resection and suturing soft tissue including skin (Kondoleon method). Coverage with skin graft after the resection (Charles method). Resection of the medial and lateral of lower extremity separately (Homan method).

4．脂肪吸引法

脂肪吸引器で四肢の脂肪を吸引する方法である[14)15)]。筆者らの経験では、術直後は改善がみられるが、圧迫を持続しても数ヵ月以内で効果が減少する傾向があった。Slavan (ハーバード大学形成外科) も脂肪性肥大症例に対する有効性は述べているが、リンパ浮腫例に対する効果に関しては否定的であった (アメリカ形成外科学会総会パネル、2010年10月、トロント)。最近ではスウェーデンのBrorsonによって積極的にこの方法がなされ、術後のシンチによってもリンパの還流障害を発生しておらず長期的にも優れた結果が得られることが報告されている。しかしながらこの方法の弱点は24時間圧迫を継続する必要があり、日本よりも南の夏の気候がある地域では継続することが難しいようである。本邦でも最近いくつかの施設でこの術式の短期経過報告が

なされ、現時点ではよい結果が得られているが血栓症が多発するようである。

5．リンパ系再建術

1）筋膜有窓術(Kondoleon 法, 1912)[12]、**筋膜弁筋内挿入術**(Thompson 法, 1962)

理論的には認容できるが、侵襲が大の割には実際の効果が出ないことが多いとされている。最近では、ほとんど適用されることはない。

2）真皮弁埋没法(Gillies & Fraser 法, 1935)(Thompson 法, 1967・1970[16][17])(**Fig. 1-3, 4**)

真皮弁によるリンパ液還流を目的としたもの。長い瘢痕が残り成績は不安定であるが、軽症浮腫例では適用されるケースもあるだろう。

3）大網移行術(Kinmonth 法, 1956、Goldsmith, 1967[18]、De Los Santos, 1967)(**Fig. 1-5**)

大網を有茎で患肢近位部の皮下に移行する方法である。子宮癌切除と同時に予防的に行われ非施行群に比べ、浮腫の発生率に優位差があったという報告もある。本邦でも旭川医科大学血管外科において行われた症例の中で5例が成功した。

4）腸管弁移行術(Kinmonth 法, 1978)

有茎腸管を腸骨窩に移行した後に腸粘膜を剥離除去し、腸管弁を患側の腸骨血管領域の腹膜に縫合固定する方法である。下肢のリンパ管が鼠径部まで開存している例が適応となる。かつて日本でも外科でなされたが成績は安定しなかったようである。手術侵襲が大き過ぎるため最近では行われない。

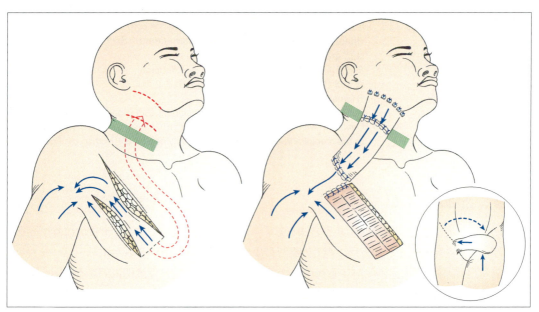

Fig. 1-3．真皮弁埋没法：Bridging procedure for head and neck(Gillies & Fraser 法, 1935)
Buried dermal flap operation：Bridging procedure for head and neck(Gillies & Fraser method in 1935)
真皮弁によるリンパ液還流を目的としたもの。頭頸部の浮腫の治療に用いられた。
This method intends to improve the lymphatic drainage through the dermal flap. It was used for the treatment of head and neck lymphedema.

1. 歴史—リンパ浮腫の外科療法

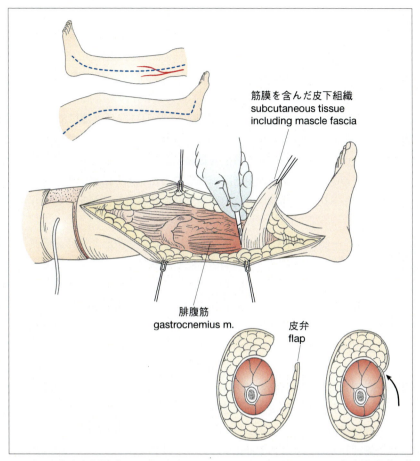

Fig. 1-4. 真皮弁埋没法：Bridging procedure for extremity（Thompson 法, 1962 & 1967）
Buried dermal flap operation：Bridging procedure for extremity（Thompson method in 1962 & 1967）
四肢の浮腫の治療に用いられた。
It was used for the treatment of extremity lymphedema.

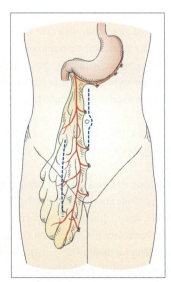

Fig. 1-5. 大網移行術（Kinmonth 法, 1956；Goldsmith, 1967；De Los Santos, 1967）
Omentum transfer（Kinmonth method in 1956；Goldsmith in 1967；De Los Santos in 1967）
有茎大網を患肢近位部の皮下に移行する方法。
This method is to transfer the pedicled greater omentum to the proximal subcutaneous region of affected extremity.

5） 筋皮弁移行術（Medgyesi, 1983）[19]

上肢のリンパ浮腫に対して、患側の広背筋皮弁を島状で移行する方法である。侵襲がやや大なため患者の同意が得られないことが多い。乳癌例では筋の栄養血管も既に結紮切断されていることが多い。筆者の数少ない経験では、術後の効果も安定しないため、第一適応とすべきではない。

6） リンパ管動静脈シャント術（Pho, シンガポール総合病院, 1989）[20]

Adipo-lymphaticovenous shunt 法は、一側性の下肢のリンパ浮腫に対しての治療法である。健側下肢の大伏在静脈を軸としてその周囲のリンパ管・リンパ組織を脂肪組織とともに有茎で患肢に移行する。大伏在静脈の遠位端を後脛骨動脈に端々吻合する。リンパ管の吻合は行わない。これによりリンパ液の還流効果を期待する術式である。ドナーに長い手術瘢痕が残るため侵襲が大で、動静脈シャントのため移植片の血行障害が発生する危険性があり結果が安定しない。

7） リンパ管静脈弁移行術（Ho, オーストラリア, 1988）[21][22]

Adipo-lymph 法は、一側性の下肢のリンパ浮腫に対しての治療法である。健側下肢の大伏在静脈を軸としてその周囲のリンパ管・リンパ組織を脂肪組織とともに有茎で患肢に移行する。次いで、患肢のリンパ管、静脈と flap のリンパ管、静脈を吻合する。これによりリンパ液の還流効果を期待する。長い瘢痕が残り侵襲が大で、移植片の血行障害が発生する危険性がある。両大腿内側面に長い瘢痕が残り、結果が安定しない。このためほとんど追加報告がなされていない。田中の報告では、下肢浮腫の2例中1例で最大10 cm の周径減少（術後1年）が得られている[23]。

8） 島状鼠径皮弁・広背筋（皮）弁（脂肪筋膜弁）移行術

下肢の浮腫例で同側の鼠径部から腰背部の浮腫がみられない症例が適応となる。有茎脂肪筋膜弁を大腿部の皮下ポケットに挿入固定する方法である。また上肢リンパ浮腫に対しては、広背筋弁または広背筋皮弁を移行することによりリンパ液を還流させる方法が報告されている。筆者の経験では、リンパ管細静脈吻合よりその効果は劣り侵襲が大である。これらの術式は、リンパ管が極めて少ない重症例においてはリンパ管静脈吻合やリンパ移植などの付加的な治療法として適応がある。

Ⅲ．The history of surgical treatment for lymphedema

The surgical procedures of lymphedema that are currently performed include lymphaticovenous anastomosis, lymphatic-lymphatic anastomosis, lymph nodes included omentum transfer, lymph nodes transfer, vascularized lymph nodes transfer, liposuction and so on. As conservative treatment, complete decongestive physiotherapy (Földi method) is well-known[9][10]. This complex lymphatic drainage therapy include compression, massage and elastic stocking, but it is difficult for radical cure. It is just an adjuvant therapy. The following methods have been reported as the surgical procedures for lymphedema (including surgical procedures that are not used currently).

1. **Lymphangioplasty** (Handrey's silk thread method, 1908)：A silk thread is placed subcutaneously, which will promote lymphangiogenesis. There is the problem of foreign body infection and the effect cannot be expected. This method is not used currently.

2. **Drainage method**：These are the subcutaneous drainage methods, in which drainage tubes and nylon mesh are placed subcutaneously to make continuous suction. These methods are partially effective to reduce severe lymphedema transiently. However, there is retrograde infection due to drainage tube and nylon mesh and these methods are not suitable for long-term improvement. So, these are not used at all currently.

3. **Skin excision and skin graft** (Charles method, 1912[11], Kondoleon method, 1912[12], Sistrunk method, 1918[13], Homan, 1936)：In Kondoleon method[12] the soft tissue including skin of affected limbs is excised for

the sake of volume reduction. After the resection, lesion is covered with skin graft (Charles method) (**Fig. 1-2**)[11]. In Homan method, excision of the medial and lateral skin of the lower limb is operated separately in two stages. These methods are effective immediately after the surgery because of extensive resection. However, from a long-term point of view, lymphedema will be exacerbated and there are many cosmetic problems such as hypertrophic scars.

4. Liposuction：This method is to aspirate subcutaneous fat in extremities with the suction instrument[14)15]. According to our experience, the improvement can be achieved immediately after the operation, but the tendency of decreased therapeutic response may be noticed within a few months despite keeping compression. Dr. Slavin (Department of Plastic surgery, Harvard University) also said that liposuction was effective to adiposity but denied its effectiveness in cases of lymphedema (the annual scientific meeting of the American Society of Plastic Surgeons, October 2010, Toronto, Canada). Dr. Broson in Sweden recently implemented this procedure actively and reported that the lymphatic drainage disorder was not observed by lymphoscintigraphy after the operation and the long-term excellent results were obtained. However, the disadvantage of liposuction is the necessity of 24-hour compression, which is unsustainable in the summer climate region in south of Japan. Recently, some facilities have reported short term results that show good therapeutic effects but thrombosis occurs frequently.

5. Lymphatic system reconstruction

1) Creation of fascial window (The Kondoleon procedure, 1912)[12], Insertion of fascial flap into the muscle (The Thompson procedure, 1962)：These methods are theoretically acceptable, but strongly invasive in most cases, with poor effect. They are no longer commonly performed recently.

2) Buried dermal flap procedure [Gillies and Fraser procedure, 1935, Thompson procedure, 1967, 1970 (**Fig. 1-3, 4**)[16)17]]：This method intends to improve the lymphatic drainage through the dermal flap. Long scar is left and the results are unstable, nevertheless, it is sometimes adaptive to some cases of mild lymphedema.

3) Omentum transfer (Kinmonth procedure, 1956；Goldsmith, 1967[18]；De Los Santos, 1967) (**Fig. 1-5**)：This method is to transfer the pedicled greater omentum to the proximal subcutaneous region of extremities with lymphedema. Some reports have shown that the incidence of lymphedema are significant lower in the group simultaneously performed this transfer with hysterectomy for uterus cancer than the control group. In Japan, 5 cases that underwent this method at the Department of Vascular surgery in Asahikawa Medical University Hospital have obtained good results.

4) Intestinal flap transfer (Kinmonth procedure, 1978)：The pedicled intestinal canal is transferred to iliac fossa and the intestinal mucosa is stripped off. The intestinal flap is fixed to the peritoneum around the iliac vessels of the affected side. This method is adaptive to the case with a patency of the lymphatic channels from lower limb till the inguinal region. The results of the operations performed in Japan were unstable. This method is too invasive and rarely performed recently.

5) Myoculocutaneous flap transfer (Medgyesi, 1983)[19]：This method is to transfer the island latissimus dorsi musculocutaneous flap at affected side for the upper limb lymphedema. It has kind of great invasion and, therefore, most patients don't accept this operation. In many cases of post mastectomy, the feeding vessels of muscle have already been ligated and excised. Depending on the author's small amount of experience, the post-operative outcomes are not stable, so this method should not be the first choice.

6) Adipose veno-lymphatic transfer (Pho, Shingapore General Hospital, 1989)[20]：Adipo-lymphaticovenous shunt method is a therapy for the treatment of unilateral lymphedema in lower limb. This technique is to transfer adipose tissue containing lymphatic vessels with the great saphenous vein as axis, from the healthy leg to the affected leg. The distal end of the great saphenous vein is anastomosed to the end of posterior tibial artery. The lymphatic anastomosis is not performed. As this procedure is invasive with long scar at donor site and has a risk of blood circulation disorder in transferred flap due to the arteriovenous shunt, the outcome is not stable.

7) Microlymphatic bypass (Ho, Australia, 1988)[21)22)] : This method is similar to the Pho's adipose veno-lymphatic transfer. It is the same for the flap transfer but different in the venous anastomosis. Venous anastomosis and lymphatic anastomosis are both performed between transferred flap and recipient site. Thus, it can be expected to obtain the effects of lymphatic circulation reconstruction. There is a risk of blood flow obstruction meanwhile long scars will be left at the internal side of bilateral thighs. Because of the great invasion and the unstable result, rarely additional cases with this method have been reported. Tanaka reported a circumference reduction up to 10 cm in 1 of 2 cases of lower limbs lymphedema 1 year after the operation[23].

8) Island groin flap, latissimus dorsi muscle or musculocutaneous flap and adipofascial flap transfer : It is adapted to cases of lower extremities lymphedema without lymphedema from the inguinal region to the ipsilateral lower back. The pedicled adipofascial groin flap is harvested and inserted into subcutaneous pocket at the affected thigh. For the upper limbs lymphedema, the latissimus dorsi muscle flap or musculocutaneous flap transfer is reported. According to the author's experience, these transfers are inferior to lymphaticovenular anastomosis because of poorer efficacy and greater invasion. Therefore, these procedures should be suitable for the rare severe cases that have little lymphatic channels and have already received lymphaticovenular anastomosis or lymphatic transfer.

Ⅳ．リンパ管吻合術

外科的治療法の鉄則として、患肢または健側肢に長い皮切を加えることはできるだけ避けたい。浮腫が改善しないのみでなく、手術創から肥厚性瘢痕、リンパ瘻、難治性潰瘍などが発生することになる。たとえ治癒しても患者の QOL を大きく障害する傷跡となる可能性がある。できる限り小皮膚切開の外科的治療にとどめるべきである。以下に述べる方法は、現在でも行われているものである。小皮膚切開で低侵襲なのが最大の利点である。

1．リンパ節-静脈吻合術 (Nielubowicz, 1966) (Fig. 1-6)

ポーランドの Nielubowicz によって極めて早期に報告され、その後 Olszewski によって継承された方法であり、リンパ管静脈吻合の基礎となった術式である。下肢の浮腫で用いられ、リンパ節を流入リンパ管とともに露出し、リンパ節の割面と皮静脈を吻合する術式である。本法は末梢側のリンパ管が近位までほぼ全長で開存している必要がある。筆者らの経験では、大腿近位部のリンパ節が残っている症例は早期例のみであり、浮腫の進行した例では既に消失している例が多い。蜂窩織炎多発例では、リンパ節が線維化して使用できない例が多い。そのためか、現在広く用いられる術式とはなっていない。

2．山田によるリンパ管静脈吻合の報告 (Fig. 1-7)

1965 年、玉井（奈良医科大学整形外科）が世界初の切断指再接着に成功した。この頃、名古屋大学血管外科でも顕微鏡下の血管吻合が行われていたようである。Laine のラットを用いたリンパ管静脈吻合（1963 年）の報告[24)]に続いて、1969 年に Yamada は、当時始まったばかりの顕微鏡下

1. 歴史—リンパ浮腫の外科療法

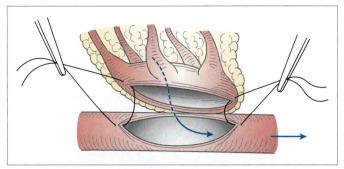

Fig. 1-6. リンパ節-静脈吻合術（Nielubowicz, 1966年）
Lymphnode-venous anastomosis（Nielubowicz in 1966）

主要リンパ節の割面と皮静脈を吻合する術式である。本法は末梢側のリンパ管がほぼ全長で近位まで開存している必要がある。また、蜂窩織炎の既往例では、リンパ節が線維化して使用できない例が多い。
The cut surface of main lymph node is anastomosed with cutaneous vein. The patency of the entire lymphatic channels from the distal side to the proximal side is necessary. In cases with repeated cellulitis, many lymph nodes cannot be used because of fibrosis.

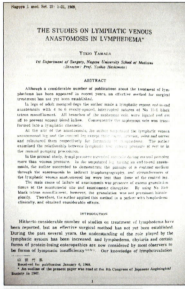
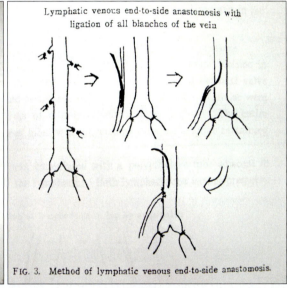

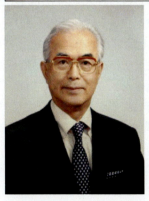

Fig. 1-7. 山田によるリンパ管静脈吻合の報告：Lymphatico-venous anastomosis（1969年）
Report of lymphatico-venous anastomosis by Yamada：Lymphatico-venous anastomosis（in 1969）
左：山田先生、左上：報告された論文、右上：論文中の図示された吻合法
Left：Photo of Dr. Yamada, upper left：The paper reported, upper right：Illustrated anastomosis method in this paper
（Yamada Y：The studies on lymphatic venous anastomosis in lymphedema. Nagoya J Med Sci 32：1-21, 1969 による）

の微小血管吻合術を応用して、イヌを用いたリンパ管と静脈の吻合を行い、リンパ浮腫の治療法になりうることを英語論文で報告した[25]。彼は、イヌを用いて端々吻合、端側吻合でリンパ管静脈吻合を行い開通度の比較を行い、また、吻合部の組織観察を行った。さらに、安静時と運動時のリンパ圧の変動を調べた。以下に彼の報告を詳述する。

[実験1、2]手術用顕微鏡を使って10-0 black tetron monofilamentで伏在静脈とそれに伴走しているリンパ管の端々吻合、端側吻合を行った。吻合の工夫として、①静脈の流入を防ぐために伏在静脈の枝をすべて結紮、②poly-ethylene tubeをsplintとしてリンパ管内に挿入して吻合後静脈壁から取り出す吻合術を行っている。吻合後の開存度はリンパ管造影で評価し、開存度（端々吻合/端側吻合）は1週後（90.9/85.7%）、8週後（72.7/55.6%）、6ヵ月後（44.4/35.7%）であった。端側吻合の方が端々吻合よりも手技が難しいことが考えられる。

[実験3]組織検査では吻合部において経過とともに壁の肥厚を認めた。

[実験4]伏在静脈と伴走リンパ管にTチューブを挿入して、安静時（at rest）、運動時（passive knee joint movement, tapping, squeezing）でのそれぞれの圧を測定した。運動時において静脈圧とリンパ圧の値は似ていた。リンパ圧に関してはat rest：4、passive knee joint movement：14、tapping：18、squeezing：26（単位：cmH_2O）であり、運動時では安静時に比べて3〜7倍の上昇を認めた。このことよりリンパ管静脈吻合の術後結果を左右するのはリンパ圧が静脈圧よりも低いということではなく、マイクロ技術によるといえる。

[臨床報告]37歳、女性、10年前に右関節結核、5年前から右下肢が腫れ始めた。伏在静脈において4端々吻合、1端側吻合を行い、術後3ヵ月後周径2〜8cmの減少を認めた（測定部位は不明）。

3．古典的リンパ管静脈吻合法(Degni法, 1974)[26][27] (Fig. 1-8)

　山田の報告から5年後に報告された。山田法によく似る方法である。この方法は1980年代に世界中に広まったリンパ管静脈吻合法であったと思われる。個人的には0.3mmの静脈の近位端を開存させるためには吻合技術が未熟であったと思われる。また、たとえ吻合部が開存したとしても太い静脈に端側吻合するため、静脈からリンパ管への逆流が生じたのではないかと思われる。

4．顕微鏡下リンパ管静脈吻合法(O'Brien法, 1976)[28]−[30]

　1976年、メルボルンの形成外科医のO'Brienは、顕微鏡下のリンパ管静脈吻合を行い良好な結果を報告した。彼の最初の論文で山田の論文が引用されている。彼は、リンパ浮腫治療のみでなく、微小血管吻合術を用いて1970〜80年代にかけて次々と新しい組織移植術を開発した形成再建外科手術のパイオニアである。その後、彼は20年にわたりその生涯をリンパ浮腫の外科治療の開発と普及に捧げた。この方法は70年代に日本でも行われたが、術後の改善率が期待したほど高くなかった。このため追従者はほとんどなかった。筆者は80〜90年代に国際微小外科学会で、たびたびO'Brienのリンパ浮腫に関する講演を聞いた。彼の最後の講演はウィーンであったが、最も印象的であった。このとき、彼は視力をほとんど失っていたようであった。自分はこれほどリンパ浮腫の治療をやってきたのに、誰もリンパのオペをやる者がいない。これが自分にとって最もつらいことだと泣きながら言い残した。その後、彼は亡くなったが、残念ながらその後オース

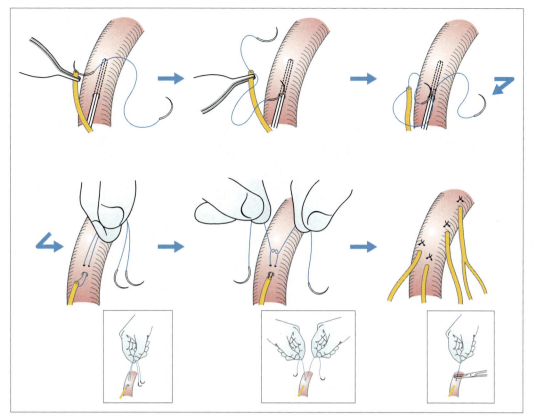

Fig. 1-8. 古典的リンパ管静脈吻合法（Degni 法） Classical lymphaticovenous anastomosis（Degni method）
太い静脈への端側吻合であり、山田の吻合法によく似ている。
This method is end-to-side anastomosis of large vein and is very similar to Yamada's method of anastomosis.

トラリアではこの術式は消滅した。現在では、新しい超微小吻合術が日本を発信基地として世界に広がりつつある。その背景には、90年前後から日本で本格的な超微小血管吻合術が完成されたことと、リンパ管の機能に関する日本の新しい知見が臨床に導入されたことがより効果的なリンパ管細静脈吻合術（lymphaticovenular anastomosis；LVA）の開発につながったことが挙げられる。

5．遊離リンパ管移植法(Fig. 1-9)

　上肢リンパ浮腫の外科治療法である。大腿部からリンパ管を採取し、鎖骨部遠位と近位でリンパ管移植することでリンパ系の再建を行う。Baumeister（ミュンヘン）は、この方法で多くの症例を治療し、良好な結果を報告している[31]。この術式は血行がないリンパ管移植なので、阻血による移植リンパ管の線維化によって内腔の閉塞が起こる可能性が危惧される。現時点では一部の外科医による利用にとどまっている。

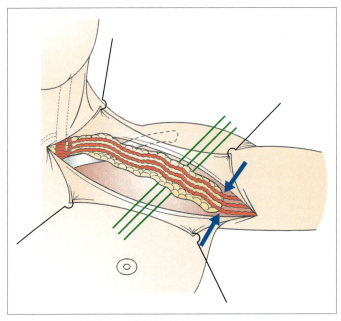

Fig. 1-9. 遊離リンパ管移植法　Free lymphatic transfer
上肢リンパ浮腫に対し、大腿部からリンパ管を採取し、鎖骨部遠位と近位でリンパ管吻合する。
For treatment of upper limb lymphedema, the lymphatic vessels were harvested from the thigh and anastomosed to the peripheral lymphatic vessels distal to the clavicle region and central lymphatic vessels proximal to the clavicle region.

6．リンパ管静脈移行(移植)法

　Campisi[32)33)]、Yamamoto[34)]らはリンパ管複合体を脂肪とともに太い静脈に移行、接合または吻合することでリンパ流を静脈に還流させる方法を報告している。Campisi は静脈移植を間に置いたりする方法も考案している。

7．超微小的リンパ管細静脈吻合法(光嶋)[35)−38)]

　山田法[25)]、O'Brien 法[28)]と異なる点は、リンパ管を同径の真皮直下の 0.3〜0.8 mm の細静脈と端々吻合することでリンパ液を静脈系に還流させることである。指尖再接着を可能とした最新のスーパーマイクロ手技が必要である。その手技の詳細は後述する。

8．血管柄付きリンパ節移植

　Shesol[39)]、Chen[40)]らが実験的に考案し、パリの女性形成外科医 Corinne Becker[41)]が報告した術式である。リンパ節は、リンパ管系を区切ることで管内の圧調節をしており、リンパ浮腫を物理的に防ぐ役割をもつと考えられている。この圧調節がうまくいかなくなると、下流のリンパ

管の内圧が上昇してポンプ機能が損なわれ、結果としてリンパ系の破綻・リンパ節の消失が起こり、リンパ浮腫が起こる。したがって、別の場所からリンパ節・リンパ管を移植することで浮腫の改善が期待される。2006年のCorinne Beckerらの報告[41]では、乳癌治療後の上肢リンパ浮腫を呈する6例にリンパ節移植を施行しており、うち5例はリンパ浮腫が消失し、全例で疼痛が消え日常生活に支障がなくなったとしている。Linらも上肢に対するリンパ節移植例について報告している[42]。その後、イヌやミニブタ、ヒツジなどでその効果が報告され、多くの臨床的な報告がなされた。その結果、リンパ節採取部のドナー肢のリンパ浮腫化や神経麻痺のリスクが報告され、特にドナーの選択にあたっては慎重さが求められている。

これまで報告されたリンパ節移植としては、鎖骨上リンパ節移植法、腋窩リンパ節移植法、鼠径リンパ節移植法などがある。

9. 血管柄付きリンパ管移植（光嶋）

2004年、LVAが無効な下肢の重度リンパ浮腫に対して第1例が行われ、11年後の現在、完治状態が続いている。そこで過去11年間LVA無効例に対しリンパ浮腫に際してこの術式がなされたが、約30%で著効が得られている。既に内外で講演・デモしている方法である。長期経過した重症のリンパ浮腫例に対して、健側から正常なリンパ管に栄養血管を付けたまま遊離血管付きリンパ管移植片として採取する。これを患肢に移植し、正常な機能をもつリンパ管移植によってリンパ液を静脈系に誘導するという方法である。片側下肢例では、対側の第1趾間部の還流機能をもつリンパ管を患肢の鼠径部に移植する。両側下肢の浮腫例では腋窩部からリンパ管を採取し、鼠径部に移植する。血管柄付きリンパ管移植片の平滑筋が生きたまま移植されるため、リンパ管のポンプ機能が復活しリンパ系の還流効果が期待される。重度リンパ浮腫に対して用いられ、完治例も出始めている。

[準備するもの]ICG蛍光リンパ管像影装置、超微小外科セット

[適応]LVAの効果がみられない重症の浮腫例。LVAに抵抗する進行性浮腫例。

[手術方法]ICG注射にて健側下肢の第1趾間部または胸壁の正常な還流機能をもつリンパ管を造影する。正常な還流機能をもつリンパ管であればICG注射後直ちにリンパ管の走行に沿って蛍光が確認でき、そのスピードによっておおよそのリンパ管の機能を推測できる。蛍光色素は短時間で消失するので7-0ナイロンや小リガクリップでリンパ管をマークしておく。移植片は挙上中出血しやすいので、丁寧に止血しながら血管茎を剥離する。最終的に、健側から正常なリンパ管に栄養血管を付けたまま遊離血管付きリンパ管移植片として採取する。

第1趾間であれば第1中足動脈と皮静脈が栄養血管茎である。腋窩部であれば外側橈動脈と皮静脈が血管茎となる。これを患肢の鼠径部または大腿内側部に移植し、正常な機能をもつリンパ管移植によってリンパ液を静脈系に誘導するという方法である。顕微鏡下の血管吻合後移植片の表面から表在出血がみられる。

[利点]手術手技が低侵襲で、すべての重症浮腫の患者に適応となる。術後完治することがある。

[欠点]移植片の採取に超微小外科手技を要するため初心者には手技が難しい。腋窩からのリンパ管（リンパ節）採取後上肢のリンパ浮腫が発生することがあるかも知れない。足背からの採取ではドナーの知覚障害が生ずる。

1）外側胸リンパ管移植法

腋窩部から外側胸動脈（胸背動脈）系の茎を付け血管柄付きリンパ管移植片を採取し、患肢の罹患部に移植する。外側胸動脈がよく発達している例では移植片を2〜3個に分割し、これを浮腫の強い部分に移植する。移植床血管は穿通枝に端々吻合あるいは主要動脈や皮静脈に端側吻合する。皮弁を付けることが望ましい。穿通枝が発達していない症例などでは脂肪リンパ管弁の血流は良好であっても皮弁は壊死となることもある。このような場合にはベッドサイドで皮弁のみ部分切除することになる。

2）第1趾間リンパ管移植法

足背の第1趾間を中心に、第1中足骨動脈の穿通枝を血管茎としたリンパ管移植片を採取し、患肢の罹患部へ移植する。

3）下腹壁リンパ管移植法

浅腸骨回旋動脈系や浅下腹壁動脈系を茎として脂肪とリンパ管を含めて採取し、移植した後移植床血管と吻合する。

Ⅳ. Lymphatic anastomosis

As an invariable principle of surgical treatment, a long skin incision on the affected limbs or the normal limbs should be avoided as much as possible. Operation with long incision might not only cannot improve lymphedema, but also lead to surgical hypertrophic scars, lymphatic fistula, intractable ulcers, and so on. Even if these can be cured, the scar will greatly reduce the patient's Quality Of Life. The skin incision should be controlled as short as possible during surgical treatment. The procedures shown below are still being performed. Small incision and low invasion are the biggest advantages.

1. Lymphnode-venous anastomosis (Nielubowicz, 1966) (**Fig. 1-6**)：Nielubowicz in Poland first reported this procedure in the very early days and Olszewski inherited it. It has become the basis for the subsequent lymphaticovenous anastomosis. For lymphedema of lower extremities, the cut surface of lymph node which is dissected along with the afferent lymph duct is anastomosed with cutaneous vein. The patency of the entire lymphatic channels from the distal side to the proximal side is necessary. In the author's experience, lymph nodes at the proximal area of a thigh only remained in cases of early stages, and disappeared in the majority of advanced lymphedema cases. In cases with repeated cellulitis, many lymph nodes cannot be used because of fibrosis. Therefore, this operation is not currently widely performed.

2. The report of lymphatic venous anastomosis by Yamada (**Fig. 1-7**)[29]：In 1965, for the first time in the world, Tamai (Department of Orthopedic Surgery, Nara Medical University, Japan) successfully performed the replantation of a totally amputated finger. Around that time, it seemed that vascular anastomosis had been performed under microscope at the department of vascular surgery in Nagoya University Hospital. Following the Laine's report of lymphatico-venous anastomosis in rats (1963)[24], Yamada performed the anastomosis of lymphatic vessels and veins in dogs by applying the microvascular anastomosis under microscope, which had just emerged at that time, and reported the possibility of using this method in the treatment of lymphedema in an English paper[25]. He compared the patency of end-to-end anastomosis with that of end-to-side anastomosis in dogs, and observed the tissue at the site of the anastomosis. Furthermore, he examined the changes of lymphatic pressure at rest and in the manual pumping procedures. The following are the details of his report.

[**Experiment 1, 2**] He performed end-to-end anastomosis and end-to-side anastomosis between saphenous vein and concomitant lymphatic vessels with 10-0 black tetron monofilament under the surgical microscope. The devices during the anastomosis include ligation of all branches of saphenous vein to avoid blood inflow and using the poly-ethylene tube as a splint which is inserted into a lymphatic vessel and then taken out of the venous wall after anastomosis. The patency at the anastomosis (end-to-end/end-to-side) was evaluated by lymphangiography after 1 week (90.9/85.7%), 8 weeks (72.7/55.6%) and 6 months (44.4/35.7%). The differences of patency rates may be precisely for this reason that end-to-side anastomosis was more difficult than end-to-end anastomosis.

[Experiment 3] The hypertrophy of vessel wall was observed at the anastomotic site by the histological examination.

[Experiment 4] By using T-tube that was inserted into the saphenous vein and the concomitant lymphatic vessels, the venous and lymphatic pressure was tested respectively at rest and during exercises (passive knee joint movement, tapping, squeezing). The lymphatic pressure during exercises was similar to the venous pressure. The lymphatic pressure at rest : 4 cmH$_2$O, passive knee joint movement : 14 cmH$_2$O, tapping : 18 cmH$_2$O, squeezing : 26 cmH$_2$O. The lymphatic pressure during exercises showed an increase up to 3 to 7 times as much as at rest. According to these results, not the lower lymphatic pressure than the venous pressure, but the microsurgical techniques controlled the effects post the lymphatico-venous anastomosis.

[Case report] A 37-year-old female contracted the right joint tuberculosis 10 years ago and had suffered lymphedema at the right lower limb for 5 years. 5 lymphatico-venous anastomoses (4 end-to-end anastomoses and 1 end-to-side anastomosis) were performed using a saphenous vein. 3 months after the operation, the circumference decreased 2～8 cm (the measurement site was uncertain).

3. Classical lymphaticovenous anastomosis (Degni procedure, 1974) (**Fig. 1-8**)[26)27)] : This procedure was reported 5 years after the Yamada's report and similar to Yamada's method. This procedure of lymphaticovenous anastomosis seemed to spread throughout the world in 1980s. As the author, I personally suspect that the anastomosis technique was immature to ensure the patency of the proximal end of the 0.3 mm vein. In addition, even if the anastomosis was patent, which was performed at the thick veins, the backflow from the vein to the lymphatic vessel would seemly occur.

4. Lymphaticovenous anastomosis under microscope (O'Brien et al. 1976)[28-30)] : In 1976, O'Brien, a plastic surgeon in Melbourne, reported good results of lymphaticovenous anastomosis under microscope. He cited Dr. Yamada's report in his first paper about this procedure. As a pioneer in plastic and reconstructive surgery, Dr. O'Brien developed not only the treatment of lymphedema, but also a novel tissue transfer method by using microvascular anastomosis in the 1970s-1980s. From then on, he devoted himself to the development and dissemination of surgical treatment of lymphedema for 20 years. The method was performed in Japan in the 1970s, but the postoperative results were not as good as expected. Because of this, there were almost no followers. The author often heard O'Brien's lectures on lymphedema in the International Society for Microsurgery in the 1980s-1990s, and was most impressed with his last speech in Vienna. At that time, he was almost blind. He cried that even though he had kept on exploring the treatment of lymphedema, no one intended to perform the operation for patients. This was the most painful thing for him. After that, he passed away ; and unfortunately, this surgical procedure in Australia disappeared. Currently, new supermicroanastomosis, originating from Japan, is spreading in the world. The background is that the full-fledged supermicrovascular anastomosis has been established in Japan since the 1990's, and the more effective lymphaticovenular anastomosis (LVA) was developed when the new knowledge about the function of the lymphatic vessels had been introduced into the clinical practice.

5. Free lymphatic transfer (**Fig. 1-9**) : This is the surgical treatment of upper limb lymphedema. In order to reconstruct the lymphatic system, lymphatic grafts were harvested from the thigh and anastomosed to the peripheral lymphatic vessels distal to the clavicle region and central lymphatic vessels proximal to the clavicle region. Baumeister, from Munich, reported good outcomes of many cases using this method[31)]. This method is a lymphatic vessel transfer without blood supply, so the possibility of the transplanted lymphatic fibrosis and occlusion due to ischemia is worried about. At this time, only a few surgeons apply this method.

6. Lymphaticovenous implantation (transfer) : Campisi[32)33)], Yamamoto[34)] et al. reported lymphaticovenous shunt by the way that the collecting lymphatics along with adipose tissue were transferred, joined or anastomosed to thick veins. Campisi also investigated the interposition vein graft.

7. Supermicrosurgical lymphaticovenular anastomosis (Koshima)[35)-38)] : The difference from Yamada procedure[25)] and O'Brien method[28)] is that lymphatic vessels are anastomosed in end-to-end style with the venules of about the same size, 0.3-0.8 mm in diameter, which are located just under the dermis to drain the lymph flow. This method requires the latest supermicrosurgical technique that used in fingertip replantation. This technique will be described in detail later.

8. Free vascularized lymph node transfer : This operation was developed experimentally by Shesol[39)], Chen[40)], et al. and was reported by Corinne Becker[41)], a female plastic surgeon in Paris. Lymph nodes, which regulate the pressure inside the lymphatic vessels by separating the lymphatic system, are believed to play a role in the prevention of lymphedema physically. If the pressure regulation fails, the inner pressure of the downstream lymphatic vessel will increase and the pumping function will be impaired, resulting in the breakdown of the lymphatic system, the disappearance of lymph nodes, and causing lymphedema. Therefore, lymph nodes and lymphatic vessels transfer from unaffected region is expected to improve lymphedema. In 2006 Corinne Becker[41)] reported six cases of the upper arm lymphedema after mastectomy. The lymphedema in 5 cases were cured after microsurgical lymph node transfer, and the pain disappeared in all the patients who returned to normal daily life. Lin et al. also reported lymph node transfer in the cases of upper extremity lymphedema[42)]. After that, experimental researches using dogs, minipigs and goats were reported and many clinical results were published. As a result, the risk of lymphedema and paralysis of the donor side extremity after lymph nodes harvest was reported. So the donor site should be chosen very carefully. The following are the normally used lymph nodes depending on different donor sites.

Supraclavicular lymph nodes transfer, axillary lymph nodes transfer, groin lymph nodes transfer are the reported lymph nodes transfer.

9. Free vascularized lymphatic vessel transfer (Koshima) : In 2004, the first transfer was performed in a case of severe lower extremity lymphedema with no efficacy to LVA and complete recovery of this case has been permanent for 11 years till now. Over the last 11 years, this operation was performed in LVA invalid lymphedema cases and about 30% of these patients achieved significant regression. The author has already shown this procedure in the form of lectures and demonstrations in Japan and other countries. In cases of severe long-term lymphedema, the vascularized normal lymphatic vessels from healthy side will be harvested as lymphatic vessel flap with free vascular pedicle. This flap, in which the lymphatic vessels have normal function, is transferred to the affected limb to lead the lymph flow drainage into veins. In cases of unilateral lower extremity lymphedema, lymphatic vessels from the first web space of the healthy foot can be transferred to the inguinal region of the affected leg. In cases with bilateral lower extremities lymphedema, lymphatic vessels can be harvested from the axillary region and transferred to the inguinal region. Because of the transfer of the live smooth muscle cells around the lymphatic vessels in the harvested tissue with vascular pedicle, the pumping function of the lymphatic vessels at the recipient site could be revived and the lymph flow can be expected. We have experienced complete recovery in some severe lymphedema cases by using this procedure.

[Preparations] ICG lymphography device, supermicrosurgical equipment

[Indications] LVA invalid severe lymphedema. LVA resistant progressive lymphedema.

[Operational technique] ICG injection is performed in order to visualize the normal lymph flow either in the first web space of the intact leg or in the axillary region. If the lymphatic vessels have normal lymphatic flow, the fluorescence can be observed immediately after the injection along the lymphatic vessels and the function of the lymphatic vessels can be speculated according to its speed. Lymphatic vessels should be marked with 7-0 Nylon or small vessel clips as the fluorescent dye will disappear in a short period of time. Vascular pedicles should be dissected carefully because it is very easy to bleed while you elevate the flap. Finally, the free vascularized lymphatic vessel flap is harvested with the vascular pedicle from the healthy side. These flaps are transferred to the groin region or the medial thigh region of the affected limb. After the

vascular anastomoses under microscope, the bleeding on the superficial surface of the flap can be observed.
[**Advantages**] The surgical technique is minimal invasive, applicable to all severe lymphedema patients.
Complete recovery can be attained.

[**Disadvantages**] Supermicrosurgical technique is required for harvesting the flap, which is difficult for beginners. Lymphedema of the upper arm might occur after the resection of the lymphatic vessels or lymph nodes from the axillary region. Donor site paresthesia could occur after harvesting from the dorsal foot.

1) Lateral thoracic lymphatic vessel transfer : The lymphatic vessel flap with vascular pedicle of the lateral thoracic artery or thoracodorsal artery is harvested from the lower axillary region and transferred to the affected zone of the extremity with lymphedema. The flap can be divided into two or three pieces if the lateral thoracic artery system is abundant and these flaps will be transferred to the severe region. End-to-end anastomosis can be performed with the perforating branches of the vessels at the recipient site or end-to-side anastomosis can be performed with the main arteries and cutaneous veins. Adding monitor skin flap is advisable. If the perforators are not rich, the skin flap might become necrotic even though the lymph-adipose flap itself is well vascularized. Under this circumstance, bedside partial resection of the monitor skin flap is needed.

2) First webspace lymphatic vessel transplantation : A lymphatic vessel graft with the penetrating branch of the first metatarsal artery as the vascular stem is collected around the first toe gap between the dorsum of the foot and transplanted to the diseased part of the affected limb.

3) Inferior epigastric lymphatic vessel transfer : Lymph-adipose flap vascularized by the superficial circumflex iliac artery system or superficial epigastric artery system is harvested, transferred and anastomosed with the vessels at the recipient site.

Ⅴ　合併外科治療：予防的リンパ管細静脈吻合術（光嶋）

　リンパ浮腫例ではリンパ郭清直後から平滑筋細胞の変性が始まるため、浮腫が出た時点で LVA を行ったとしても還流機能はもとに戻らないという考えに立って考案された治療法である（**Fig. 1-10**）。この concept は筆者によって提案され、90 年代中頃以後、海外を含めて多数の講演で発表された。武石＆高橋ら（慈恵会医科大学形成＆産婦人科）は、この concept をもとにして婦人科領域の癌切除と同時の即時的骨盤内 LVA を試み、術後長期の良好な経過を報告している[43]。この方法は、骨盤内での癌切除と同時のバイパス作成であるため、癌細胞の転移の可能性が危惧される。筆者は、浮腫発生後数ヵ月以内に局麻にて四肢の遠位部で LVA をできるだけ多く作成する予防的 LVA を考案した。癌切除後 ICG 検査でリンパのうっ滞が認められ、その後下肢浮腫に発展する可能性がある例を適応としている。追加 LVA も容易にでき、現時点では良好な結果が得られている。なお、IVG で異常所見がみられる例は、子宮癌切除術前からうっ滞がみられることが多い（大島梓：東京大学形成外科, 日本マイクロ学会, 2010 年 11 月）。これは癌のリンパ節転移によるものというよりも先天的または遅発性リンパ流障害がある可能性が考えられる。リンパ浮腫発生因子としてはいろいろ考えられているが、リンパ郭清、放射線治療、後腹膜閉鎖などに加えて、先天的な潜在性リンパ還流障害が存在する可能性が出てきている。

（辛川　領、伊藤太智、水田栄樹、森下悠也、森脇裕太、光嶋　勲）

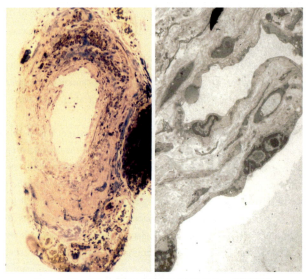

Fig. 1-10. リンパ管の電顕像（上肢リンパ浮腫例）
Electron microscopic findings of lymphatics (upper arm lymphedema)
変性後に再生した小型平滑筋細胞が中膜にみられる。これが集合リンパ管の収縮能消失の原因と思われるリンパ管硬化症。リンパ管拡張、リンパ管壁の肥厚、中膜平滑筋細胞の小型化と密度の不均一がみられる。
The small smooth muscle cells that regenerated after degeneration can be seen in tunica media. Lymphangiosclerosis seems to cause the loss of the contractive function of lymphatic vessels. Dilation of the lymphatic vessels, thickening of the tunica media, miniaturization and imbalanced distribution of smooth muscle cell in tunica media can be seen.
(Koshima I, Kawada S, Moriguchi T, et al : Ultrastructural observation of lymphatic vessels in lymphedema in human extremities. Plast Reconstr Surg 97 : 397-405, 1996 による)

V. Combined surgical treatments : Prophylactic lymphaticovenular anastomosis (Koshima)

This operation was invented based on the notion that smooth muscle cell degeneration begins immediately after the lymphadenectomy and LVA performed at the point of the appearance of lymphedema cannot lead to the complete recovery of the lymphatic function (**Fig. 1-10**). This concept has been proposed by the author and presented in many lectures all over the world since mid-1990s. Based on this concept, Takeishi, Takahashi et al. (Department of Plastic and Reconstructive Surgery, Department of obstetrics and gynecology, Jikei University School of Medicine) reported long-term good outcomes after gynecologic cancer resection and immediate intrapelvic LVA[43]. There is the possibility of cancer cell metastases because this method is the simultaneous LVA with the intrapelvic cancer resection. The author performed prophylactic LVAs under local anesthesia as many as possible at the distal part of the extremities within a few months after lymphedema appeared. Indication is set to cases in which lymph flow congestion is observed and there is the possibility of leg lymphedema progression. Additional LVAs can be performed easily and good results have been obtained at the present time. If the abnormal ICG patterns are observed, lymph flow congestion tends to exist before hysterectomy (Azusa Oshima, Department of Plastic and Reconstructive Surgery, University of Tokyo. Japan society of microsurgery, November 2011). In these cases, there is the possibility of congenital or late-onset lymphatic flow disorder rather than the lymph node metastasis of cancer cells. The cause of lymphedema is considered to be the lymph node resection, radiation therapy, close of the retroperitoneum and the presence of congenital latent lymph flow reflux disorder.

〔*Ryo Karakawa, Taichi Ito, Haruki Mizuta, Yuya Morishita, Yuta Moriwaki, Isao Koshima*〕

1) Kanter MA：The lymphatic system；An historical perspective. Plast Reconstr Surg 79：131-139, 1987.
2) 小谷正彦：リンパ管研究の歴史．リンパ管；形態・機能・発生，大谷　修，ほか（編），pp311-320，西村書店，東京，1997.
Kotani M：The History of Lymphatic study. Otani O, et al（eds），pp311-320, Nishimura-shoten, Tokyo, 1997.
3) Funaoka S：Untersuchungen uber die physiologie der lymphbewegung. Heft 1. Die rontgenographie des lymphgefasses. 京都帝国大学解剖学第3講座論文集, The paper collection of the 3rd lecture, department of anatomy, Kyoto Imperial University, 1930.
4) Suami H, Taylor GI, Pan WR：A new radiographic cadaver injection technique for investigating the lymphatic system. Plast Reconstr Surg 115：2007-2013, 2005.
5) Suami H, Taylor GI, Pan WR：The lymphatic territories of the upper limb；Anatomical study and clinical implications. Plast Reconstr Surg 119：1813-1822, 2007.
6) Suami H, Pan WR, Taylor GI：Changes in the lymph structure of the upper limb after axillary dissection；Radiographic and anatomical study in a human cadaver. Plast Reconstr Surg 120：982-991, 2007.
7) Suami H, O'Neill JK, Pan WR, et al：Perforating lymph vessels in the canine torso；Direct lymph pathway from skin to the deep lymphatics. Plast Reconstr Surg 121：31-36, 2008.
8) Narushima M, Mihara M, Azuma R, et al：Intraoperative lymphography using indocyanine green dye for near-infrared fluorescence labeling in lymphedema. Ann Plast Surg 59：180-184, 2007.
9) Földi E, Földi M, Clodius L：The lymphedema Chaos；A lancet. Ann Plast Surg 22：505-515, 1989.
10) Földi M：Discussion for Koshima's paper "Ultrastructural observations of lymphatic vessels in lymphedema in human extremities". Plast Reconstr Surg 97：406-407, 1996.
11) Charles RH：Elephantiasis Scroti. Churchill, London, 1912.
12) Kondreon E：Die operative Behandlung der elephantiastischen Odema. Zentralbl Chir 39：1022, 1912.
13) Sistrunk WE：Contribution to plastic surgery；Removal of scars by stages；an open operation for extensive laceration of the anal sphincter；the Kondreon operation for elephantiasis. Ann Surg 85：185-193, 1927.
14) Illouz YZ：Body contouring by lipolysis；A 5-year experience with over 3000 cases. Plast Reconstr Surg 72：591-597, 1983.
15) O'Brien BM, Khazanchi RK, Kumar PA, et al：Liposuction in the treatment of lymphoedema；a preliminary report. Br J Plast Surg 42：530-533, 1989.
16) Thompson N：The surgical treatment of chronic lymphedema of the extremities. Surg Clin North Am 47：445-503, 1967.
17) Thompson N：Buried dermal flap operation for chronic lymphedema of the extremities；Ten-year survey of results in 79 cases. Plast Reconstr Surg 45：541-548, 1970.
18) Goldsmith HS, De los Santos R, Beattie EJ Jr.：Relief of chronic lymphedema by ometal transposition. Ann Surg 166：573-585, 1967.
19) Medgyesi S：A successful operation for lymphoedema using a myocutaneous flap as a "wick". Br J Plast Surg 36：64-66, 1983.
20) Pho RWH, Bayon P, Tan L：Adipose veno-lymphatic transfer for management of post-radiation lymphedema. J Reconstr Microsurg 5：45-52, 1989.
21) Ho LC, Lai MF, Kennedy PJ：Micro-lymphatic bypass in the treatment of obstructive lymphedema of the arm；Case report of a new technique. Br J Plast Surg 36：350-357, 1983.
22) Ho LC, Lai MF, Eates M, et al：Microlymphatic bypass in obstructive lymphoedema. Br J Plast Surg 41：475-484, 1988.
23) 田中嘉雄，田嶋定夫，今井啓介，ほか：一側二次性リンパ浮腫のAdipo-lymphatico venous transferによる治療の試み．マイクロサージャリー 4：126-132，1991.
Tanaka K, Tajima S, Imai K, et al：The treatment of secondary lymphedema using adipo-lymphaticovenous transfer. Microsurgery 4：126-132, 1991.
24) Laine JB：Experimental lymphatico-venous anastomosis. Surg Forum 14：111-112, 1963.

25) Yamada Y : The studies on lymphatic venous anastomosis in lymphedema. Nagoya J Med Sci 32 : 1-21, 1969.

26) Degni M : New technique of lymphatic-venous anastomosis (buried type) for the treatment of lymphedema. Vasa 3 : 479-483, 1974.

27) Degni M : New technique of lymphatic-venous anastomosis for the treatment of lymphedema. Cardiovasc Surg (Trino) 19 : 577-580, 1978.

28) O'Brien MB, Sykes P, Threlfall GN, et al : Microlymphaticovenous anastomoses for obstructive lymphedema. Plast Reconstr Surg 60 : 197-211, 1977.

29) O'Brien BM, Shafiroff BB : Microlymphaticovenous and resectional surgery in obstructive lymphedema. World J Surg 3 : 3-15, 121-123, 1979.

30) O'Brien MB, Mellow CG, Khazanchi RK, et al : Long-term results after microlymphaticovenous anastomoses for the treatment of of obstructive lymphedema. Plast Reconstr Surg 85 : 562-572, 1990.

31) Baumeister RG, Siuda S : Treatment of lymphedema by microsurgical lymphatic grafting ; What is proved? Plast Reconstr Surg 85 : 64-74, 1990.

32) Campisi C : Use of autologous interposition vein graft in management of lymphedema ; Preliminary experimental and clinical observations. Lymphology 24 : 71-76, 1991.

33) Campisi C : Lymphoedema ; modern diagnostic and therapeutic aspects. International Angiology 18 : 14-24, 1999.

34) Yamamoto Y, Sugihara T : Microsurgical lymphaticovenous implantation for the treatment of chronic lymphedema. Plast Reconstr Surg 101 : 157-161, 1998.

35) Koshima I, Kawada S, Moriguchi T, et al : Ultrastructural observation of lymphatic vessels in lymphedema in human extremities. Plast Reconstr Surg 97 : 397-405, 1996.

36) Koshima I, Inagawa K, Urushibara K, et al : Supermicrosurgical lymphaticovenularanastomosis for the treatment of lymphedema in the upper extremities. J Reconstr Microsurg 16 : 437-442, 2000.

37) Koshima I, Nanba U, Tsutsui T, et al : Long-term follow-up after lymphaticovenular anastomosis for lymphedema in the legs. J Reconstr Microsurg 19 : 209-215, 2003.

38) Koshima I, et al : Minimal invasive lymphaticovenular anastomosis under local anesthesia for leg lymphedema. Is it effective for Stage III and IV? Ann Plast Surg 53 : 1-6, 2004.

39) Shesol BF, Nakashima R, Alavi A, et al : Successful lymph node transplantation in rats, with restoration of lymphatic function. Plast Reconstr Surg 63 : 817-823, 1979.

40) Chen HC, O'Brien MC, Rogers IW, et al : Lymph node transfer for the treatment of obstructive lymphoedema in the canine model. Br J Plast Surg 43 : 578-589, 1990.

41) Becker C, Assouad J, Riquet M, et al : Postmastectomy lymphedema ; Long term results following microsurgical lymph node transplantation. Ann Surg 243 : 313-315, 2006.

42) Lin CH, Ali R, Chen SC, et al : Vascularized groin lymph node transfer using the wrist as a recipient site for management of postmastectomy upper extremity lymphedema. Plast Reconstr Surg 123 : 1265-1275, 2009.

43) Takeishi M, Kojima M, Mori K, et al : Primary intrapelvic lymphaticovenular anastomosis following lymph node dissecdtion. Ann Plast Surg 57 : 300-304, 2006.

Important Reference

■ リンパ節郭清後のリンパ節の再生と リンパ道の回復について

Regeneration of lymph nodes and recovery of the lymphatic tract after lymph node dissection

1 リンパ節の再生

　リンパ節郭清後、リンパ節は再生しない。その理由はまだわかっていない。個体発生学的[1)-3)]にみると、リンパ節原基は囊性原基にしろ、管性原基にしろ、間葉性細胞の小さな集合からなり、胎生2ヵ月の末（深頸、腰、腋窩、鼠径リンパ節など）から3ヵ月（腸間膜、気管気管支、顎下リンパ節など）にかけて出現し始め、遅くても3ヵ月の末（膝窩リンパ節など）から4ヵ月にかけてすべて出揃う。リンパ節原基からリンパ節への発育過程をみると、胎生4ヵ月で線維性の被膜が形成されて、周囲組織との境が明瞭になり、胎生5ヵ月に入ると辺縁洞の形成が認められる。また、ほとんどのリンパ節に髄洞、髄索が形成され、皮質と髄質が区別される。胎生6～7ヵ月頃、皮質に初めて二次小節が出現する。その出現は深頸、腋窩、腸骨リンパ節に始まり、漸次ほかのリンパ節にも出現する。腸間膜根リンパ節には特に多い。ただし、胚（または芽）中心を備えた二次小節は生後出現する。これを要するに、リンパ節は抗原刺激のない胎生期から生体防御のために準備された**器官（organ）**である。脾臓、肺、腎臓などの器官に比べると小さくて、身体のあちこちに分散しているが、各リンパ節のひとつひとつが生体防御の**器官**であり、ほかの器官と同じように、完全に摘出されると再生しない。身体のあちこちに分散していると述べたが、実際はリンパ節の出現する場所、そこに出現する数はヒトを含めどの動物でも決まっている。なお、系統発生学的[1)-3)]にみると、リンパ節が出現するのは、哺乳動物と鳥類の一部（アヒルなどの水禽類）だけである。多くの鳥類や爬虫類、両棲類にはリンパ節はないが、リンパ管内皮下にリンパ球浸潤やリンパ小節が出現する。リンパ球浸潤やリンパ小節はヒトのリンパ管にも存在するので、このような小さいリンパ装置に癌が転移した場合は発見が困難で、ここから再発する可能性もあると思われる。

1. Regeneration of lymph nodes

　Lymph nodes never regenerate after complete surgical dissection. The reason remains still unclear. Ontogenically[1)-3)], the lymph node anlage consisting of a small aggregate of mesenchymal cells begin to appear from the second month of the embryo (including the deep cervical, lumbar, axillary, and inguinal lymph nodes) to the third month (including the mesenteric, tracheobranchial, and submandibular lymph nodes). The anlage of all other lymph nodes appear from the end of the third month (including the poplitial lymph nodes) to the fourth month at the latest. Focusing on the development process from the lymph node anlage to the lymph node, the fibrous capsule is formed around the anlage in the fourth month of the embryo and the subcapsular marginal sinus in the fifth month. The formation of nodular cord and sinus occur successively in the most developing lymph nodes. The secondary (also termed cortical) nodules appear in the cortex for the first time around the sixth to seventh month of the embryo. This appearance begins from the deep cervical, axillary, and iliac lymph nodes, in addition, to also gradually appearing in other lymph nodes. It is particularly common in the lymph nodes at the root of the mesentery. It should be noted that the germinal centers are absent in the fetus. In short, the lymph node is an **organ** prepared for biological defence from the prenatal period without antigen stimulation. Although lymph nodes are smaller than organs such as the spleen, lung and kidney and are dispersed throughout the body, every single lymph node is an **organ** for biological defense and does not regenerate in the same way as other so-called organs do not regenerate after complete surgical dissection. Although I mentioned that lymph nodes are dispersed throughout the body, the sites where lymph nodes appear and the number that appears there are actually fixed in all animals including human beings.

Phylogenically[1)-3)], lymph nodes only appear in mammals and some birds (aquatic birds such as ducks). Although lymph nodes absent in many birds, reptiles, and amphibians, the subendothelial lymphoid tissues such as lymphocyte infiltrations and lymph nodules appear commonly in their lymphatics. These lymphoid tissues also appear in the human lymphatics. When cancer metastasis occur in such small lymphoid tissues, discovery is difficult and the possibility of recurrence is also conceivable.

2 リンパ道の回復

リンパ節郭清後、やがてリンパ道は開通する。そのメカニズムに次の2つの方法が考えられる。

①リンパ節剔出部は間葉性の細網線維と線維芽細胞で埋められる。リンパ管内皮細胞になる潜在能をもつ。あるいは潜在能を獲得した間葉性細胞は小隙を挟み扁平に並び、リンパ管を形成する。新生リンパ管は剔出部周辺のリンパ管に連なり、リンパ道が開通する。これはまさに胎生初期のリンパ管系形成における求心説[3)]を思わせるものである。

②リンパ節剔出部の周辺に残ったもとの輸入リンパ管からリンパ管内皮の発芽が起こり、剔出部を越えて中枢側に向かって延び、もとの輸出リンパ管に連なり、リンパ道が開通する。リンパ節摘出時に結紮された輸入リンパ管に強いリンパのうっ滞が起こり、それがリンパ管内皮の発芽を促進する。

(小谷正彦)

2. Recovery of the lymphatic tract

The lymphatic tract recovers after lymph node dissection. The following two mechanisms are conceivable.

①Recovery of the lymphatic tract occur by differentiation of mesenchymal cells filling up the excised part of lymph nodes to the lymphatic endothelial cells. This is precisely what brings to mind the centripetal theory[1)] of embryonal lymphatic development.

②Recovery of the lymphatic tract occur by sprouting of remaining afferent lymphatic endothelial cells in a centripetal direction. Budding off from afferent lymphatic endothelial cells is accelarated by lymph stasis.

(*Masahiko Kotani／Ryo Karakawa*)

1) Kotani M：The lymphatics and lymphoreticular tissues in relation to the action of sex hormones. Arch Histol Cytol 53(Suppl)：1-76, 1990.
2) Kotani M：Development of lymphoid tissues. Jap J Lymphology 28：64-66, 2005.
3) Kotani M：Seven mysteries of the lymphatics. Jap J Lymphology 35：66-80, 2012.

| CHAPTER 2 | 解 剖
Anatomy
1. 頭頸部領域におけるリンパ解剖
Lymphatic anatomy in head and neck region |

■はじめに

　頭頸部には多数のリンパ節が存在し、また左頸部下方は全身のリンパ液を集めた胸管が静脈角に流入する部位でもあることから、その解剖学的知識は重要である。頭頸部悪性腫瘍では頸部リンパ節に転移を生じることが多く、頸部リンパ節郭清がしばしば行われるが、時に顔面のリンパ浮腫を生じる。一方で、頸部の豊富なリンパ節を血管柄付きリンパ節移植のドナーとして用いることも可能である。

■ Introduction

　There are multiple lymph nodes (LN's) in the head and neck region. In the left lower neck region, thoracic duct collects lymph from most parts of the body and drains into the venous-angle, so its anatomical knowledge is clinically important. Metastasis of the head and neck cancer often occur in this region, therefore the neck dissection is often performed which may result in facial lymphedema. On the other hand, harvesting LN's from this region as a donor for free vascularized LN's transfer has also been reported.

I　頭部のリンパ節

　浅在性と深在性に大別される。浅在性のものとしては以下が挙げられる。
・耳前リンパ節（浅耳下腺リンパ節）……耳下腺の表面に存在し、顔面上部、前頭部からのリンパ液を集める。
・耳後リンパ節…………側頭部からのリンパ液を集める。
・後頭リンパ節…………外後頭隆起の外側に存在し、後頭部のリンパ液を集める。

　深在性のものとしては以下のものがある。
・深耳下腺リンパ節……耳下腺の内部に存在し、顔面上外側部や側頭部から流入。
・頬リンパ節……………顔面深部からのリンパ液を集める。
・オトガイ下リンパ節…下口唇、口腔前方などから集める。
・顎下リンパ節…………口唇、鼻腔、歯肉、口腔、舌前方など広範囲からリンパ液を集める。

I.　LN's in head and neck region

　These are classified as superficial and deep LN's.
・Superficial LN's includes：Preauricular LN's is situated on the Parotid gland, collecting lymph from upper face and forehead.
・Postauricular LN's collect lymph from temporal region.
・Occipital LN's are situated lateral to the external occipital protuberance, collecting lymph from occipital

27

region.

- Deep LN's includes : Deep parotid LN's is situated in the Parotid gland, draining the lateral upper face and temporal regions.
- Buccal LN's drains lymph from the deep part of the face.
- Submental LN's drains the lower lip and the front part of the face.
- Submandibular LN's widely collects lymph from lip, nasal cavity, gingiva, oral cavity and front part of tongue.

II 顔面、頭部のリンパ流(Fig. 2-1-1)

顔面、頭部のリンパ流は、主に、
・耳介より前方のリンパ流は耳前部リンパ節へ流入する。
・耳介より後方のリンパ流は耳後部リンパ節に流入する。
・頬部や口腔前方からのリンパ流は顎下リンパ節に流入する。

このほかにも一部、迂回路を経て還流している。正中部の病変では左右のリンパ管が交通しているため、両側のリンパ節に転移が生じうる。また、手術などの影響で本来のリンパ流が途絶、閉塞した場合、逆流をきたすなどの変化が生じうる。

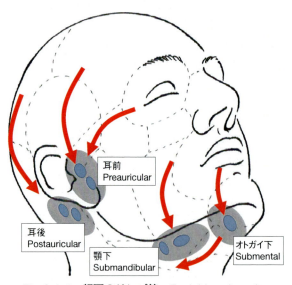

Fig. 2-1-1. 顔面のリンパ節　Facial lymph nodes
・耳介より前方のリンパ流は耳前部のリンパ節へ流入。
・耳介より後方からのリンパ流は耳後部に流入。
・頬部からのリンパ流は下顎部に向かう。
・後頭部、うなじ部は側頸部に向かう。
・Preauricular lymph drains into the preauricular lymph nodes.
・Postauricular lymph drains into the postauricular lymph nodes.
・Lymph from the buccal region drains towards the mandible.
・The occipital and nuchal lymph drains towards temporal region.

2-1. 頭頸部領域におけるリンパ解剖

II. Lymphatic flow in head and facial regions（Fig. 2-1-1）

・Preauricular lymph drains into the preauricular lymph nodes.
・Postauricular lymph drains into the postauricular lymph nodes.
・Lymph from the buccal region and anterior aspect of the oral cavity drains towards the mandible.
・The occipital and nuchal lymph flows towards temporal region.

There are some collateral pathways. The cancer in medial region can metastasize to bilateral LN's through the lymph vessel communication of both sides. The lymphatic flow interruption due to the surgical invasion also can result in the lymph back flow.

Ⅲ　頸部のリンパ節

　頸部のリンパ流は主として内頸静脈に沿って進むが、ほかにも多くのリンパ節があり、浅層と深層に分けられる。浅層のリンパ節としては以下が挙げられる。
・浅頸リンパ節………胸鎖乳突筋表面で外頸静脈に沿って存在する。耳下腺、耳介から流入。
　深層のリンパ節は、内頸静脈、副神経、頸横動脈に沿った三角形の領域に3つのリンパ節群が存在する（**Fig. 2-1-2**）。
・内深頸リンパ節……内頸静脈に沿って存在する頸部で最も重要なリンパ節群である。上、中、下に細分される。
・副神経リンパ節……副神経に沿って存在。後頭部、耳下腺などから流入し、鎖骨上へ流出する。
・鎖骨上リンパ節……頸横動脈に沿って鎖骨上窩に存在する。主に中内深頸、副神経リンパ節から流入するが、胸部や腋窩からのリンパ液も流入する。左側の鎖骨上窩リンパ節は胸腹部悪性腫瘍が胸管を経由して転移すると腫脹する（Virchowリンパ節）。
　顔面から頸部へのリンパの流れは以下のとおりである。
・オトガイ下リンパ節は顎下リンパ節を経て上内深頸リンパ節へ流入する。
・耳下腺リンパ節も上内深頸リンパ節へ流入する。
　頸部でのリンパの流れは以下のとおりである。
・上→中→下内深頸リンパ節の順でリンパ液は下降する。
・副神経リンパ節は、鎖骨上リンパ節を経て下内深頸リンパ節に注ぐ。
・前頸部のリンパ液からは中、下内深頸リンパ節へ流入する。
・最終的には、下内深頸リンパ節から、静脈角や鎖骨下静脈に直接流入するか、左側では胸管に合流した後に静脈に流入する。

Ⅲ. LN's in neck region

　Although the neck lymph mainly drains along Internal Jagular Vein, There are lots of LN's classified to superficial and deep regions.
　・The superficial region：Superficial neck LN's is situated along External Jagular Vein on Sternocleidomastoid muscle collecting lymph from Parotid gland and Auricle.
　The deep region is classified into three LN groups which make triangle along Internal Jagular Vein, Accessory Nerve and Transverse Cervical Artery（**Fig. 2-1-2**）.

29

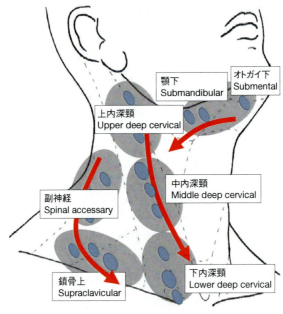

Fig. 2-1-2. MSKCC 分類
Memorial Sloan-Kettering Cancer Center(MSKCC) Classification
内頸静脈リンパ節は頭頸部の最も主要なリンパ節群である。
Internal jugular chain is a group of the most important nodes in the Head and Neck.
[Level]
Ⅰ　オトガイ下、顎下リンパ節　Submental and submandibular lymph nodes
Ⅱ　上内深頸リンパ節　Upper deep cervical lymph nodes
Ⅲ　中内深頸リンパ節　Middle deep cervical lymph nodes
Ⅳ　下内深頸リンパ節　Lower deep cervical lymph nodes
Ⅴ　後頸三角部(副神経リンパ節、鎖骨上窩リンパ節など)　Posterior triangle (the spinal accessory nodes, supraclavicular nodes, etc.)
Ⅵ　前頸部(気管傍リンパ節など)　Anterior compartment (paratracheal nodes, etc.)

- Medial deep neck LN's are the most important LN's in the neck region, which is situated along Internal Jagular Vein, classified to the upper, middle and lower regions.
- Accessory Nerve LN's present along Accessory Nerve, draining from the occipital region and Parotid gland to supraclavicular region.
- Supraclavicular LN's present along Transverse Cervical Artery, draining mainly from the median deep neck and Accessory Nerve LN's and partly from Thoracic duct and axillary region. Thoracicoabdominal cancer can metastasize to the left supraclavicular LN's through thoracic duct (Virchow's LN).
 Lymphatic flow from face to neck;
- Submental lymph drains into upper median deep neck LN's through submundible LN's.
- Lymph in Parotid gland LN's drains into upper median deep neck LN's.
 Lymphatic flow in neck region;
- Lymph drains in order of the upper, middle and lower median deep neck LN's.
- Lymph in Accessory Nerve LN's drains into the lower median deep neck LN's through the supraclavicular LN's.
- Lymph in anterior cervical region drains into middle and lower median deep neck LN's.
- Lymph in the lower median deep neck LN's directly drains into Venous-angle or Subclavicular Vein. In left side lymph drains from thoracic duct into Venous-angle.

2-1. 頭頸部領域におけるリンパ解剖

IV MSKCC(Memorial Sloan-Kettering Cancer Center)分類

　頭頸部外科領域で最も一般的に用いられている頸部リンパ節の臨床的分類として MSKCC 分類がある。

Level
I　オトガイ下、顎下リンパ節
II　上内深頸リンパ節
III　中内深頸リンパ節
IV　下内深頸リンパ節
V　後頸三角部（僧帽筋、胸鎖乳突筋、鎖骨で囲まれた区域。副神経リンパ節、鎖骨上窩リンパ節などが含まれる）
VI　前頸部（総頸動脈より内側の区域。気管傍リンパ節などを含む）

　II〜IVは内頸静脈リンパ節である。IIとIIIの境界は舌骨の高さ、IIIとIVの境界は肩甲舌骨筋である（**Fig. 2-1-3**）。

IV. Memorial Sloan- Kettering Cancer Center(MSKCC) Classification of the cervial lymph nodes

　The regional classification of the cervical lymph nodes proposed by MSKCC is now widely used in the field

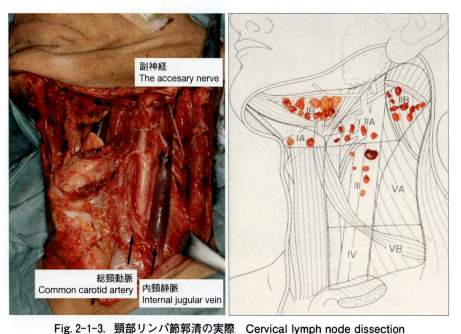

Fig. 2-1-3. 頸部リンパ節郭清の実際　Cervical lymph node dissection
左頸部リンパ節郭清後の状態と、摘出されたリンパ節。
Operative field after the left cervical lymph node dissection and the dissected nodes.

of Head and Neck Surgery.

> **Level**
> Ⅰ Submental and submandibular lymph nodes.
> Ⅱ Upper deep cervical lymph nodes.
> Ⅲ Middle deep cervical lymph nodes.
> Ⅳ Lower deep cervical lymph nodes.
> Ⅴ Regional lymph nodes in the posterior triangle demarcated by the trapezius muscle, sternocleidomastoid muscle, and the clavicle. The spinal accessory nodes and supraclavicular nodes are included in this group.
> Ⅵ Regional lymph nodes in the anterior compartment between the left and right common carotid arteries which include paratracheal nodes.

　　Level Ⅱ to Ⅳ indicate internal jugular chain. The boundary of level Ⅱ and Ⅲ is hyoid bone, level Ⅲ and Ⅳ omohyoid muscle (**Fig. 2-1-3**).

Ⅴ　頭頸部のリンパに関する臨床との関係

　　頭頸部領域は重力によってリンパ液の還流が促されるため、リンパ節郭清後も顔面リンパ浮腫は下肢に比べると生じにくい。しかし、時に顔面の浮腫が1年を超えて残存することがあり、われわれはICGを用いて耳前部や鼻唇溝などでリンパ流を確認し、LVA（リンパ管細静脈吻合術）

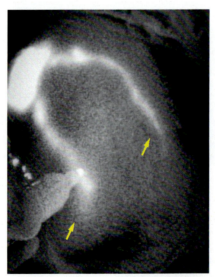

Fig. 2-1-4.　インドシアニングリーンを用いた頭部のリンパ流の観察
Lymphatic flow observed under indocyanine green lymphography
頭部正中にインドシアニングリーンを皮下注射し、Photo-Dynamic Eye を用いて観察すると、耳前部や眼窩上部に向かうリンパ流を確認できる。
Lymph flow towards preauricular and supraorbit region can be observed under Photo-Dynamic Eye by subcutaneously injecting indocyanine green in the middle of the neck.

を用いた治療も行っている（**Fig. 2-1-4**）。

　また頭頸部の豊富なリンパ節をリンパ節移植のドナー部とした報告もある。Hung-Chi Chen らは右頸横動脈に沿ったリンパ節（MSKCC Level Ⅴ）を足背に移植し、浮腫軽減がみられたとしている。また、Ming-Huei Cheng らは顔面動脈の枝であるオトガイ下動脈を茎としたオトガイ下リンパ節（MSKCC Level Ⅰa）を足関節部に移植して有効であったと報告している。

（飯田拓也）

V. The cervical lymph nodes in clinical practice

Lymph drainage from the cervical region is enhanced by the gravity which makes the facial lymphedema following the lymph node dissection less frequent than the lower leg lymphedema. However facial lymphedema sometimes persists for over a year and in those cases we observe lymphatic flow with ICG injected subcutaneously in the preauricular region or nasolabial fold, and then the Lymphatico-venous anastomosis is planned（**Fig. 2-1-4**）.

Some lymph node transplantations using the abundant nodes in the neck as the donor sites are reported. Hung-Chi Chen et al. transplanted MSKCC level Ⅴ nodes along the right transverse cervical artery to the dorsum of foot and lymphedema is reported to be alleviated. Additionally, Ming-Huei Cheng et al. reported the effective result in wchich they employed MSKCC level Ⅰ submental nodes with submental artery pedicle which is the branch of the facial artery for the transplantation to the ankle joint.

（*Takuya Iida*）

CHAPTER	2	解 剖

解 剖
Anatomy

2. 四肢のリンパ管解剖

Anatomy of the lymphatic vessels in the limbs

■**はじめに**

　四肢のリンパ浮腫の患者では、リンパ液の貯留、線維化、脂肪組織の増生が進行性に進んでいく。これらの病態を改善させるために近年リンパ管細静脈吻合術（LVA）などのリンパ外科治療が開発されている。リンパ管の解剖を知ることはLVAにおいて非常に役立ち、またその他のリンパ外科治療においてもリンパ管の解剖を知ることは欠かせないことと思われる。

■**Introduction**

　Patients with lymphedema in the limbs experience progressively advancing growth in adipose tissue with fibrosis and build up of lymphatic fluid. Lymphatic surgical treatments have been developed in recent years such as lymphatic venous anastomosis(LVA) to improve such clinical conditions. Knowing the anatomy of the lymph vessels is extremely useful in LVA and is indispensable to other lymphatic surgical treatments.

Ⅰ　四肢リンパ管のミクロ解剖

　四肢のリンパ管は、表皮直下に存在する毛細リンパ管から始まり、前集合リンパ管を通り脂肪層内の浅集合リンパ管に至る。これらは浅リンパシステムと呼ばれ、深筋膜より下には深集合リンパ管が存在しこれは深リンパシステムと呼ばれる。これらの浅リンパシステムと深リンパシステムはリンパ管穿通枝を通して互いに交通していると考えられている。

1. 毛細リンパ管

　表皮直下に網目状に存在し、起始は盲端である。1層のリンパ管内皮細胞からなり、周細胞や平滑筋細胞をもたない。通常基底膜もない。管径は 30～80 μm である。

　毛細リンパ管は断続的で間隙をもち、これにより浸透性を高め、微小分子や白血球を容易に脈管系に取り込むことができる。

2. 前集合リンパ管

　真皮内から脂肪層にかけて網目状に存在し、毛細リンパ管と浅集合リンパ管をつないでいる。毛細リンパ管と違い不完全ながら平滑筋細胞に覆われており、弁構造をもつのが特徴である。

3. 集合リンパ管

全集合リンパ管が集合リンパ管に流れ込み四肢を長軸方向に走る。いわゆるリンパ管と呼ばれるもので、集合リンパ管がリンパ節へとつながる。平滑筋細胞をもち、基底膜が存在する。また弁構造をもつ。

浅集合リンパ管と深集合リンパ管に分かれ、浅集合リンパ管は深筋膜より浅い脂肪層に存在する。深集合リンパ管は深筋膜下に存在し、四肢の動脈に伴走することが多い。

4. リンパ管のポンプ作用

血管系と違い、リンパ管ではリンパ液は心臓のポンプ作用で動くわけではない。リンパ液を押し運ぶ力としては2つあり、1つ目はリンパ管の平滑筋の収縮による自動運動である。リンパ管は平滑筋をもち、これが毛細リンパ管の内圧上昇に伴い自発収縮することでリンパ液が流れる。2つ目は周囲の動脈の動きや骨格筋の収縮によるポンプ作用である。これらの自動運動と他動運動によりリンパ液は中枢へと運ばれる。

リンパ浮腫の患者ではその進行とともに平滑筋細胞の変性が起こり、リンパ管の収縮作用が失われると考えられている。

I. Micro-anatomy of lymph vessels in the limbs

The lymph vessels of the limbs start from the lymphatic capillaries located just below the epidermis, travel through the front collecting lymph vessels, and extend to the superficial collecting lymph vessels located in fat layers. This network of vessels is known as the superficial lymphatic system, and the deep collecting lymph vessels, which are located below deep fascia is known as the deep lymphatic system. The superficial and deep lymphatic systems are thought to be interconnected through lymphatic trunks.

1. Lymphatic capillaries：The lymphatic capillaries form a web-like mesh just below the epidermis, and the origin of the lymphatic capillaries are blind-ended. The lymphatic capillaries are composed of a single layer of lymphatic vessel endothelial cells with no pericytes or smooth myocytes and do not have usual basal membranes.

The diameter of the capillaries are between 30 and 80 micrometers.

The lymphatic capillaries have intermittent gaps which elevate permeability, thereby enabling micro-molecules and white blood cells to be drawn into the vascular system easily.

2. Anterior collecting lymphatic vessels：The anterior collecting lymphatic vessels exist in a web-like mesh from the dermis to the adipose layer and connect the lymphatic capillaries to the superficial collecting lymphatic vessels. As opposed to the lymphatic capillaries, the anterior collecting lymphatic vessels are partially covered in smooth myocytes and stand out for their valve structure.

3. Collecting lymphatic vessels：The anterior collecting lymphatic vessels empty into the collecting lymphatic vessels and run through the limbs in a longitudinal direction. Also known as lymph vessels, the collecting lymphatic vessels connect to the lymph nodes. They feature smooth myocytes and have a basal membrane. The collecting lymphatic vessels also have a valve structure.

Divided into the superficial lymph vessels and deep lymph vessels, the superficial lymph vessels are located in shallow layers of fat above deep fascia. The deep lymph vessels exist below deep fascia and often parallel arteries in the limbs.

4. Pumping mechanism of the lymph vessels：Unlike the vascular system, lymphatic fluid is not pushed through the lymph vessels by the pumping mechanism of the heart. There are two forces that pump lymphatic fluid : one is spontaneous movement prompted by the contraction of smooth muscles in the lymphatic vessels. The lymph vessels have smooth muscles that spontaneously contract as internal pressure in the lymphatic capillaries rises, thereby pumping lymphatic fluid. The second force is the pumping effect induced by the movement of surrounding arteries and the contraction of skeletal muscles. Lymph is carried to the core as the result of these spontaneous and passive movements.

In patients with lymphedema, it is thought that this contracting mechanism of the lymphatic vessels is lost with progression of the disease since lymphedema progression is associated with a degeneration of the smooth myocytes.

Ⅱ 上肢リンパ管のマクロ解剖

1. 指

指のリンパ管は末節部の毛細リンパ管より起こり、各指の外側内側の2本の集合リンパ管となる。径は約0.2mmである。指動脈神経に平行に沿って指に並走する。

その後隣接する指同士のリンパ管は指間部で合流し、その後手背を放射状に走行する。

2. 手 背

手背レベルでは約15本の集合リンパ管が互いに分岐と合流をしながら走行している。径は0.2～0.6mmであり、母指から中指より走行している橈側のグループと環指と小指より走行している尺側のグループの主に2つが存在する。

3. 前 腕

前腕レベルでは約25本の集合リンパ管が存在し、径は0.3～0.5mmである。

これらの集合リンパ管は主に橈側皮静脈や尺側皮静脈に沿って走行している。

前腕では手関節背側の橈側から外側肘窩に向かって走行する橈側グループと、手関節背側の尺側から内側肘窩に向かって走行する尺側グループと、手関節前面より生じ、前腕腹側を走行し肘窩に向かって走行する手掌側グループがある。

これらは肘部内側前面で集合し、その後、主に尺側皮静脈に沿って走行する。

4. 上 腕

上腕では約20本の集合リンパ管が存在し、径は0.3～1.2mmである。そのほとんどは内側に存在し、外側にはない。腋窩リンパ節に流入する前に合流し、より太い集合リンパ管となる。

5. 腋窩リンパ節に流入しない経路

　上肢の集合リンパ管のほとんどは肘部で前面内側に集合し、その後尺側皮静脈に沿って上腕前面内側を走行し、腋窩リンパ節群の最外側に存在する比較的大きなリンパ節に流入する。

　それ以外の経路として、以下の2つのものが知られている。

・橈側皮静脈に沿って平行に走行し、肩関節前面で三角筋と大胸筋の間を通って深部へ向かい三角胸筋リンパ節へ流入するもの。

・前腕で尺側皮静脈に沿って走行し、肘窩リンパ節へ流入して深部リンパ管へと合流するもの。

　これらのルートは腋窩リンパ節を郭清しても障害されないため、リンパ浮腫の治療に利用できる可能性がある。

6. 上肢の深部リンパシステム

　上肢の深集合リンパ管は主要な動脈に沿って走行し、総掌側指動脈から前腕では橈骨動脈・尺側動脈、上腕では上腕動脈に沿って走行する。深集合リンパ管は腋窩外側の優位なリンパ節に接続せず、腋窩動脈に近接するため、通常の腋窩リンパ節郭清では障害されないことが多い。

II. Macro-anatomy of the lymph vessels in the upper limbs

　1. Fingers：The lymph vessels of the fingers originate from the lymphatic capillaries in the distal ends of the fingers and are made up of two collecting lymph vessels on the inner and outer side of each finger. These lymph vessels are approximately 0.2 millimeters in diameter. The lymph vessels in the finger run parallel to the arteries, nerves of the finger.

　Subsequently, these lymph vessels in the finger converge with the lymph vessels of neighboring fingers in the interdigital area, then run in a radial fashion along the dorsum (back) of the hand.

　2. Dorsum of the hand：Upon reaching the dorsum (back) of the hand, approximately 15 collecting lymphatic vessels run along the hand, branching from and converging with one another. The lymph vessels here are between 0.2 and 0.6 millimeters in diameter and are composed primarily of two groups：the radial side group that runs from the thumb to the middle finger and the ulnar side group that runs from the ring finger to the little finger.

　3. Forearm：At the forearm level, there are approximately 25 collecting lymph vessels that range from between 0.3 and 0.5 millimeters in diameter.

　These collecting lymph vessels primarily run along the cephalic and basilic veins.

　The lymph vessels in the forearms are composed of the radial side group that runs toward the outer cubital fossa from the radial side of the dorsal wrist, the ulnar side group that runs toward the inner cubital fossa from the ulnar side of the dorsal wrist, and the palmar group running toward the cubital fossa on the ventral side of the forearm from the anterior wrist.

　These converge in front of the medial side of the elbow and subsequently run along the basilic vein.

　4. Upper Arm：There are approximately 20 collecting lymph vessels in upper arm that range from 0.3 to 1.2 millimeters in diameter. The majority of these lymph vessels are on the inner side of the upper arm, whereas there are very few on the outer side. These vessels converge into thicker collecting lymph vessels prior to flowing into the axillary lymph nodes.

　5. Routes not flowing into the axillary lymph nodes：Most of the collecting lymph vessels in the upper limbs converge on the front inner side of the limbs in the cubital region and subsequently flow along the inner side of the upper arm along the basilic vein, flowing into the relatively large lymph nodes that exist in the outermost end of the axillary lymph nodes.

Aside from these, there are two other known routes :

· Those running parallel to the cephalic vein, traveling between the deltoids and pectoralis major muscles in front of the shoulder joints, and flowing into the deltopectoral lymph nodes toward the deep lymphatic region.

· Those running parallel to the basilic vein in the forearms and flowing into the cubital lymph nodes, converging with the deep lymphatic vessels.

These routes are unaffected even when the cubital lymph nodes are dissected, and therefore may have applications in the treatment of lymphedema.

6. The deep lymphatic system of the upper limbs : The deep collecting lymph vessels of the upper limbs run along the primary arteries, traveling from the palmar digital arteries and running along the radial and ulnar arteries in the forearms and the brachial arteries in the upper arm. The deep collecting lymph vessels encroach on the axillary arteries without connecting to the superior lymph nodes on the outer side of the axillary fossa, and are therefore often unaffected by standard dissection of the axillary lymph nodes.

Ⅲ 下肢リンパ管のマクロ解剖

1. 足 趾

それぞれの足趾は外側・内側に 2 本の集合リンパ管をもち、midaxial line に沿って走行する。径は約 0.5 mm である。隣接する足趾同士のリンパ管は趾間部で合流する。その後、足背を放射状に走行する。

2. 足 部

約 15 本の集合リンパ管が存在し、径は約 0.5 mm である。

足趾より起こり足背前面を走行するグループと、足部の内側から起こり足部の内側を走行するグループと、足部の外側から起こり足部の外側を走行するグループとがそれぞれ互いに分岐・合流しネットワークを形成している。

3. 足関節

足関節レベルでは約 12 本の集合リンパ管が存在しており、その径は約 0.5 mm ほどである。大部分は足関節前面を走行している。足関節後面ではアキレス腱の両側に少数の集合リンパ管が存在する。

4. 下 腿

下腿レベルでは約 15 本前後の集合リンパ管が存在しており、その径は約 0.5 mm である。

ほとんどは大伏在静脈とその枝に近接して走行している。前面外側を走行するものは比較的散

在しており、下腿近位 1/3 の内側前面へ向かって走行する。下腿後面では小伏在静脈に並走して1 本か 2 本の集合リンパ管が走行する。

5．膝

径は約 0.5 mm である。大部分は膝関節内側を走行する。前面を走行するものは比較的少数であり、大腿前面内側に向かって斜めに走行している。

後面では小伏在静脈に並走する少数のリンパ管のみが存在し膝リンパ節へ流入する。

6．大　腿

大腿レベルでは約 30 本の集合リンパ管が存在し、その径は約 0.6 mm である。

内側を走行するものは下腿の内側を走行するものから続いており、大伏在静脈に近接して走行し浅鼠径リンパ節群の中央部のリンパ節に流入する。

その他に、大腿前面外側から起こり大腿前面を斜めに走行し外側の浅鼠径リンパ節に流入するもの、大腿後面外側から起こり大腿後面を斜めに走行し内側の浅鼠径リンパ節に流入するものがある。

7．下肢の深リンパシステム

下肢の深集合リンパ管は上肢と同様に主要な動脈に沿って走行する。前脛骨動脈・後脛骨動脈・腓骨動脈に沿って下腿を走行し、大腿では大腿動脈に沿って走行する。

（播摩光宣）

Ⅲ．Macro- anatomy of the lymph vessels in the lower limbs

1．Toes：Each toe has two collecting lymph vessels on the inner and outer side that run along the mid-axial line. The vessels are approximately 0.5 millimeters in diameter. The lymph vessels of adjacent toes converge together in the interdigital toe region. Subsequently, the vessels run radially along the dorsal （back） of the foot.

2．Foot region：There are approximately 15 collecting lymph vessels in the foot region, each of which is approximately 0.5 millimeters in diameter.

The group originating in the toes and running along the dorsal of the foot, the group originating on the inner side of the foot region and running along the inner side of the foot, and the group originating on the outer side of the foot and running along the outer side of the foot form a network, branching off and converging with one another.

3．Ankles：At the ankle level, there are approximately 12 collecting lymph vessels, each of which is approximately 0.5 millimeters in diameter.

The majority of them run along the front side of the ankle. There are a few collecting lymph vessels on both sides of the Achilles tendon on the posterior side of the ankle.

4．Lower leg：At the level of the lower leg, there are approximately 15 collecting lymph vessels, more or less, each of which is approximately 0.5 millimeters in diameter.

Most of these lymph vessels run adjacent to the great saphenous vein and its tributaries. The collecting lymph vessels running on the front outer side of the lower leg are relatively sparse and one-third run toward the inner front side of the proximal lower leg. On the posterior side of the lower leg, one or two collecting lymph vessels run parallel to the small saphenous vein.

5. Knees: The lymph vessels in the knees are approximately 0.5 millimeters in diameter. The majority of them run on the inner side of the knee joint. There are relatively few lymph vessels running on the front side, and they run diagonally toward the front inner side of the thigh.

On the back side of the knee, only a few lymph vessels running parallel to the small saphenous vein exist and flow into the popliteal lymph nodes.

6. Thighs: At the thigh level, there are approximately 30 collecting lymph vessels, each of which are approximately 0.6 millimeters in diameter.

The lymph nodes that run along the inner side of the thigh continue from those that run along the inner side of the lower leg and run adjacent to the great saphenous vein, flowing into the central lymph nodes of the superficial inguinal lymph node cluster.

Additionally, there are collecting lymph vessels that originate in the front lateral side of the thigh and run diagonally along the anterior aspect of the thigh, flowing into the the outer side of the superficial inguinal lymph nodes, as well as vessels that originate in the outer anterior thigh and run diagonally along the pesterior aspect of the thigh, flowing into the inner side of the superficial inguinal lymph nodes.

7. The deep lymphatic system of the lower limbs: Like in the upper limbs, the deep collecting lymph vessels of the lower limbs run along the primary arteries. The deep collecting lymph vessels run through the lower legs along the anterior and posterior tibial arteries and the fibular artery, and run along the femoral artery in the thigh.

(Mitsunobu Harima)

1) Suami H, et al : The lymphatic territories of upper limb ; anatomical study and clinical implications. Plast Reconstr Surg 119 : 1813-1822, 2007.
2) Suami H, et al : Changes in the lymph structure of the upper limb after axillary dissection ; Radiographic and anatomical study in human cadaver. Plast Reconstr Surg 120 : 982-991, 2007.
3) Suami H, et al : The lymphatic anatomy of the breast and its implications for sentinel lymph node biopsy ; a human cadaver study. Ann Surg Oncol 15 : 863-871, 2008.
4) 須網博夫：マクロ所見(四肢リンパ解剖)．リンパ浮腫のすべて，光嶋　勲(編)，永井書店，大阪，2011.
Suami H : Macro observations (lymphatic anatomy of the limbs). All about lymphedema, Koshima I (ed), pp19-27, Nagai-Shoten, Osaka, 2011.
5) Yoffey JM, et al : Lymphatics, Lymph and Lymphomyeloid complex. Academic Press, London, 1970.
6) Rusznyak IF, et al : Lymphatics and lymph circulation. Pergamon Press, Oxford, 1967.
7) 大橋俊夫：リンパの吸収と輸送機構．リンパ管；形態・機能・発生．大谷　修，ほか(編)，pp1-9, 西村書店，東京，1997.
Ohashi T : Lymph absorption and transportation mechanisms. The form, function, and development of lymph vessels, Otani S, et al (eds), pp1-9, Nishimura-Shoten, Tokyo, 1997.
8) Suami H, et al : A new radiographic cadaver injection technique for investigating the lymphatic system. Plast Recnstr Surg 115 : 2007-2013, 2010.
9) Pan WR, et al : Alternative lymphatic drainage routes from the lateral heel to the inguinal lymph nodes ; anatomic study and clinical implications. ANZ J Surg 81 : 431-435, 2010.
10) Pan WR, et al : Superficial lymphatic drainage of the lower extremity ; anatomic study and clinical implications. Plast Reconstr Surg 132 : 696-707, 2013.
11) Pan WR : Changing concepts in lymphatic pathways. Lymphedema, Peter C. Neligan, et al (eds), pp61-96, CRC press, Washington DC, 2015.

CHAPTER **3**

分 類
Classification
1. リンパ浮腫の分類

Classification of lymphedema

■ **はじめに**

　リンパ浮腫は、特発性リンパ浮腫と続発性リンパ浮腫とに大別される。人類の歴史において、リンパ浮腫の原因として最も多いのはフィラリアによる続発性リンパ浮腫であり、現代でもフィラリア撲滅が行われていない途上国におけるフィラリア保虫率の高さが、世界におよそ2.5億人ともいわれるリンパ浮腫患者の数を押し上げている。近年の医学の進歩により、新たに発生するリンパ浮腫の多くは、乳癌・婦人科癌術後の続発性リンパ浮腫であり、先進国においては患者の大部分を占めている。これに対し、特発性リンパ浮腫は比較的稀である。

■ **Background**

　Lymphedema is classified into primary lymphedema and secondary lymphedema by etiology. Worldwide, the most common cause of lymphedema is a secondary lymphedema due to filariasis. At present, high prevalence of filariasis in developing countries continues to give rise to lymphedema, a population of approximately 250 million in the world. With the recent advances in medicine, the majority of lymphedema in developed countries occurs secondary to cancer treatment including breast cancers and gynecologic cancers. In contrast, primary lymphedema is relatively rare.

I　特発性リンパ浮腫

　特発性リンパ浮腫は6,000～10,000人に1人の有病率とされ、浮腫発症の時期により、①先天性リンパ浮腫（出生から2歳頃までに発症）、②早発性リンパ浮腫（2～35歳までに発症）、③遅発性リンパ浮腫（35歳以降に発症）、の3つに分類される（**Table 3-1-1**）。

　またKinmonthらは、リンパ管造影の検査結果をもとに特発性リンパ浮腫をaplasia、hypoplasia、hyperplasiaの3つに分類し（**Table 3-1-2**）、さらに臨床病理的分類として特発性リンパ浮腫を6種類に分類した[1]（**Table 3-1-3**）。

　生下時よりなんらかの形態で浮腫を発症していると考えられるaplasiaやリンパ管弁不全が原因と考えられる疾患以外では、浮腫の発症時期やリンパ管の形態はさまざまであるが、いずれにおいてもリンパ灌流が破綻した時点で浮腫が症状として出現し、リンパ浮腫の発症に至ると考えられる。そして、いったん発症したリンパ浮腫は、自然に軽快することはほぼない。

　リンパ灌流の破綻の原因としては、①時間経過（成長とともに増大したリンパ流入量の増加にリンパ灌流能が追い付かない、または加齢によるリンパ管灌流能の低下）、②accident、の両者が複合的要因として働くと考えられる。ここでいうaccidentとはリンパ灌流能の低下を引き起こしうるものすべてを指し、もともとのリンパ流入量に対し、ギリギリの状態で灌流を行えていたリンパ灌流能が、なんらかのaccidentにより低下することでリンパのうっ滞が始まるものと

41

Table 3-1-1. 特発性リンパ浮腫の発症時期による分類
Clinical classification of primary lymphedema

先天性リンパ浮腫 Congenital onset	出生〜2歳頃までに発症したもの Before 2 years after birth
早発性リンパ浮腫 Lymphedema precox	2歳頃〜35歳までに発症したもの Onset between 2 and 35 years old
遅発性リンパ浮腫 Lymphedema tarda	35歳以降に発症したもの Onset after 35 years old

Table 3-1-2. リンパ管形態による Kinmonth 分類
Kinmonth's classification of primary lymphedema by lymphangiogram

Aplasia
Hypoplasia
Hyperplasia

Table 3-1-3. 特発性リンパ浮腫の臨床病理的分類 Kinmonth 分類
Kinmonth's clinicopathological classification of primary lymphedema

Lymphoedema with unilateral hyperplasia of lymph vessels (megalymphatics)
Lymphoedema with bilateral hyperplasia
Lymphoedema with gonad dysgenesis (Turner's and other syndromes)
Lymphoedema with pes cavus
Milroy's disease (congenital familial lymphoedema)
Primary hypoplastic lymphoedema

考えられる。さらに、一度うっ滞したリンパ自体がリンパ管の変性を引き起こし、元来機能低下に陥っていたリンパ管の局所リンパ灌流能をさらに低下させることで、浮腫は自然治癒することなく、一般的に進行する。当然重力に抗してリンパを灌流しなければならない下肢でのリンパ浮腫発症は、上肢と比べて圧倒的に多い。

　浮腫を増悪させる trigger となる accident としては、些細なものを含めた外傷（足首を捻る、足を打撲する、などから交通外傷までのあらゆる外傷）、虫刺症（局所の炎症によるリンパ灌流能の低下）、医療行為（腫瘍切除などが局所リンパ管灌流へ負荷を与える）、感染症（丹毒などの炎症がリンパ灌流能を低下させる）、長時間の同一姿勢（飛行機などでの同一姿勢によるリンパうっ滞が、局所リンパ管灌流能で代償できず、そのリンパうっ滞自体が局所の炎症やリンパ管変性の原因となり、リンパ浮腫へと至る）、などさまざまである。時間経過と accident が複合的に作用することで、元来リンパ灌流能の低い個体では、人生のいずれかの段階でリンパ浮腫を発症するものと考えれば、発症時期の患者分布や、患者の浮腫発症 episode にも合致し、本疾患を理解しやすい。

　最新の研究によると、早発性リンパ浮腫の中でも、特に 11 歳未満での浮腫発症例ではリンパ管細静脈吻合術（LVA）の治療効果が得られにくいことが報告されている[2]。これは、低年齢でのリンパ浮腫の発症例では、リンパ管機能不全よりもリンパ管低形成例（hypoplasia）や弁の機能障害例が多いことが原因と考えられ、実際にリンパ管低形成の患者群では、術中に状態のよいリン

パ管が同定できずに、有効な LVA を行えないことも多い。われわれが LVA 手術時に同定したリンパ管の評価からも、術中所見でリンパ管の低形成を認めた患者群では、若年発症が多く、LVA の効果も低い傾向にある。

I. Primary lymphedema

Primary lymphedema can be caused by a genetic abnormality of the lymphatic system, however it can also arise sporadically and occurs in one of every 6000-10000 of the general population. Primary lymphedema is classified into three groups as per the time of edema onset ; ①congenital (developing until around 2 years after birth), ②lymphedema praecox (develop from 2 to 35 years), and ③lymphedema tarda (develop over the age of 36 years) (**Table 3-1-1**).

Other classification of primary lymphedema was made by Kinmonth et al. based upon lymphangiography and divided into aplasia, hypoplasia, and hyperplasia (**Table 3-1-2**). They also classified primary lymphedema in six categories based upon clinical pathological classifications (**Table 3-1-3**).

Aplasia type lymphedema develops from birth, and can manifest a variable spectrum of symptoms. Other types of primary lymphedema usually have a specific time of onset. This is considered the start point of lymphatic perfusion disruption, which ultimately leads to the development of extremity lymphedema. Once lymphedema developes, it continues to worsen over time with as the degeneration of lymphatic vessels progresses.

The cause of lymph congestion at the point of onset is considered to occur due to an interplay of underlying condition of the lymphatic system and events of injury. Problem of underlying condition of lymphatic system differs in each patient. In young generation, insufficient lymph perfusion ability to keep up with increased lymph flow with growth can trigger lymphedema. In contrast, gradual deterioration of lymph perfusion over time can initiate the onset of lymphedema in lymphedema tarda.

Injury refers to all events that can cause a reduction of lymph perfusion capacity. Once lymph perfusion is compromised, the congestion of the lymph itself leads to the degeneration of lymphatic vessels. Because degenerated lymphatic smooth muscles are inadequate to propel lymph, this exacerbates the lymphedema with no chance for spontaneous recovery. Lower extremity lymphedema develops more readily than upper extremity lymphedema, because the smooth muscles of lymphatic vessels in the lower extremity must propel lymph against gravity, there is a tendency for early decline of lymph perfusion.

Events that can trigger lymphedema include trauma (such as road traffic accidents, trivial trauma like an ankle sprain or minor foot confusion), insect bites and stings (decreased lymph perfusion due to local inflammation), iatrogenic (*ex.* tumor resection, etc.), infection (cellulites etc.), and postural (*ex.* precipitates the pooling of lymph in lower limbs which might cause inflammation in the presence of underlying degeneration of lymphatic vessels).

Recognising the trigger for lymphedema development helps us to understand the classification of primary lymphedema into three groups as follows, "Patients, who have genetically low lymph perfusion, are susceptible to lymphedema at any stage of life, due to a complex interplay of genetic and environmental factors".

According to the latest research, very young patients with primary lymphedema do not experience significant improvement following lymphaticovenular anastomosis (LVA). It is difficult to treat Lymphedema praecox with LVA, particularly when the onset of edema occurres before 11 years of age[2]. We hypothesize that the reason for this difficulty seen in early onset lymphedema is caused by lymphatic hypoplasia or valve dysfunction rather than lymphatic dysfunction. In our experience performing LVA's, lymphatic vessels with hypoplasia are usually seen in young patients. In such cases, hypoplastic lymphatic vessels with low lymph flow are difficult to identify and extremely fragile to anastomose accurately. Which could explain the less than desirable results obtained.

Ⅱ　続発性リンパ浮腫

　続発性リンパ浮腫も、基本的な疾患理解は原発性リンパ浮腫での考え方と矛盾しない。近年の ICG リンパ管造影を用いた続発性下肢リンパ浮腫の前向き研究の報告によると、山本らの LDB（Leg Dermal Backflow）分類における Stage Ⅰ以上の続発性下肢リンパ浮腫の病態を呈する患者は、骨盤部リンパ節郭清を伴う婦人科癌術後の患者全体の 4 割以上に及んでいる[3][4]。実際の臨床経験においても、軽症例を含めれば婦人科癌術後の患者の多くにリンパ浮腫を認め、この数字に矛盾しないと考えられる。上肢において続発性上肢リンパ浮腫を呈する患者は、腋窩リンパ節郭清を伴う乳癌術後の患者の 1～3 割程度と推察される。

　続発性においても原発性と同様に、リンパ灌流が破綻した時点で浮腫が症状として出現してリンパ浮腫の発症に至る。そして、いったん完成したリンパ浮腫は、自然に軽快することはほぼない。上肢よりも下肢で浮腫発症の割合が多いのは、重力の影響によると考えられる。

　ここでもやはり、リンパ灌流の破綻の原因としては、①時間経過、②accident の両者の複合的要因と考えられる。続発性リンパ浮腫における最大の accident は、リンパ節郭清を伴う当該癌手術治療である。標準化された近代医学の癌治療手術手技において、術後にリンパ浮腫をまったく呈さない患者と、術後リンパ浮腫に至る患者が存在する原因は、個々の患者のリンパ灌流能の違いに起因すると考えるしかない。癌治療を行う各施設間での、細かい手術の作法、組織愛護を含めた手技の丁寧さは異なるであろうが、どんなに丁寧に同じ術式で手術をしても、リンパ浮腫という合併症をほとんど生じていないという施設は存在していないのである。

　つまり、施設間による手術侵襲の多少の差はあるにしても、術後にリンパ浮腫を生じてしまうかどうかは、特発性リンパ浮腫と同様に、患者のリンパ灌流能に起因すると考えられる。当該癌の手術直後にリンパ浮腫が完成してしまう患者は、リンパ灌流能がもともと低く、浮腫の増悪も比較的早いことが多い。ここではリンパ節というリンパ路の消失を、残存したリンパ路で代償できなかったことによりリンパ液のうっ滞が生じ、そのリンパうっ滞がリンパ管硬化を引き起こし、さらに浮腫が進行するという悪循環に至る。この場合でも、浮腫の進行に患者間で大きな差がある理由は、新生リンパ路の増生能を含めた側副リンパ路の違いであろう。新生リンパ路の増生と側副リンパ路の成立が遅ければ、あっという間に浮腫は完成する一方で、比較的高いリンパ路の増生能と側副リンパ路の成立を認めるケースでは進行は緩徐である（ICG リンパ管造影において、新生リンパ路を含めた側副リンパ路を示すと考えられる Splash パターンを多く認めるケースがこれに該当する）。最も新生リンパ路と側副リンパ路への移行が際立っているものが、腋窩リンパ節郭清を伴う乳癌術後患者で認める事象である「癌術後に一過性の患側上肢の浮腫を認めたが、時間経過で自然に浮腫が消失した」というものである。これは常に重力に抗す必要のない、上肢でしかみられない現象と考えられ、下肢リンパ浮腫患者においては、一度発生した術後リンパ浮腫を新生リンパ路と側副リンパ路のみで代償できるケースは存在しないと思われる。

　一般的に続発性リンパ浮腫の症例では、リンパ管低形成の患者は少なく（リンパ管低形成群の患者は当該癌発症よりも早期の段階で特発性リンパ浮腫を発症していると考えられる）、リンパ外科治療を行った場合に、吻合可能な状態のリンパ管が同定できるケースがほとんどであり、LVA の治療効果が得られやすい。

また、癌治療後の続発性リンパ浮腫の重症度に関係する重要な accident 要因としては、放射線療法が挙げられる。放射線療法を行った患者では、放射線療法を行っていない患者よりもリンパ管変性が進行していることが多く、リンパ浮腫も重症化しやすい。しかし、当該癌の治療が最優先されるべきであり、リンパ浮腫発症の恐怖から放射線療法を思いとどまるべきではない。発症早期であれば、LVA を含めたリンパ外科療法の治療効果はより高まるため、放射線療法を行っている続発性リンパ浮腫の患者では、より早期にリンパ外科療法を行っている専門家へ紹介することが推奨される。

浮腫を増悪させる trigger となる他の accident 要因としては、原発性と同様に、些細なものを含めた外傷、虫刺症、医療行為、感染症、長時間の同一姿勢などが挙げられる。

（関 征央）

II. Secondary lymphedema

Understanding the etiology of secondary lymphedema is simple to recognize based on the same concept of "Underlying condition of the lymphatic system and events of injury". According to a recent prospective study of secondary lower extremity lymphedema using ICG lymphography, 44% of patients who underwent gynecological cancer surgery with lymphadenectomy developed secondary lower extremity lymphedema with Leg Dermal Backflow Stage I to V (Yamamoto's Leg Dermal Backflow Stage I is considered as lymphedema). Secondary upper extremity lymphedema occurres in approximate 10 to 30% of breast cancer patients following axillary lymph node dissection.

Same as primary lymphedema, secondary lymphedema developes following the reduction of lymph perfusion capacity, degeneration of lymphatic vessels with no spontaneous recovery of normal lymph flow. Lower extremity lymphedema develops more readily compared to upper extremity lymphedema, because of gravity's effect.

The main trigger for secondary lymphedema is lymph node dissections performed as part of cancer diagnosis or treatments.

In standardized modern surgical procedures, we have to think that secondary lymphedema is not caused by the surgeons' handling of the tissue, but rather the resultant defect in lymph perfusion. No matter how carefully the surgical procedures are performed, there is no facility that has shown reduced occurrence of secondary lymphedema.

Patients, who experience a reduction in lymphatic perfusion early after lymph node dissection, tend to develop severe lymphedema even in the very early stage of lymphedema progression. They cannot compensate for lymph return by using alternative pathways of lymph instead of the major route of the dissected lymph node. Once lymphedema is established, lymphedema itself causes sclerosis of the lymphatic vessels. This accelerates progression of lymphedema, because degenerated smooth muscles cannot generate sufficient power to propel lymph proximally and the resultant stagnant lymph fluid causes regional inflammation. The reason why progression of lymphedema is varied in each patient must be the difference of ability to make alternative new pathway for lymph outflow. When the formation of new lymphatic pathways is slow, lymphedema develops in the very early stage and is rapidly progressive. This is why each patient has a different latency of lymphedema onset and progression. Lower extremity lymphedema patients with slow disease progression tend to have plenty of splash patterns seen in the groin region with ICG lymphography (Splash patterns are considered to be alternative new lymph pathways). Total compensation of lymphedema by alternative formation of new lymph pathways can be observed in some cases of early stage secondary upper extremity lymphedema after a short latency period, where spontaneously recovery occurs because of the emergence of new lymph pathways and regeneration of lymphatic vessels. This phenomenon is not typically seen in cases of lower extremity lymphedema, because the new pathway's ability to propel lymph is not strong enough against gravity.

Excellent therapeutic effect of LVA is more readily achieved in instances of secondary lymphedema compared to primary lymphedema cases. This is mainly due to the absence of aplasia of lymphatic vessels in secondary lymphedema, which is more typically seen in some cases of primary lymphedema.

Another important factor relating to the severity of secondary lymphedema after cancer treatment is the additional injury caused by radiation therapy. Following radiation therapy, patients usually show degeneration of lymphatic vessels compared to cases without radiation therapy. Sclerosis of lymphatic vessels is a major reason for the early progression of lymphedema in patients who receive radiation therapy. Therefore, early LVA treatment should be considered for cases of radiation induced lymphedema in order to prevent the rapid degeneration of lymphatic vessels.

The same can be considered in primary lymphedema, events of injury can trigger exacerbation of edema such as trauma, insect bites and stings, iatrogenic, infection, and postural (*ex.* precipitates the pooling of lymph in lower limbs which might cause inflammation in the presence of underlying degeneration of lymphatic vessels).

(Yukio Seki)

1) Kinmonth JB, Eustace PW : Lymph nodes and vessels in primary lymphoedema. Their relative importance in aetiology. Ann R Coll Surg Engl 58(4) : 278-284, 1976.
2) Hara H, Mihara M, et al : Indication of lymphatico-venous anastomosis for lower limb primary lymphedema. Plast Reconstr Surg 136(4) : 883-893, 2015.
3) Yamamoto T, Matsuda N, et al : The earliest finding of indocyanine green lymphography in asymptomatic limbs of lower extremity lymphedema patients secondary to cancer treatment ; the modified dermal backflow stage and concept of subclinical lymphedema. Plast Reconstr Surg 128 (4) : 314e-321e, 2011.
4) Akita S, Mitsukawa N, et al : Early diagnosis and risk factors for lymphedema following lymph node dissection for gynecologic cancer. Plast Reconstr Surg 131(2) : 283-290, 2013.

CHAPTER 3

分類
Classification

2. リンパ浮腫症候群
Lymphedema syndrome

■はじめに

　先天性リンパ浮腫の概念が確立されたのは、Allen[1]が 1934 年に Congenital と Praecox を報告してからである。その後、Kinmonth[2]が 1957 年に遅発性の先天性リンパ浮腫を Tarda として報告し、先天性リンパ浮腫は発症時期により、Congenital（生下時より浮腫を認める）、Praecox（生後早期に浮腫を認める）、Tarda（35 歳以降に浮腫を認める）に分類されてきた。また、先天性リンパ浮腫の疫学は、6,000 人に 1 人発症するといわれている[3]。一方で、これまでに多くの原因遺伝子が解明されており（**Table 3-2-1**）、本章では、代表的なリンパ浮腫症候群について説明する。

■Introduction

　Allen (1934)[1] classified the primary lymphedema into Congenita and Praecox, and Kinmonth (1957)[2] later reported on delayed onset lymphedema as Tarda. Primary lymphedema is divided into three broad groups according the age of onset; 'Congenita' in which the swelling is present at birth, 'Praecox' in which the swelling appears after birth, and 'Tarda' in which the swelling is develops after the age of 35 years. The prevalence of primary lymphedema is estimated as 1/6000[3]. On the other hand, mutations in several genes are recognized to cause primary lymphedema (**Table 3-2-1**). The purpose of this chapter is to describe several representative lymphedema syndromes.

Table 3-2-1. リンパ浮腫症候群とその原因遺伝子
Lymphedema syndrome and the responsible gene

症候群　Syndrome	原因遺伝子　Responsible gene
Hennekam syndrome	CCBE1
Hypotrichosis-lymphoedema-talangiectasia	SOX18
Lymphedema distichiasis syndrome	FOXC2
Macrocephaly-capillary-malformation	PIK3CA
ミルロイ病　Milroy disease	FLT4
MCLMR	KIF11
ヌーナン症候群　Noonan syndrome	PTPN11 KRAS SOS1
Oculo-dento-digital syndrome	GJA1
Prader Willi syndrome	15q11 microdeletion or maternal UPD 15
Proteus syndrome	AKT1
ターナー症候群　Turner syndrome	45X

I　ターナー症候群

　ターナー症候群は、45,X を代表とする性染色体異常であり、その他にも i(Xq)、Xp-、Yp-や

種々のモザイク型などが存在する[4]。臨床症状は、低身長、原発性無月経(60〜90%)、先天性心疾患(〜50%、大動脈狭窄、大動脈縮窄、大動脈弁閉鎖不全症)、四肢リンパ浮腫、翼状頸、盾状胸、腎奇形(〜39%、馬蹄腎)などがある[5)-7)]。

リンパ浮腫は 60%に認め、手背や足背に生下時より出現するため、新生児における早期診断に役立っている。また、リンパ浮腫を認めるターナー症候群のほとんどが non-mosaic 45,X karyotype である。リンパ浮腫は、ほとんどが 2 歳までに自然軽快するが、中には生涯継続する場合やいったん自然軽快したものが成人期に再発する場合もある。ターナー症候群 42 例を対象にしたリンパ浮腫の経過観察では、リンパ浮腫発症例は 76%あり、19%は浮腫が自然消失(87%は 2 歳までに消失)し、31%が改善、10%が増悪し、40%が不変であり、浮腫発症例の約半数の症例では浮腫は継続することがわかっている[8]。

I. Turner syndrome

Turner syndrome is a complex disorder caused by sex chromosome monosomy(45,X), with the remaining cases caused by a structurally abnormal X-chromosome(i(Xq), Xp-, Yp-) or mosaicism[4]. Clinical manifestations vary, but they usually include short stature, primary amenorrhoea, congenital heart disease, congenital lymphedema, webbed neck, renal complication(〜39%, horseshoe kidney)[5)-7)].

Lymphedema of the hands and feet is present in more than 60% of infants with Turner syndrome which facilitates an early diagnosis. Lymphedema is most commonly found in Turner syndrome patients with a non-mosaic 45,X Karyotype that usually resolves by 2 years of age, although it can persist through life and recur. A retrospective study focusing on the progression of lymphedema in 42 Turner syndrome patients, found that 76% patients had swelling at birth and 55% had swelling of the hands and feet. Swelling resolved in 19%, improved in 31%, worsened in 10% and was unchanged in 40%. Lymphedema continues in a half of the patients[8].

Ⅱ ヌーナン症候群

ヌーナン症候群は、RAS/MAPK シグナル伝達経路の構成分子である *PTPN11*、*KRAS*、*SOS1* などの遺伝子異常により発症する。これらの遺伝子異常の頻度は *PTPN11*(40%)、*SOS1*(8〜14%)、*KRAS*(5% >)となっている。遺伝形式は常染色体優性遺伝であり、低身長、思春期遅発、心奇形、眼間乖離、翼状頸、外反肘などを特徴とする症候群である[9]。また、知能低下、難聴、男児外性器形成障害、胎児水腫、白血病、固形腫瘍なども時に出現する。疫学は、1,000〜2,500 人に 1 人である[10]。診断確定は遺伝子診断により行うが、遺伝子変異は約 40%の患者では遺伝子異常を認めないため **Table 3-2-2** の診断基準が用いられることが多い[11]。

20%にリンパ管の異形成や低形成、そして無形成を認める。症状は、全身性リンパ浮腫、四肢リンパ浮腫、肺リンパ管拡張症、腸リンパ管拡張症、乳び胸水などさまざまである[12]。最も一般的な症状は、四肢背側に生じるリンパ浮腫であるが幼少時に消失する場合が多い。胎児期には、妊娠初期に嚢胞性リンパ管腫を生じることがあり、自然退縮するが生後翼状頸として残る。また、胎児期の浮腫の影響で、停留精巣や特異的顔貌(後方回転した耳介低位、両眼隔離など)を呈する。

48

3-2. リンパ浮腫症候群

Table 3-2-2. ヌーナン症候群の診断基準　Scoring system for Noonan syndrome

症状　Feature	A＝主症状　Major	B＝副次的症状　Minor
1　顔貌 Facial	典型的な顔貌 Typical face dysmorphology	示唆的な顔貌 Suggetive face dysmorphology
2　心臓 Cardiac	肺動脈狭窄および／または典型的な心電図所見 Pulmonary valve stenosis, HOCM and/or ECG typical of NS	その他の異常 Other defect
3　身長 Height	3 パーセンタイル未満 ＜P3	10 パーセンタイル未満 ＜P10
4　胸郭 Chest wall	鳩胸／漏斗胸 Pectus carinatum/excavatum	広い胸郭 Broad thorax
5　家族歴 Family history	第 1 度近親者に確実な NS*あり First degree relative with definite NS	第 1 度近親者に NS の可能性 First degree relative with suggestive NS
6　その他 Other	次のすべてを満たす（男性）：精神遅滞、停留精巣、リンパ管形成異常 Mental retardation, cryptochidism and lymphatic dysplasia	精神遅滞、停留精巣、リンパ管形成異常のうち 1 つ One of mental retardation, cryptochidism, lymphatic dysplasia

HOCM：hypertrophic obstructive cardiomyopathy
*確実な NS：1A と、2A〜6A のうち 1 項目、または 2B〜6B のうち 2 項目；1B と、2A〜6A のうち 2 項目または は 2B〜6B のうち 3 項目。
Definitive NS：1″A plus one other major sign or two minor signs；1″B plus two major signs or three minor signs.
（文献 2）より改変 adapted from Ref. 2）

II．Noonan syndrome

Noonan syndrome is caused by the mutations in PTPN11, KRAS, and SOS1. It is an autosomal dominant disorder characterized by short stature, delayed puberty, congenital heart disease, hypertelorism, webbed neck, and cubitus valgus[9]. Other features are mental retardation, deafness, fetal hydrops, acute leukaemia, and solid tumor. The incidence of Noonan syndrome is between 1 in 1000 and 1 in 2500 live births[10]. Establishing the diagnosis can be difficult, as gene mutations are not shown in 40％ of the Noonan syndrome patients. Noonan syndrome is clinically diagnosed by the scoring system like **Table 3-2-2**[11].

Lymphatic vessel dysplasia, hypoplasia, or aplasia is common findings in 20％ of the Noonan syndrome patients. They lead to generalized lymphedema, peripheral lymphedema, pulmonary lymphangiectasia or interstinal lymphangiectasia[12]. The most common manifestation is dorsal limb edema, which usually disappears during childhood. A cystic hygroma is found in early pregnancy, and this welling subsequently regresses and results in webbed neck. Other features are cryptorchidism and specific facial configuration （low-set posteriorly rotated ears, hypertelorism）.

III　ミルロイ病

ミルロイ病は、1892 年に William Milroy が報告した家族性先天性下肢リンパ浮腫である[13]。
Brice は、ミルロイ病 71 例を解析しその表現型を以下のようにまとめた[14]。浮腫は、足部に対称性に認めるが、稀に下腿まで浮腫を認めることがある。その他には、爪床の浮腫による影響で ski-jump 爪変形となることがある。また、成人期には静脈瘤を認め、1/3 の男性には陰囊水腫を認める。浮腫は自然軽快するが、足部に残ることもある。また、胎児水腫が進行し子宮内胎児死

49

亡となることがある。遺伝形式は常染色体優性遺伝であるが、*de novo* 変異も認める。原因遺伝子は *FLT4* であり、ミルロイ病の 70%に認められる[15]。

III. Milroy disease

William Milroy (1892) first described Milroy disease in a family with congenial lower limb lymphedema[13]. Brice summarized the clinical features as follows[14]. Lymphedema is confined to the bilateral feet, and rarely reach the lower leg. 'Ski-jump' toenails due to disturbance of the nail bed by edema are present. Varicose veins have been reported in adults. A third of affected males have hydroceles. The swelling may regress and remain confined to the feet, or the hydrops may progress and result in intrauterine death. Inheritance is autosomal dominant, but *de novo* mutations may occur. Mutations in FLT4 are found in 70% of patients with Milroy disease[15].

IV Milroy-like lymphedema

生下時から下肢リンパ浮腫を認め、ミルロイ病と同様の症状や家族歴をもつものの中には、*FLT4* 遺伝子変異を認めないものがあり、特に、Milroy-like lymphedema と呼んでいる。*VEGFC* のフレームシフト変異が原因である[16]。

IV. Milroy-like lymphedema

Patients with congenial lower limb lymphedema who screen negative for FLT4 mutations are classified as Milroy-like lymphedema. Frame shift mutations in VEGFC are causative for Milroy-like lymphedema[16].

V MCLMR 症候群

小頭症に先天性リンパ浮腫を合併する疾患を Leung (1985 年)が報告し[17]、microcephaly-lymphedema-chorioretinal dysplasia (MLCRD) と chorioretinal dysplasia-microcephaly-mental retardation (CDMMR) が統合され、現在では MCLMR 症候群となっている。臨床症状は、小頭症、下肢リンパ浮腫、網脈絡膜症、精神遅滞が認められる。原因遺伝子は *KIF11* である[18]。

V. MCLMR syndrome

Leung (1985) reported syndromic microcephaly and congenial lymphedema[7]. Microcephaly-lymphedema-chorioretinal dyplasia (MLCRD) and chorioretinal dysplasia-microcephaly-mental retardation (CDMMR) are united as MCLMR syndrome. Clinical features include microcephaly, lower limb lymphedema, chorioretinopathy, and mental retardation. Causative gene is *KIF11*[18].

3-2. リンパ浮腫症候群

VI Lymphedema distichiasis syndrome

　思春期頃に発症する下肢リンパ浮腫と生下時より認める二重睫毛は、Lymphedema distichiasis syndrome に特徴的な臨床症状である[19]。リンパ浮腫と二重睫毛の組み合わせは Neel の報告が最初である[20]。二重睫毛は 95％に認められ、その他にも、眼瞼下垂（35％）、口蓋裂、先天性心疾患（8％）などが認められる。遺伝形式は常染色体優性遺伝である。原因遺伝子は *FOXC2* であり、Lymphedema distichiasis syndrome の 95％に認められる[21]。

VI. Lymphedema distichiasis syndrome
　Patients with lymphedema distichiasis syndrome develop lower limb lymphedema and distichiasis[19]. Onset of lymphedema is during puberty and that of distichiasis is at birth[20]. Other characteristics of this syndrome are ptosis (35%), cleft palate, and congenital heart disease (8%). This syndrome is inherited in an autosomal dominant manner. The causative gene is *FOXC2* and the mutation can be identified in more than 95% of patients[21].

VII メージュ病

　メージュ病は、最も頻度の高い先天性リンパ浮腫であり、1898 年に Meige が 4 世代 8 例の浮腫例を報告した[22]。下腿に限局した浮腫が特徴で、幼少時には認められないが青年期以降に発症する[23]。

VII. Meige disease
　Meige disease is the most prevalent subtype of primary lymphedema and was originally described in 1898 by Henry Meige who reported lower limb lymphedema of 8 cases in 4 generations[22]. In Meige disease, the lymphatic system abnormalities are present from birth, although the swelling is not usually apparent until puberty[23].

VIII Hennekam 症候群

　Hennekam 症候群は、四肢リンパ浮腫にリンパ管拡張症（腸、肺）を伴う全身性リンパ浮腫を特徴的症状とする疾患である[24]。その他、精神遅滞や胎児期の浮腫の影響でさまざまな特徴的顔貌を呈する。遺伝形式は常染色体劣性遺伝である。原因遺伝子は *CCBE1* であるが、23％にしか認められず遺伝的異質性が示唆されている[25]。

VIII. Hennekam syndrome
　Hennekam syndrome includes four limb lymphedema and lymphangiectasia[24]. Other characteristics of this syndrome are learning difficulties and characteristic facies due to hydrops fetalis. It is an inherited autosomal recessive disorder with mutations in *CCBE1*. However, *CCBE1* mutations were present in 23% of cases[25].

51

IX WILD 症候群

　WILD 症候群は、4つの主要症状(Warts、Immunodeficiency、Lymphedema、anogenital Dysplasia)の頭文字を合わせた疾患である。非対称性のリンパ浮腫、結膜浮腫、外性器浮腫、表皮母斑などを生じる[26]。

（山下修二）

IX. WILD syndrome
　Warts, immunodeficiency, lymphedema, and anogenital dysplasia characterized WILD syndrome. Other characteristics include asymmetrical lymphedema, conjunctival edema, swelling of the genitalia, and dermal nevi[26].

（*Shuji Yamashita*）

文 献
Reference

1) Allen E：Lymphedema of the extremities. Classification, etiology and differential diagnosis；a study of three hundred cases. Arch Intern Med 54：606-624, 1934.
2) Kinmonth JB, Taylor GW, Tracy GD, et al：Primary lymphedema；clinical and lymphangiographic studies of a series of 107 patients in which the lower limbs were affected. Br J Surg 45：1-9, 1957.
3) Dale RF：The inheritance of primary lymphedema. J Med Genet 22：274-278, 1985.
4) Wolff DJ, Vam Dyke DL, Powell CM：Working Group of the ACMG Laboratory Quality Assurance Committee；Laboratory guideline for Turner syndrome. Genet Med 12：52-55, 2010.
5) Zhong Q, Layman LC：Genetic considerations in the patient with Turner syndrome-45,X with or without mosaicism. Fertil Steril 98：775-779, 2012.
6) Matura LA, Ho VB, Rosing DR, et al：Aortic dilatation and dissection in Turner syndrome. Circulation 116：1663-1670, 2007.
7) Sybert VP, McCauley E：Turner's Syndrome. N Engl J Med 351：1227-1238, 2004.
8) Welsh J, Todd M：Incidence and Characteristics of lymphedema in Turner's Syndrome. Lymphology 39：152-153, 2006.
9) Allanson JE：Noonan syndrome. J Med Genet 24：9-13, 1987.
10) Sharland M, Burch M, McKenna WM, et al：A clinical study of Noonan syndrome. Arch Dis Child 67：178-183, 1992.
11) Van der Burgt I, Berends E, Lommen E, et al：Clinical and molecular studies in a large Dutch family with Noonan syndrome. Am J Med Genet 53：187-191, 1994.
12) Nisbet DL, Griffin DR, Chitty LS：Prenatal features of Noonan syndrome. Prenat Dign 19：642-647, 1999.
13) Milroy W：An undescribed variety of hereditary edema. NY Med J 56：505-508, 1892.
14) Brice G, Child AH, Evans A, et al：Milroy disease and the VEGFR-3 mutation phenotype. J Med Genet 42：98-102, 2005.
15) Connell FC, Ostergaard P, Carver C, et al：Analysis of the coding regions of VEGFR3 and VEGFC in Milroy disease and other primary lymphedema. Hum Genet 124：625-631, 2009.
16) Gordon K, Schulte D, Brice G, et al：Mutation in vascular endothelial growth factor-C, a ligand for vascular endothelial growth factor receptor-3, is associated with autosomal dominant milroy-like primary lymphedema. Circ Res 112：956-960, 2013.
17) Leung AKC：Dominantly inherited syndrome of microcephaly and congenital lymphedema. Clin Genet 27：611-612, 1985.
18) Ostergaard P, Simpson MA, Mendola A, et al：Mutations in KIF11 cause autosomal-dominant

microcephaly variably associated with congenital lymphedema and chorioretinopathy. Am J Hum Genet 90：356-362, 2012.

19) Kuhnt H Ⅳ：Ueber distichiasis（congenital）vera. Ophthalmologica 2：46-57, 1899.

20) Neel JV, Schull WJ：Human Heredity. pp50-51, University of Chicago Press, Chicago, 1954.

21) Brice G, Mansour S, Bell R, et al：Analysis of phenotypic abnormalities in lymphedema-distichiasis syndrome in 74 patients with FOXC2 mutations or linkage to 16q24. J Med Genet 39：478-483, 2002.

22) Meige H：Dystrophie oedemateuse hereditaire. Presse Med 6：341-343, 1898.

23) Rezaite T, Ghoroghchian R, Bell R, et al：Primary non-syndromic lymphedema（Meige disease）is not caused by mutations in FOXC2. Eur J Hum Genet 16：300-304, 2008.

24) Hennekam RCM, Geerdink RA, Hamel BCJ, et al：Autosomal ressesive intestinal lymphangiectasia and lymphedema, with facial anomalies and mental-retardation. Am J Med Genet 34：593-600, 1989.

25) Alders M, Hogan BM, Gjini E, et al：Mutations in CCBE1 cause generalized lymph vessel dysplasia in humans. Nat Genet 41：1272-1274, 2009.

26) Kreuter A, Hochdorfer B, Brockmeyer NH, et al：A human papillomavirus-assciated disease with disseminated warts, depressed cell-mediated immunity, primary lymphedema, and anogenital dysplasia-WILD syndrome. Arch Dermatol 144：366-372, 2008.

CHAPTER 4

病態・重症度評価
Assessment of clinical condition and severity

1. リンパ浮腫の病態
Pathophysiology of lymphedema

I　むくみとリンパ

　長時間の立ち仕事で足がむくむ、身体をぶつけて腫れる。「むくみ」と「腫れ」は体表に起こる変化として使われるが、それぞれ病態は別である。すなわち「むくみ（＝浮腫）」とは過剰なリンパ液が間質に貯留し、結果として膨れた状態になることであり、一方で「腫れ（＝腫脹）」は血液成分が血管外で貯留し、体積が増加した状態である。本題のリンパ浮腫とはリンパ機能の低下などが原因となって浮腫を起こした状態である。

　体液の循環は主に動静脈・リンパ管が担っており、それぞれ血管系、リンパ管系と呼ばれている。血管系では動脈が毛細血管に移行し、約90％が直接静脈に流入して循環する。これら動静脈は閉鎖した脈管内を血液が通行するため、閉鎖血管系といわれている。一方、毛細静脈に直接回収されなかった体液は間質内で間質液となりリンパ管に吸収される。吸収された間質液は毛細リンパ管から集合リンパ管、リンパ管本管を経て胸管に合流し、さらには静脈角で中心静脈に流入する。リンパの流れは起始側である間質内では開放的であり、一方向性であるため半環状のリンパ輸送といわれ、循環とは表現しない。リンパ液は成人で約1 L/日の流量があり、体液の循環に大きな役割を担っている。

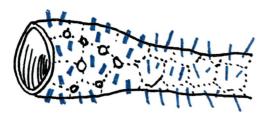

Fig. 4-1-1. 毛細リンパ管
Capillary lymph vessels
左側（管腔側）：拡張した状態
右側（閉鎖側）：収縮した状態
Left (luminal)：expanded state
Right (closed side)：contracted state

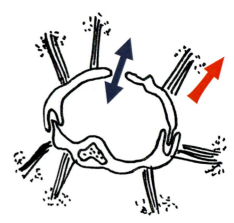

Fig. 4-1-2. 毛細リンパ管：断面図
Capillary lymph vessels：sectional view
係留フィラメントが収縮して側孔が開くとリンパ管内外が交通しリンパ液が通過する。
When filaments contract (red arrow), foramens on the side walls open up to transport lymphatic fluid between lymph vessels and the stroma (lymph flow depicted in blue arrow).

リンパ管起始側は毛細リンパ管と呼ばれ、内皮細胞の間隙が多数あり、内皮細胞は係留フィラメントを有している(**Fig. 4-1-1, 2**)。これら毛細リンパ管が集合し、集合リンパ管になると中層に平滑筋細胞を有した3層構造となり、能動的な輸送が行われる(**Fig. 4-1-3**)。すなわち間質内圧が上昇すると係留フィラメントが働き、内皮細胞間隙が開く。続いてリンパ管内に間質液が流入し、これらを集めた集合リンパ管を通り、リンパ本管・胸管へと流れていく。通常では集合リンパ管より中枢では弁構造があり一方向性の流れをつくっている。

リンパ浮腫はリンパ管のリンパ液回収・輸送能力に異常をきたした状態であり、その原因は次項に挙げるように多岐にわたる。

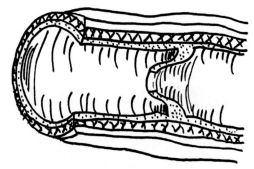

Fig. 4-1-3. 集合リンパ管
Collecting lymph vessels
3層構造で中層には平滑筋細胞を有する。弁構造もみられる。
Collecting lymph vessels have a three-layer structure, with smooth muscle cells in the middle layer. Furthermore, vessels have a valve structure, which prevents reverse flow.

I. Edema and Lymph

There are several terms to describe a swelling state, such as dependent swelling that occurs on long haul flights, or swelling secondary to localized trauma. "Edema" and "Swelling" are different entities based on their pathophysiology. "Edema" consists of excessive interstitial lymph fluid accumulation, while "Swelling" is a state that causes blood constituents to be trapped outside of blood vessels, leading to an increase in volume localized to that area.

The main topic of this chapter is to deal with "lymphedema"; a condition where the edema results from lymphatic malfunctions.

Circulation of body fluids occurs mainly within arteries, veins, or lymphatic vessels, which make up the vascular and or lymphatic systems, consecutively. In the vascular system blood flows from arteries into capillaries, 90% of which then flows into veins; thus, establishing a circulation. These arteries and veins pass the blood in a closed intravascular system "closed vascular system". On the other hand, the residual fluid that is not passed directly into venules is collected by the lymphatic vessels, and make up the lymphatic fluid. This interstitial fluid collected into capillary lymph vessels flows through the collecting lymphatic vessels and then into the thoracic duct, which further flows into the central vein at the vein angle. In the stroma, capillary lymph flows freely and uni-directionally, therefore it is called semi-annular lymphatic transport, and is not considered a circulatory system. About 1 L of lymph flows through an adult in a day, and plays a significant role in the circulation of body fluids.

Lymph originates within lymph capillaries. In the wall of lymph capillaries, there are many gaps between endothelial cells that have multiple filaments (**Fig. 4-1-1 and 2**). These lymphatic capillaries converge and become collecting lymphatic vessels, which are a three-layered structure with smooth muscle cells in the middle layer that involves an active transport of lymphatic fluid (**Fig. 4-1-3**). When the interstitial pressure is increased, the filaments enlarge the gaps of capillaries to open. Subsequently interstitial fluid flows into the capillary lymph vessels and through collecting lymph vessels, then flows into the main lymphatics and/or thoracic duct. Lymph ducts that are downstream of collecting lymph vessels have valve structure to keep the unidirectional flow.

Lymphedema is a condition of an abnormality in lymph fluid collection and transport capacity of the lymphatic vessels. Its causes may be multitude, as described below.

Ⅱ　リンパ浮腫の種類

リンパ浮腫は発症の原因の有無、発症の時期、部位によって種類が分類されている。

1.　一次性(原発性)リンパ浮腫

先天的なリンパ管低形成や過形成が一因と考えられているが、いまだに原因は不明である。下肢に発症することが多く、顔面や上肢に発症することは稀である。浮腫の発症時期もさまざまであり、幼少期から発症するものや晩発性と呼ばれる小児・思春期より徐々に発症するものもある。

先天性リンパ浮腫は 2 歳以前に発症し、常染色体優性遺伝による家族性の報告例もある。ミルロイ病は *VEGF3* の変異が確認されており、胆汁うっ滞性黄疸や蛋白漏出性胃腸症と関連する。

早発性リンパ浮腫は 2〜35 歳、晩発性は 35 歳以降に発症するとされる。家族性・散発性のものがある。

そのほか、症候群に併発するリンパ浮腫として、メージュ病、ヌーナン症候群、ターナー症候群、Hennekam 症候群、黄色爪症候群、モノマック症候群などがある。近年、各遺伝子と疾患群の関係が明らかになってきた(**Table 4-1-1**)。

Table 4-1-1.　遺伝子が関係する疾患群　Diseases in which genes are involved

原発性リンパ浮腫関連症候群 Primary lymphedema related syndrome			他の疾患名 Alternative titles	遺伝様式 Inheritance	MIM #	遺伝子座 Location	遺伝子 Gene/Locus
遺伝性リンパ浮腫 Lymphedema, Hereditary	Ⅰ A	LMPH1A	ミルロイ病 Milroy disease	AD	# 153100	5q53.3	FLT4
	Ⅰ B	LMPH1B		AD	% 611944	6q16.2-q22.1	LMPH1B
	Ⅰ C	LMPH1C		AD	# 613480	1q42.13	GJC2
	Ⅰ D	LMPH1D		AD	# 615907	4q34.3	VEGFC
	Ⅱ	LMPH2	メージュ病 Meige disease	AD	% 153200	Not Maped	LMPH2
Hennekam リンパ管拡張症-リンパ浮腫症候群 Hennekam lymphangiectasia-lymphedema syndrome	1	HKLLS1		AR	# 235510	18q21.32	CCBE1
	2	HKLLS2		AR	# 616006	4q28.1	FAT4
免疫不全 21 AML/MDS Immunodeficiency 21 AML/MDS		IMD21	モノマック症候群 MonoMAC syndrome	AD	# 614172	3q21.3	GATA 2
ヌーナン症候群 1 Noonan syndrome 1		NS1	男性ターナー症候群 Male turner syndrome	AD	# 163950	12q24.13	PTPN11
黄色爪症候群 Yellow nail syndrome		YNS			% 153300	16q24	FOXC2
リンパ浮腫二列睫毛症候群 Lymphedema-Distichiasis syndro.me				AD	# 153400	16q24.1	FOXC2

AML：acute myeloid leukemia 急性骨髄性白血病
MDS：myelo dysplastic syndrome 骨髄異形成症候群
AD：autosomal Dominant 常染色体優性遺伝
AR：autosomal Recessive 常染色体劣性遺伝

2．二次性（続発性）リンパ浮腫

リンパ浮腫発症の要因として、手術（放射線治療）・腫瘍・感染・外傷・静脈性などがある。リンパ管の通過障害が主体となり、集合リンパ管における内圧が上昇する。続いて浅在性リンパ管（毛細リンパ管）へリンパ液が逆流し、間質への液体貯留が起こる。浅層への逆流や間質への液体貯留を Dermal Backflow と呼び、画像検査において特徴のある所見となる。検査の章（Chap. 5「術前評価」）を参照されたい。

a．術後（放射線）

成人のリンパ浮腫で最も患者数が多い。主に下肢では子宮や付属器切除・骨盤内リンパ節郭清術を受けた患者に発症し、放射線治療の併用で増悪することが多い。同様に上肢では乳房切除・腋窩リンパ節郭清の術後に多い。

b．リンパ節生検

乳癌の治療・診断の一環としてセンチネルリンパ節生検が行われるが、術後（放射線）同様にリンパ浮腫をきたすことがある。

c．悪性腫瘍・リンパ節転移

悪性腫瘍が直接リンパの通過路を圧迫することがある。特に後腹膜腫瘍では脂肪成分の多い乳び腹水をきたすことがある。その他、悪性腫瘍がリンパ節に転移をきたした場合にも腹水やリンパ浮腫となることがある。

d．リンパ管炎

体内に侵入した細菌や白癬菌などがリンパ管に取り込まれて炎症を起こした場合、皮膚表面にリンパ管に沿った線条発赤を認める。直接リンパ管内でリンパ流を阻害するほか、細菌性2次感染による浮腫の悪化も起こる。リンパ管炎を繰り返すことでリンパ管内に塞栓が形成され、炎症後の瘢痕による収縮・狭窄・閉塞を起こし、浮腫が悪化し、さらに感染が増悪することがある。

e．寄生虫感染（フィラリア感染）

バンクロフト糸状虫やマレー糸状虫が蚊を媒体として感染し、リンパ節炎やリンパ管炎を起こす。急性炎症期には再発性の発熱・リンパ管炎やリンパ節炎・急性副睾丸炎が起こる。慢性期に入るとリンパ浮腫・象皮病・陰嚢水腫を発症する。近代日本では九州南部・四国に発症例が多かった。衛生状態の向上と防圧活動の成果で1970年代以降に日本での感染はみられなくなったが、いまだに58の国々で1億2,300万人以上が罹患している。西郷隆盛が罹患していたことが知られている。

f．外傷

四肢・陰部の外傷後や術後にリンパ浮腫をきたすことがある。原因として血管運動神経の反射機構の変化が考えられているが不明である。

g．静脈血栓症

静脈血栓から静脈循環障害が起こり、間質液が増加するためにリンパ管系に負荷が増大することでリンパ浮腫が起こるとされる。下肢に多く、皮膚が赤紫色になることが特徴である。

II. Types of lymphedema

Lymphedema is categorized based on, timing of onset, or site of occurrence.

1. Primary lymphedema : Congenital lymphatic hypoplasia or hyperplasia is considered to be the main contributing factor of primary lymphedema ; however, its cause is largely unknown.

It often develops in the lower extremities, and is rarely seen in the face and upper limbs. Onset of edema varies ; some of which occurs in infancy, or gradually progress from childhood or adolescence.

Congenital lymphedema develops in 2 year-old's or younger. There are also some familial cases with an inheritance pattern of autosomal dominant. Such as Milroy's disease, with a known mutation in VEGF3 gene, and is associated with cholestatic jaundice and a protein-losing gastrointestinal disorder.

A common onset of precocious lymphedema is between 2 and 35 years old, whereas the tardive type develops after the 35-years of age. These can be either familial or sporadic cases.

Other syndromic lymphedemas includes Meige, Noonan, Turner, Hennekam, Yellow nail, MonoMAC syndromes. The relations of gene and lymph-related syndromes are getting clear, recently (**Table 4-1-1**).

2. Secondary lymphedema : There are factors that trigger lymphedema, such as surgery (radiation therapy), tumor, infection, trauma, and venous congestion. Obstructions or stenoses of lymphatic vessels from these factors lead to an increase of internal pressure in the collecting lymph vessels, followed by a reversal flow of lymph into superficial lymph ducts (lymphatic capillaries), resulting in accumulation of lymph fluid within the stroma.

The backflow to the superficial dermis is called dermal backflow, which can be observed as a typical findings when evaluating indocyanin-green lymphagraphy imaging. See chapter related to lymphatic imaging (Chap. 5).

a. Post-operative (Post Radiation therapy) : The majority of adult lymphedema patients are classified to this. Lymphedema develops in the lower limbs of patients who undergo hysterectomy or oophorectomy combined with lymph node dissection. Concomitant radiation therapy often exacerbates the edema.

Similarly, many patients after mastectomy and lymph node dissection can develop lymphedema in the upper limb.

b. Lymph node biopsy : Sentinel lymph node biopsy is commonly performed as part of diagnosis and treatment of breast cancer, which may lead to lymphedema post-operatively.

c. Malignant tumor, lymph node metastasis : Malignant tumors could directly compress the passage of lymph and cause lymphedema. A retroperitoneal tumor in particular may cause chyle ascites rich in fat. Furthermore, when malignant tumors metastasize to the lymph nodes, ascites and lymph edema can occur.

d. Lymphangitis : When bacteria or fungus enter the body through skin and lymphatic system, inflammation of the lymphatic vessels can occur. The inflammation can cause the streak redness along the lymphatic vessels on the skin surface. The infection-driven edema could inhibit lymph flow directly, and exacerbate the edema by secondary bacterial infection. Repetitive lymphangitis could cause embolus formation in the lymphatic channels, which leads to contraction, stenosis, and obstruction of lymphatic vessels. The edema further aggravated from additional or worsening infection, which establishes a negative loop.

e. Parasitic infections (filarial infection) : Bancroft heartworm and Murray heartworm infect mosquitos as a medium, and cause lymphadenitis and lymphangitis in humans. Recurrent fever, lymphadenitis and acute epididymitis occur in the acute inflammatory phase. In the chronic phase, lymphedema, elephantiasis and hydrocele of the testis may develop. In modern Japan many cases in the southern Shikoku or Kyushu have occurred reported in the past. Although no case in Japan has been reported after the 1970s due to an improvement of sanitary conditions and a prevention campain, and yet more than 123 million people in 58 countries are suffering from this type of lymphedema.

f. Trauma : Post-trauma or post-surgery on the extremities or the genital regions may lead to lymphedema. Changes in the reflection mechanisms of vasomotor are thought to be a cause, but the detailed mechanisms are yet to be revealed.

g. Venous thrombosis : Venous circulatory disorder followed by venous thrombosis can increase interstitial fluid pressure, which loads the lymphatic system and can lead to lymphedema. Many cases are seen in the lower limbs, typically with changes in skin color to red-purple.

III　リンパ浮腫の病態

　リンパ管は末梢部分で目の粗い構造になっている。多数の係留フィラメントが周辺の組織間をつなぎ、間質とのリンパ液の流入・流出にかかわる。間質液が増加すると係留フィラメントが収縮し、毛細リンパ管の側壁に穴が空くことによりリンパ液がリンパ管内に流入する。これら毛細リンパ管は合流して皮下組織レベルまで達すると集合リンパ管となり、3層構造となる。集合リンパ管より近位では平滑筋による能動的なリンパ液の輸送能力が加わる。さらに弁構造がみられ、リンパ液の逆流が防止される(**Fig. 4-1-4**)。

　リンパ浮腫はリンパ管の閉塞や狭窄が起こるため、通過障害部位の末梢側にリンパ液がうっ滞する。うっ滞が進行すると末梢の毛細リンパ管(集合リンパ管の前段階で真皮内に多く存在する)の内圧が高まり拡張する。間質圧を超えると係留フィラメントが収縮し、毛細リンパ管の側孔が開いて間質にリンパ液が漏出する。この間質にリンパ液が貯留した状態をリンパ浮腫と呼ぶ(**Fig. 4-1-5**)。さらに内圧が亢進すると集合リンパ管内で弁による逆流防止機能を超越し、リンパ液の逆流をきたす。持続的な内圧亢進と周囲の炎症の影響を受け、次第にリンパ管は平滑筋の蠕動運動機能が廃絶しリンパ液輸送機能を失う。ついには線維化し、内腔が狭窄・閉塞する。線維化し

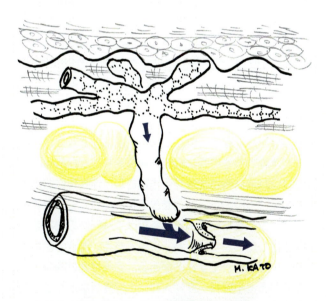

Fig. 4-1-4. リンパ浮腫がない状態
Normal state of lymph system (The absence of lymphedema)
毛細リンパ管で回収されたリンパ液は集合リンパ管へ流入し一方向性に近位へ向かう。
Lymph fluid collected at the capillary lymph vessels flows thorough to the collecting lymph vessels that run between fat cells (yellow) unidirectionally (blue arrows).

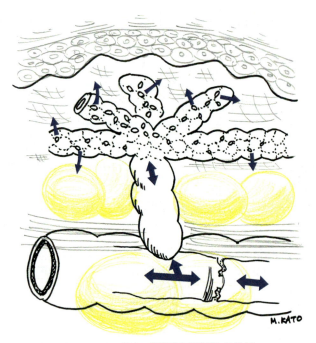

Fig. 4-1-5. リンパ浮腫（可逆性）の状態
Reversible lymphedema state of the lymph system
弁構造の機能不全が起こり集合リンパ管でリンパ液が逆流する。毛細リンパ管での内圧が高まり側孔が開いて真皮・皮下組織にリンパ液が漏出・貯留する。
Lymph fluid backflow into the collecting lymph vessels (large bidirectional blue arrows) occurs due to dysfunction of the valve structure. The internal pressure of capillary lymph vessels is increased, leading to lymph fluid leaked (small unidirectional blue arrow) and its accumulation in the dermis and subcutaneous tissues.

たリンパ管はリンパ輸送能を失う。
　リンパ管は免疫系を司るリンパ液を多く含んでおり、間質内でリンパ液が貯留すると局所炎症を起こす。悪化したリンパ浮腫の患者に蜂窩織炎を繰り返すことがあるのはこのためである。
　さらに間質に貯留したリンパ液は脂肪沈着を引き起こし、浮腫部における脂肪組織の肥大化をきたす。肥大化した脂肪組織は患肢のリンパ流を改善したとしても残存するため、進行した患者ではリンパ管静脈吻合術やリンパ移植術による治療だけでは四肢の左右差が残ることがある。
　リンパ浮腫は四肢を中心とした体表で起こる一現象である。同様の病態で胸管や乳び槽などからリンパ液が漏出し、胸水・腹水をきたすことがある。先天性乳び胸腹水であるが、リンパ浮腫に対する外科治療が有効であると小児科・産婦人科・小児外科などから近年注目されている。内科的加療での難治例に対して、四肢におけるリンパ管静脈吻合術が奏効した症例報告が散見される。漏出部位よりも末梢レベルでリンパ液を静脈に流すことで、胸管や乳び槽への内圧負荷が減少し、胸水・腹水の量を減少させると考えられている。病態を理解することでリンパ浮腫の外科治療を新領域に応用できた点が興味深い。

III. The pathology of lymphedema

The lymphatic vessels have many foramens at the periphery. A number of filaments connect the surrounding tissues, and modulate inflow and outflow of lymph fluid between the lymph vessels and the stroma. An increase of interstitial fluid drives filament contraction, then lymph fluid flows into the lymphatic through expanded foramens on the sidewall of the capillary lymph vessels. These capillary lymph vessels become collecting lymph vessels in the subcutaneous layer, and obtain a three-layered structure. Proximal to the collecting lymph vessels, lymphatics become capable of active transport driven by smooth muscles. Furthermore, vessels have a valve structure, which prevents a reversal flow(**Fig. 4-1-4**).

Lymphedema is caused by blockage or constriction of lymph vessels, followed by lymph congestion. When the congestion progresses, internal pressure of capillary lymph vessels increases and causes a dilation of vessels(often exist in the dermis). When the internal pressure exceeds the interstitial pressure, the filaments contract. The foramens of capillary lymphatic vessels are opened and lymph fluid leaks into the stroma. When this lymph fluid accumulates within the interstitial space it is called lymphedema(**Fig. 4-1-5**). Prolonged high pressure may overwhelm the valve capacity and prolonged high pressure could destroy the valve system and cause lymph backflow in the collecting lymph vessels. Under the influence of sustained hypertension and the surrounding inflammation, smooth muscle function is gradually damaged, and impede lymph vessel transport functions. This may eventually lead to fibrosis, where the lumen becomes narrow and obstructed. Fibrotic lymphatic vessels loose lymph transport ability.

Lymphatics contain a lot of lymph fluid that controls the immune system, and an accumulation of lymph fluid in the stroma causes local inflammation ; thus, patients with advanced lymphedema are prone to repetitive bouts of cellulitis.

Long-term congestion of lymph fluid in the stroma causes fat deposition, which may lead to hypertrophy of adipose tissue in the edematous area. Bloated adipose tissue remains even after improvement of lymphatic flow ; thus, lymphatic venous anastomosis and lymph transplantation should be performed in combination with other therapies(to decrease the adipose tissue, such as liposuction)to improve the laterality.

Lymphedema is one phenomenon that occurs in the body surface following lymph transporting error. Lymph fluid leakage from thoracic duct and/or cisterna chyli may cause a pleural effusion or ascites. Congenital chylothorax or ascites could be effectively treated with the same surgical method for lymphedema, because their pathophysiologies are quite similar. Many experts in the field of pediatrics, OB/GYN, and pediatric surgery are interested in this new approach. Contrary to the medical challenges to treat congenital chylothorax or ascite, several successful cases of lymphatic venous anastomosis in the limbs have been reported. By creating a bypass from the lymph to veins at the peripheral to the leakage site, the innernal pressure load on the thoracic duct and cisterna chyli decrease, and it is believed to reduce the amount of pleural effusion and/or ascites. Note that this approach to treat these conditions is relatively new, and it is absolutely interesting that surgical intervention used for lymphedema can be applied to treat other disorders, which have shed light to a new level of understanding in the pathophysiology.

Ⅳ リンパ浮腫の進行・ステージ分類

リンパ浮腫は全身のさまざまな部位に起こり、前述した病態を経て発症・進行する。症状が出現する前段階から、徐々に進行し重篤化した状態まで、身体所見などの臨床像がさまざまに変化する。以下にその分類と臨床像、ミクロレベルでの変化について述べる。

1. 潜在性リンパ浮腫

臨床的に浮腫の所見がない状態。自覚症状として局所が腫れた感じを訴えることがある。リンパ管の側副路が発達し、リンパ液は迂回して局所貯留することなく流出できるため、間質での液体貯留は認めない。リンパ管造影では異常を確認されることがあり、真皮内の浅在性・深在性リンパ管・皮下組織内の集合リンパ管が拡張していることが多い。

この時期にリンパ管の側副路で処理し切れないほど負荷が増大した場合、特に虫刺されや小さな外傷からの炎症を契機に血管外への水分・蛋白の漏出が増加した場合などに病態が進行することがある。

2. 可逆性リンパ浮腫

片側または局所の浮腫が起こり始めた状態。四肢の場合、挙上や圧迫により軽快することが多い。間質にリンパ管で処理し切れない液体が貯留し始めた状態。リンパ管造影では dermal backflow の所見が明確となる。組織の硬さは変化せず、軟らかいままのことが多い。リンパ管は拡張期から進行に従って徐々に線維化をきたす。

3. 非可逆性リンパ浮腫

浮腫が圧迫や挙上によって軽快しない状態。皮膚の硬度も上昇し、圧痕を残さない浮腫となる（non-pitting edema）。間質に貯留したリンパ液から蛋白や脂肪などが変性・沈着した状態。皮下組織・リンパ管の線維化が著明となる。

毛細リンパ管の内圧が上昇し拡張がみられると、リンパ漏をきたすことがある。体表からリンパ液が持続的に排出され、創傷治癒が遅延する。

4. 象皮症

皮膚の表面まで硬さが著明となり、象の皮膚のように変化した状態。非可逆性リンパ浮腫がさらに進行・悪化し、蛋白は線維網を形成し脂肪も沈着する。皮下組織の膠原線維が異常に増殖した状態。

（加藤　基）

IV. Stage classification of lymphedema

Lymphedema can occur in various parts of the body, emerge and progress in aforementioned manner. From a pre-symptomatic to an advanced stage ; clinical manifestations and physical findings dramatically change over time. Its classification, the clinical picture, and micro-level changes are described below.

1. Subclinical lymphedema : It is a state in which there is no evidence of clinical edema. Patients may complain feeling partial swelling as a subjective symptom. As collateral lymph vessels develop and a bypass for lymph flow is formed, local fluid accumulation does not occur. Lymphangiogram imaging in theses cases may show some abnormality, as lymph vessels in dermis or adipose tissue are often expanded.

If, at this stage, the lymph load overwhelms the flow capacity of collateral lymphatics due to inflammation, for example, after an insect bite or even small trauma, an increase in leakage of lymph fluid and/or extravasated proteins from blood can accelerate clinical progression.

2. Reversible lymphedema: It is a state whereby local or unilateral edema begins to emerge. In the case of the extremities, it is often alleviated by elevation or compression. It is also a state in which the lymph fluid starts to accumulate in the stroma because this fluid excess cannot be drained into the lymphatic vessels. Findings of dermal backflow become clear by lymphangiogram. On palpation the tissue does not change and usually remains soft. The lymph vessels become fibrous as edema progresses from the diastolic stage.

3. Irreversible lymphedema: This is a state in which edema does not improve by compression or elevation. The skin is also harder than normal, and edema does not leave an impression (non-pitting edema). At this stage, the diffused and accumulated protein and fat in the stroma become denatured and deposited.

When the internal pressure of the capillary lymph vessels increases and the vessels are dilated, it may cause a leakage of the lymph. Therefore, lymph fluid is continuously discharged from the body surface, leading to a delay in wound healing.

4. Elephantiasis: This is a state that causes hardening of the skin surface, similar to elephant skin. Lymphedema is further advanced compared to the irreversible stage, and may be characterized by deposition of protein forming fibrous network and fat. Furthermore, collagen fibers in the subcutaneous tissue are abnormally enlarged.

(Motoi Kato)

1) 加藤征治：リンパの科学．講談社，東京，2013．
   Kato S：Science of the Lymph. Kodansha, Tokyo, 2013.
2) 大谷 修，ほか(編)：リンパ管；形態・機能・発生．西村書店，新潟，1997．
   Otani O, et al (eds)：Lymph vessels；The feature, function and the occurrence. Nishimura-shoten, Niigata, 1997.
3) 加藤征治，ほか：新しいリンパ学．金芳堂，京都，2015．
   Kato S, et al：New lymphology. Kinpodo, Kyoto, 2015.
4) Northup KA, et al：Syndromic classification of hereditary lymphedema. Lymphology 36：162-189, 2003.
5) The Merck Manuals (http://merckmanual.jp/mmpej/sec07/ch081/ch081h.html).
6) 藤田紘一郎：リンパ性フィラリア症．日本における寄生虫学の研究，第7巻，目黒寄生虫館，東京，1999．
   Fujita K：Lymph filariasis. The study of palasitology in Japan, vol. 7, Meguro Parasitological Museum, Tokyo, 1999.
7) 加藤 基：先天性乳び胸腹水に対する外科治療；リンパ管静脈吻合術の可能性．周産期新生児学会雑誌 51(2)：638，2015．
   Kato M：Lymph surgery for corgenital chylothorax and chylo abdomen；Possibility of lymphatic venous anastomosis. J Jan Soc Perin Neon Med 51(2)：638, 2015.
8) 血管腫・血管奇形・リンパ管奇形診療ガイドライン2017．第2版，平成26-28年度厚生労働科学研究費補助金難治性疾患等政策研究事業，2017．
   Japanese clinical guideline of vascular tumors, vasular malformations, lymph duct malformations. 2nd ed, 2017.
9) NCBI database OMIM (www.omim.erg) 2017.3.13.

CHAPTER 4

病態・重症度評価
Assessment of clinical condition and severity

2. リンパ管変性・硬化
Lymphatic vessels' degeneration and sclerosis

I　リンパ流閉塞によるリンパ循環の変化

　リンパ浮腫はリンパ循環障害により間質液が貯留する疾患で、浮腫による形態変化のみならず局所リンパ循環の異常による免疫異常から炎症・感染・悪性腫瘍の発生といったさまざまな病態による障害をきたす難治性の疾患である。多くはがん治療などによるリンパ流閉塞が原因となる二次性リンパ浮腫であり、リンパ流閉塞によるリンパ管・リンパ流の変化を理解することがリンパ浮腫の治療に極めて重要である。

　リンパ流閉塞により閉塞部位より遠位のリンパ管内圧が上昇しリンパ管が拡張する。リンパ管拡張により弁の機能不全が生じ逆行性リンパ流が生じることで、前集合リンパ管・毛細リンパ管が拡張するが、この拡張したリンパ管は側副路としても機能する。側副路がリンパ流負荷を代償し切れないと、間質液のリンパ管へのドレナージが不十分となり浮腫をきたすようになる。また、リンパ管への内圧による負荷はリンパ管変性・硬化をもたらしリンパ漏出をきたすようになる（Fig. 4-2-1〜3）。

I. Lymphodynamics after lymph flow obstruction

　Lymphedema is an intractable chronic disease due to abnormal lymph circulation, which ultimately leads not only to morphological changes resulting from the edema but also to various functional disabilities due to inflammation, infection, and malignancy resulting from local abnormality of lymphodynamics. Most cases are secondary to lymph flow obstruction as a consequence of cancer or its treatments. For better management of lymphedema, it is critical to understand the pathophysiology of lymphatic vessels and flow changes after lymph obstruction.

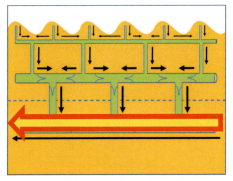

Fig. 4-2-1.　正常のリンパ流　Normal lymph flow

4-2. リンパ管変性・硬化

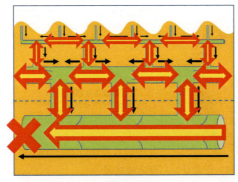

Fig. 4-2-2. リンパ管弁不全によるリンパ管の拡張と逆行性リンパ流
Lymphatic valvular insufficiency causes dilatation of lymphatic precollectors and capillaries, leading to retrograde lymph flows

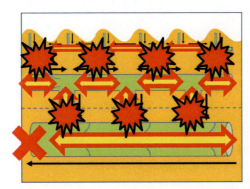

Fig. 4-2-3. リンパドレナージ不全・漏出による浮腫の顕在化
Manifestation of edema due to insufficient lymph drainage and/or lymph extravasation

　Obstruction of lymph flow increases the internal pressure of distal collecting lymphatic vessels, and leads to dilatation of the vessels. Retrograde lymph flows takes place due to lymphatic valvular insufficiency caused by the dilated lymphatic vessels, which act to further dilatate lymphatic precollectors and capillaries. These dilated lymphatics act as collateral pathways. When the collaterals fail to compensate for lymph fluid overload, lymphedema becomes clinically evident because of insufficient drainage of interstitial fluid. Lymphatic hypertension causes degenerative and sclerotic changes of the lymphatic vessels, resulting in extravasation of lymph from the degenerated sclerotic lymphatic vessels (**Fig. 4-2-1 to 3**).

II　リンパ浮腫の進行とリンパ管変性・硬化

　リンパ流閉塞により内圧が上昇することでリンパ管は拡張するが、内圧上昇・拡張はリンパ管内皮・平滑筋に負荷がかかり変性をきたすこととなる。平滑筋は分化した収縮型平滑筋から合成型平滑筋へと形質転換して増殖し、リンパ管中膜が肥厚することで内腔が狭くなっていく。リンパ管内皮はデスモゾームによる内皮間接着が緩んでいき、個々のリンパ管内皮細胞が離れて内膜

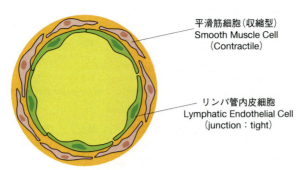

Fig. 4-2-4. 正常リンパ管の模式図
A schematic drawing of normal lymphatic vessel

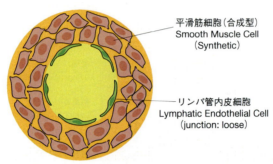

Fig. 4-2-5. 変性・硬化したリンパ管の模式図
A schematic drawing of a degenerated/sclerotic lymphatic vessel

下のコラーゲン線維が内腔にむき出しとなる(**Fig. 4-2-4, 5**)。この過程でリンパ管内より間質へリンパ液が漏出しリンパ管内を流れるリンパ液は減少して、ますます間質液のドレナージ能が低下し浮腫が悪化する。圧迫療法はリンパ浮腫の重要な治療法であるが、リンパ流閉塞という根本原因は改善しないためリンパ管変性・硬化は保存療法にもかかわらず進行していく。最終的にはリンパ管内腔および内腔を流れるリンパ液が確認できなくなり、リンパドレナージ能が廃絶する。

II. Degenerative and sclerotic changes with progression of lymphedema

Lymphatic hypertension and dilatation, resulting from lymph flow obstruction, causes lymphatic vessel degeneration and sclerosis. The smooth muscle cells in lymphatic vessels change from contractile type to synthetic type, and the tunica media of the lymphatic vessels becomes thicker and decreases the lumen space. The inter-lymphatic ligands between endothelial cells and the desmosomes are weakened, which results in the separation of each lymphatic endothelial cell and exposure of the collagen fibers beneath the endothelium (**Fig. 4-2-4 & 5**). Lymph flow within the lymphatic vessel becomes sluggish due to extravasation of lymph as a result of this degeneration/sclerosis. This deterioration of lymph drainage function exacerbates worsening of the lymphedema. Although compression is a mainstay of lymphedema treatment, lymphatic degeneration/sclerosis further progresses in spite of conservative treatments because of the underlying lymph flow obstruction. Eventually, there is complete obstruction of lymph drainage function with no lymph flow within lymphatic vessels due to severe degeneration/sclerosis.

Ⅲ　ICGリンパ管造影所見によるリンパ管硬化の評価

　リンパ浮腫の進行とともにリンパ管変性・硬化も進行するが、リンパ管の状態を評価し適切な治療方針を立てることがリンパ浮腫の管理では極めて重要である。リンパ管の状態は身体診察のみでは評価ができないため、適切なリンパ流評価を用いることで、リンパ管変性・硬化の進行によるリンパドレナージ能が廃絶するのを見過ごさないよう注意が必要である。特に、根治的な低侵襲外科治療であるLVAの治療効果が期待できるのは、リンパ管内にリンパ流が認められる病期までであり、治療適応判断にリンパ循環評価は必須である。

　リンパシンチグラフィなどさまざまな画像評価が用いられているが、リンパ管の状態との関連が明らかになっているのはICGリンパ管造影のみである。ICGリンパ管造影所見はリンパ浮腫の進行とともにLinearパターン、Splashパターン、Stardustパターン、Diffuseパターンと変化するが、これらの所見がリンパ管の状態をよく表しているため、リンパ管の状態の予測およびLVA治療適応の判断に有用である（**Fig. 4-2-6**, Chap. 4-3、5-4参照）。Linearパターンの部位（L領域）ではリンパ管径は0.44 mmでリンパ管硬化はほとんど認めないが、Splash・Stardustパターンの部位（S領域）ではリンパ管径は0.45 mm程度であるものの軽度-中等度のリンパ管硬化を認め、Diffuseパターンの部位（D領域）ではリンパ管径は0.26 mmと細くリンパ管硬化も高度であることがほとんどとなる（**Fig. 4-2-7**）。D領域のリンパ管は高度な変性・硬化を伴っている可能性が高いため、L領域・S領域でのLVAが望ましい。保存療法による経過観察中でもICGリンパ管造影でS領域やD領域の拡大がないことを慎重にフォローする必要がある。

〔山本　匠、山本奈奈、林　明辰〕

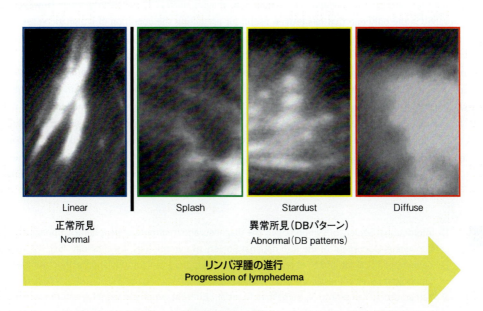

Fig. 4-2-6. ICGリンパ管造影所見の変化　ICG lymphography findings

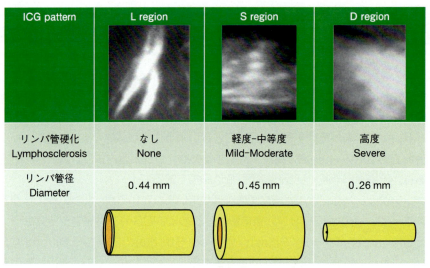

Fig. 4-2-7. ICG リンパ管造影所見とリンパ管の状態
ICG lymphogrtaphy findings and lymphatic vessel's conditions

III. Evaluation of lymphosclerosis using ICG lymphography

Lymphatic vessels become degenerative and sclerotic with lymphedema progression. For optimal lymphedema management, it is critical to adequately evaluate lymphatic vessels to devise optimal therapeutic strategy. Because the underlying condition of the lymphatic vessels cannot be assessed by physical examination, lymph flow imaging is important to evaluate lymph flow function and lymphatic vessel condition. Minimally invasive treatment with LVA's works best to treat and even cure lymphedema, at an early stage of the disease process. Therefore, evaluating the underlying lymph circulation is essential for assessing the indication of lymphedema management.

Although there are several modalities for lymph flow imaging such as lymphoscintigraphy. However, ICG lymphography is the only one that has proven useful for predicting the condition of lymphatic vessels. ICG lymphography findings change from Linear, to Splash, Stardust, and finally to a Diffuse pattern with progression of lymphedema. These findings are well associated with lymphatic vessel conditions, and useful for considering the indication of LVA (**Fig. 4-2-6**, see Chap. 4-3 & 5-4). In a region with Linear pattern (L region), lymphatic vessel diameter is 0.44 mm, and lymphosclerosis is usually not present. In a region with Splash/Stardust pattern (S region), diameter is 0.45 mm, and lymphosclerosis is mild-moderate. In a region with Diffuse pattern (D region), diameter is 0.26 mm, and lymphosclerosis is usually severe (**Fig. 4-2-7**). LVA should be performed on L/S regions, because lymphatic vessels in D region are unlikely to respond to treatment with LVA. It is important continue management of S/D regions with conservative treatments.

(Takumi Yamamoto, Nana Yamamoto, Akitatsu Hayashi)

1) International Society of Lymphology : The diagnosis and treatment of peripheral lymphedema ; 2013 Consensus Document of the International Society of Lymphology. Lymphology 46(1) : 1-11, 2013.
2) Yamamoto T, Yamamoto N, et al : LEC score ; A judgment tool for indication of indocyanine green lymphography. Ann Plast Surg 70(2) : 227-230, 2013.
3) Yamamoto T, Yamamoto N, Yamashita M, et al : Efferent lymphatic vessel anastomosis (ELVA) ; supermicrosurgical efferent lymphatic vessel-to-venous anastomosis for the prophylactic

treatment of subclinical lymphedema. Ann Plast Surg 76(4)：424-427, 2016.

4) Lee BB, Antignani PL, et al：IUA-ISVI consensus for diagnosis guideline of chronic lymphedema of the limbs. Int Angiol 34(4)：311-332, 2015.

5) Yamamoto T, Yamamoto N, Yoshimatsu H, et al：Indocyanine green lymphography for evaluation of genital lymphedema in secondary lower extremity lymphedema patients. J Vasc Surg：Venous and Lym Dis 1(4)：400-405, 2013.

6) Ogata F, Fujiu K, Koshima I, et al：Phenotypic modulation of smooth muscle cells in lymphoedema. Br J Dermatol 172(5)：1286-1293, 2015.

7) Mihara M, Hara H, Hayashi Y, et al：Pathological steps of cancer-related lymphedema；histological changes in the collecting lymphatic vessels after lymphadenectomy. PLoS One 7(7)：e41126, 2012.

8) Koshima I, Kawada S, Moriguchi T, et al：Ultrastructural observations of lymphatic vessels in lymphedema in human extremities. Plast Reconstr Surg 97：397-405, 1996.

9) Yamamoto T, Narushima M, Yoshimatsu H, et al：Indocyanine green velocity；Lymph transportation capacity deterioration with progression of lymphedema. Ann Plast Surg 71(5)：591-594, 2013.

10) Yamamoto T, Narushima M, Yoshimatsu H, et al：Dynamic indocyanine green lymphography for breast cancer-related arm lymphedema. Ann Plast Surg 73(6)：706-709, 2014.

11) Yamamoto T, Koshima I：Supermicrosugical anastomosis of superficial lymphatic vessel to deep lymphatic vessel for a patient with cellulitis-induced chronic localized leg lymphedema. Microsurgery 35(1)：68-71, 2015.

12) Yamamoto T, Yamamoto N, Hayashi A, et al：Supermicrosurgical deep lymphatic vessel-to-venous anastomosis for a breast cancer-related arm lymphedema with severe sclerosis of superficial lymphatic vessels. Microsurgery 37(2)：156-159, 2017.

13) Yamamoto T, Yamamoto N, et al：Indocyanine green (ICG)-enhanced lymphography for upper extremity lymphedema；a novel severity staging system using dermal backflow(DB) patterns. Plast Reconstr Surg 128(4)：941-947, 2011.

14) Yamamoto T, Narushima M, et al：Characteristic indocyanine green lymphography findings in lower extremity lymphedema；the generation of a novel lymphedema severity staging system using dermal backflow patterns. Plast Reconstr Surg 127(5)：1979-1986, 2011.

15) Yamamoto T, Yamamoto N, Yoshimatsu H, et al：Indocyanine green lymphography for evaluation of genital lymphedema in secondary lower extremity lymphedema patients. J Vasc Surg：Venous and Lym Dis 1(4)：400-405, 2013.

16) Yamamoto T, Iida T, et al：Indocyanine green (ICG)-enhanced lymphography for evaluation of facial lymphoedema. J Plast Reconstr Aesthet Surg 64(11)：1541-1544, 2011.

17) Yamamoto T, Yamamoto N, Narushima M, et al：Lymphaticovenular anastomosis with guidance of ICG lymphography. J Jpn Coll Angiol 52：327-331, 2012.

18) Yamamoto T, Narushima M, et al：Minimally invasive lymphatic supermicrosurgery(MILS)；indocyanine green lymphography-guided simultaneous multi-site lymphaticovenular anastomoses via millimeter skin incisions. Ann Plast Surg 72(1)：67-70, 2014.

19) Yamamoto T, Yamamoto N, Azuma S, et al：Near-infrared illumination system-integrated microscope for supermicrosurgical lymphaticovenular anastomosis. Microsurgery 34(1)：23-27, 2014.

20) Yamamoto T, Yoshimatsu H, Narushima M, et al：Indocyanine green lymphography findings in primary leg lymphedema. Eur J Vasc Endovasc Surg 49：95-102, 2015.

21) Yamamoto T, Matsuda N, Doi K, et al：The earliest finding of indocyanine green(ICG) lymphography in asymptomatic limbs of lower extremity lymphedema patients secondary to cancer treatment；the modified dermal backflow(DB) stage and concept of subclinical lymphedema. Plast Reconstr Surg 128(4)：314e-321e, 2011.

CHAPTER 4

病態・重症度評価
Assessment of clinical condition and severity

3. ICG リンパ管造影による病態生理的重症度評価
Pathophysiological severity staging using dynamic ICG lymphography

---

■ I ■ リンパ循環動態の変化と身体所見による評価

　がん治療などによりリンパ流が閉塞すると閉塞部位より遠位のリンパ管内圧が上昇し、リンパ管が拡張する。リンパ管拡張により弁の機能不全が生じて逆行性リンパ流が生じ、前集合リンパ管・毛細リンパ管が拡張し、側副路を形成する。側副路がリンパ流負荷を代償し切れないと、リンパ管硬化・変性を生じリンパ漏出をきたすようになる。リンパ漏出により増えた間質液は長期経過により脂肪沈着をきたし、炎症により線維化を生じていく。

　リンパ浮腫の進行にはさまざまな現象が生じているが、身体所見により評価可能となるのは、リンパ漏出をきたし間質液が増え pitting edema として所見が得られるようになってからである。古典的な教科書では「リンパ浮腫は non-pitting edema」が特徴的とされるが、non-pitting edema となるのは長期経過により脂肪沈着をきたした段階での状態である。象皮病と呼ばれる状態は、長期の炎症性変化により皮膚が粗造になった状態で、リンパ浮腫が相当進行しないとみられない所見である。

　現在、最もよく用いられているのが国際リンパ学会（International Society of Lymphology；ISL）のリンパ浮腫病期分類である（**Table 4-3-1**）。ISL 0 期は浮腫はなくリンパ循環障害がある状態である。ISL 1 期では患肢挙上により軽減する pitting edema を認める。ISL 2 期前期では患肢挙上で軽減しない pitting edema を認め、ISL 2 期後期では non-pitting edema を認めるようになる。ISL 3 期は皮膚変化をきたすようになる状態で、その終末期が象皮病である。わかりやすい分類ではあるが、分類に用いられる指標は基本的に身体所見での pitting edema、non-pitting edema と皮膚変化と患肢挙上により軽減するかどうかの自覚症状である。ISL 0 期で言及されている「リンパ循環障害」はリンパシンチグラフィの所見によるが、リンパシンチグラフィはリンパ循環障害の検出感度・特異度共に後述の ICG リンパ管造影に比較して低いのが難点である。

I. Lymphodynamics and physical examinations

　Lymphadenectomy or irradiation obstructs lymph flow, which leads to lymphatic hypertension, lymphatic vessel dilation, lymphatic valvular insufficiency, and ultimately retrograde lymph flows. Retrograde lymph flows stimulates the formation of collateral lymph pathways. When the collateral pathways are not enough to compensate lymph overload, lymphatic vessel sclerosis and degeneration, and lymph extravasation take place. Extravasated lymph in the interstitial space results in fat deposition and tissue fibrosis via inflammation.

　Although various dynamic phenomena take place with development and progression of lymphedema, medical professionals note lymphedematous change such as pitting edema with physical examinations only

Table 4-3-1. ISL 病期分類　ISL stage

stage 0	リンパ循環不全あり 臨床症状なし no edema, abnormal lymphoscintigraphy
stage 1	患肢挙上で改善する浮腫 pitting edema improved by elevation
stage 2	患肢挙上では改善しない圧痕性浮腫 pitting edema not improved by elevation
stage 3	非圧痕性浮腫 non-pitting edema

after development of lymph extravasation via sclerotic lymphatic vessels. Non-pitting edema, a characteristic finding of lymphedema mentioned in classical textbooks, is evident only in significantly advanced lymphedema with fat deposition. Elephantiasis is only seen in the end stage of lymphedema with fibrous changes of the skin.

The most commonly used staging system is International Society of Lymphology (ISL) staging (**Table 4-3-1**). Although the ISL staging system is easy to understand, indices to classify the different stages are based on subjective symptoms and physical examinations. Abnormal lymph circulation mentioned in the ISL stage 0 refers to lymphoscintigraphy findings. However, lymphoscintigraphy has lower sensitivity and specificity compared with ICG lymphography.

Ⅱ　ダイナミック ICG リンパ管造影によるリンパ循環動態の評価

　自覚症状は個人差があまりにも大きく、身体所見による評価ではリンパ循環動態を間接的に評価しているに過ぎず、進行してからでないと所見が得られない。リンパ浮腫は“リンパ循環異常による浮腫性疾患”であり、リンパ循環動態を可視化し評価することが重要である。国際的にはリンパシンチグラフィが標準検査として普及しているが、異常リンパ流の検出感度・特異度が低く評価者により評価が異なることがある。また、放射性物質を用いるため被曝のリスクがある。

　ICG リンパ管造影は、肝臓機能検査として長年使用され安全性が認められている色素 ICG を皮下・皮内注射し、近赤外線デバイスを用いて観察することで浅い（体表から 1〜2 cm までの）リンパ流を可視化する検査法で、リンパシンチグラフィと比較するとかなり明瞭にリンパ流を可視化できる。2007 年に本邦で開発・報告され、リンパシンチグラフィと異なり被曝リスクがなくリアルタイムでリンパ流を可視化できることから、リンパ浮腫の評価法として広まりつつある（**Table 4-3-2**）。リアルタイム評価である利点を活かした、ダイナミック ICG リンパ管造影により、リンパ循環動態とリンパ管のポンプ機能が 1 回の注射で評価できる。

　ダイナミック ICG リンパ管造影は 1 回の注射、2 回の観察（遷移相と定常相での観察）で行われる（**Fig. 4-3-1**）。まず、注射前に仰臥位で 15 分安静にしてもらい（注射前の軽度の運動も ICG 移動速度に影響するため。会話は問題ないのでこの間に問診するとよい）、0.25% の ICG 溶液を 0.05〜0.2 mL 注射する。下肢・陰部では第二趾間部とアキレス腱外側に 0.2 mL ずつ、上肢では第二指間部と長掌筋腱尺側に 0.1 mL ずつ、顔面では人中・眉間・前頭部正中生え際に 0.05 mL

Table 4-3-2. ICG リンパ管造影とリンパシンチグラフィ
ICG lymphography and lymphoscintigraphy

	ICG-L	LSG
被曝 radiation exposure	−	＋
深部評価 deep evaluation	−	＋
画像 image quality	鮮明 sharp	不鮮明 obscure
検出感度・特異度 sensitivity/specificity	高い high	低い low

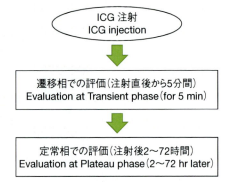

Fig. 4-3-1. ダイナミック ICG リンパ管造影
Dynamic ICG lymphography

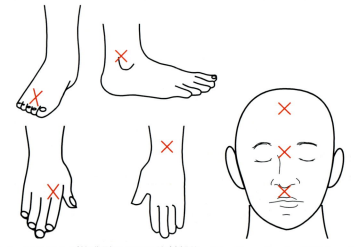

Fig. 4-3-2. ICG リンパ管造影における注射部位　Injection sites for ICG lymphography

ずつ皮内注射する（**Fig. 4-3-2**）。注射後 5 分間臥位で安静にしてもらい、ICG の移動を近赤外線カメラで観察する。ICG 注射 5 分後の移動距離から ICG の移動速度（ICG velocity；ICGv）を計測し、リンパ管のポンプ機能を評価する。リンパ浮腫の進行によりリンパ管のポンプ機能は廃絶していき ICGv（ICG velocity）は低下していく（**Fig. 4-3-3**）。リンパ浮腫早期ではマッサージや軽い運動刺激によるリンパ流亢進がみられるため、評価前から安静にしておかないと評価誤差が生じやすい。臨床経過とともに経時的にフォローしポンプ機能の推移を評価することが重要である。術前検査として ICG リンパ管造影を行う際は、このときにマッピングを行っておくとよい。Linear パターン（後述）の一部は定常相で Dermal Backflow パターンにより見えなくなることがあるためである。

　注射後 5 分で遷移相の評価が終了し、その後は患者に弾性着衣を装着して自由に動いてもらう。ICG は注射後にリンパ管に吸収され中枢へと移動し、また、逆流を介して皮膚に拡散していく。ICG が評価部位に行き渡ったときに 2 回目の観察を行う（定常相での観察）。定常相ではリンパ循環動態を評価するが、後述のとおり 4 つの造影所見の領域を記録する。正常肢では 5 分以内に中

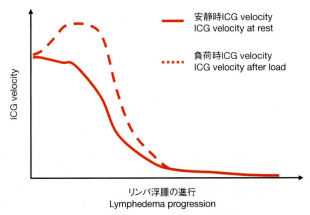

Fig. 4-3-3. ICG velocity とリンパ浮腫の進行
ICG velocity and lymphedema progression

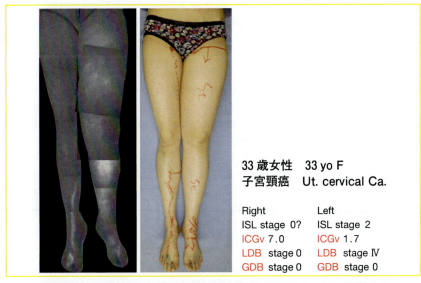

Fig. 4-3-4. ダイナミック ICG リンパ管造影によるリンパ浮腫評価の例
Comprehensive lymphedema evaluation with dynamic ICG lymphography

枢まで ICG が移動するが、リンパ浮腫肢では有意に ICG の取り込み・移動が遅れている。弾性着衣を装着して患肢を動かしてもらうと重症例でも 2 時間で定常相に達する。定常相に達した後は徐々に ICG が拡散し造影所見が不明瞭になっていく。造影所見が不明瞭になる 72 時間以内に評価する必要があるため、定常相における評価は ICG 注射後 2〜72 時間で行う。外来では午前に ICG 注射し午後に定常相の観察、入院時では ICG 注射翌日に定常相の観察をすると、1 回の ICG 注射ですべての評価ができるため効率的である（**Fig. 4-3-4**）。

II. Dynamic ICG lymphography for evaluation of lymphodynamics

Subjective symptoms and physical examination findings are unreliable or likely to underestimate lymphedema progression. Lymph flow imaging is the most important evaluation. Because this is an edematous disease with abnormal lymph circulation. Lymphoscintigraphy is currently used as a gold standard for lymph imaging, but has lower sensitivity and specificity to detect early abnormal lymph flows. Other disadvantages include variability of inter-observer evaluation and risk of radiation exposure.

ICG lymphography visualizes superficial (1-2 cm from body surface) lymph flows far more clearly than lymphoscintigraphy. In ICG lymphography, a safe dye ICG is injected intradermally or subcutaneously, and the target tissue is observed with a near-infrared camera. Since 2007 when it was developed and reported as an evaluation method of lymphedema in Japan, ICG lymphography has become popular, because it can clearly visualize lymph flows in real-time without the risk of radiation exposure (**Table 4-3-2**). Dynamic ICG lymphography allows evaluation of lymph pump function and lymph circulation with a single injection.

Dynamic ICG lymphography consists of 1 injection and 2-phase observations ; early transient phase for evaluation of lymph pump function, and late plateau phase for evaluation of lymph circulation (**Fig. 4-3-1**). An examinee is kept still for 15 minutes, and 0.05-0.2 ml of ICG is intradermally injected (at the 2nd web space for extremity and genital lymphedema, and at the glabella, median frontal, and the philtrum for facial lymphedema (**Fig. 4-3-2**). Immediately after ICG injection, fluorescent lymph flow images are obtained using an infrared camera system (transient phase). Examinees are kept still in supine position during lymph pump function measurement. At 5 minutes after injection, ICG velocity (ICGv) is calculated ; distance (cm) from the injection site to the most distal ICG enhanced point is divided by time (min). ICGv decreases with progression of lymphedema disease condition (**Fig. 4-3-3**). It is important to follow changes in ICGv before and after interventions.

A subject is allowed to move freely with elastic garments after completion of ICGv measurement. When ICG movement reaches a plateau, the second observation is performed (plateau phase). In the plateau phase, lymph circulation is assessed based on ICG lymphography findings as mentioned in the next paragraph. ICG reaches a plateau in an intact limb within 5 minutes, whereas it takes a longer time in a lymphedematous limb. For more rapid and convenient assessment, patients are instructed to move their extremity rigorously. When patients move their extremity rigorously, ICG can reach a plateau 2 hours after ICG injection. Plateau phase continues until 72 hours after ICG injection. Thus, evaluation of lymph circulation in the plateau phase should be done between 2-72 hours after ICG injection. In an outpatient setting, ICG is injected in the morning, and plateau-phase observation is done in the afternoon. During hospitalization, plateau-phase observation is done the day after ICG injection (**Fig. 4-3-4**).

Ⅲ　ICG リンパ管造影所見と DB stage

　定常相の ICG リンパ管造影所見により、観察部位におけるリンパ循環動態を知ることができる。ICG リンパ管造影所見は正常の Linear パターンと異常な Dermal Backflow(DB)パターンに分けられ、DB パターンはさらに Splash パターン、Stardust パターン、Diffuse パターンに細分化される。リンパ浮腫の進行とともに、造影所見は Linear→Splash→Stardust→Diffuse の順に変化していく(**Fig. 4-2-6**、67 頁参照)。遷移相でも DB パターンを認めることがあるが、遷移相では Splash・Stardust・Diffuse いずれの造影所見とも異なる、網状に造影された領域 Reticular パターンとして観察される。Reticular パターンは定常相においていずれかの DB パターンに変化するため、遷移相で DB を評価してはならない(**Fig. 4-3-5**)。

　Linear パターンは正常時にみられる所見で、リンパ集合管を流れるリンパ管が造影された所見である(**Fig. 4-3-6**)。リンパ流の閉塞により前集合リンパ管や毛細リンパ管が拡張し側副路を形成するが、ICG リンパ管造影では Splash パターンとして蛇行する線状の造影所見として観察

74

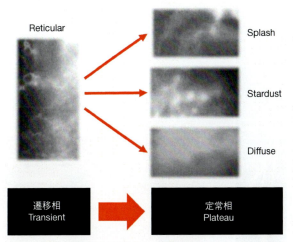

Fig. 4-3-5. 遷移相と定常相における DB パターンの変化
DB pattern change in an early transient phase and a late plateau phase

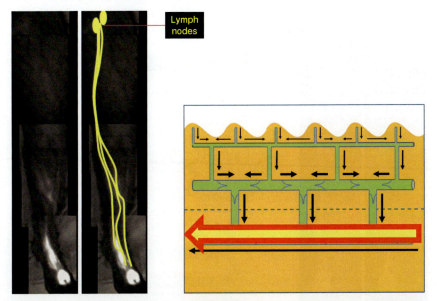

Fig. 4-3-6. Linear パターン部のリンパ循環動態　Lymphodynamics in a Linear region

される(**Fig. 4-3-7**)。側副路がリンパ負荷を代償し切れずリンパ漏出をきたすと、Stardust パターンとして多数の点を伴う造影領域が観察される(**Fig. 4-3-8**)。リンパ漏出が高度になると点状の漏出点が認識できないほど多くなり、Diffuse パターンとして一様に造影された領域が観察されるようになる(**Fig. 4-3-9**)。後述のとおり、これら 4 パターンではリンパ管の状態が異なるため、DB パターンを細分化して評価することが極めて重要である。

　定常相における ICG リンパ管造影所見での DB パターンの種類・分布から、閉塞性リンパ浮腫の病態生理的重症度分類 DB stage を評価する。DB stage には上肢リンパ浮腫用の arm DB (ADB) stage、下肢リンパ浮腫用の leg DB (LDB) stage、陰部リンパ浮腫用の genital DB

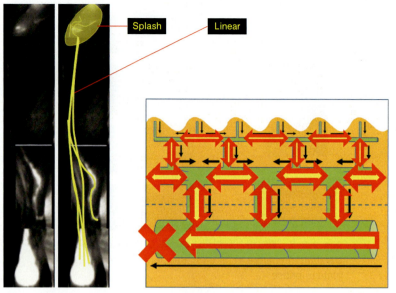

Fig. 4-3-7. Splash パターン部のリンパ循環動態　Lymphodynamics in a Splash region

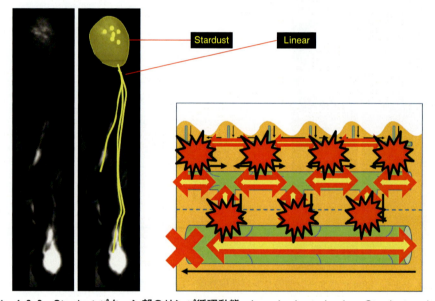

Fig. 4-3-8. Stardust パターン部のリンパ循環動態　Lymphodynamics in a Stardust region

(GDB) stage、顔面リンパ浮腫用の facial DB（FDB）stage がある（**Fig. 4-3-10〜12**）。いずれにおいても、stage 0 では DB パターンを認めず、stage Ⅰ では閉塞部位周辺に Splash パターンを認め、stage Ⅱ 以降で Stardust パターンを認め（進行により Stardust パターンが近位から遠位に拡大する）、最終 stage（stage Ⅳ/Ⅴ）で Diffuse パターンを認める（**Table 4-3-3**）。

　DB stage の違いにより予後が異なるため、治療方針の決定に有用である。ISL stage 0 と診断されていたリンパ浮腫は ICG リンパ管造影により、DB stage 0、stage Ⅰ、stage Ⅱ と異なる 3 つの stage に分類される（**Fig. 4-3-13**）。DB stage 0 はリンパ浮腫でないため治療が不要

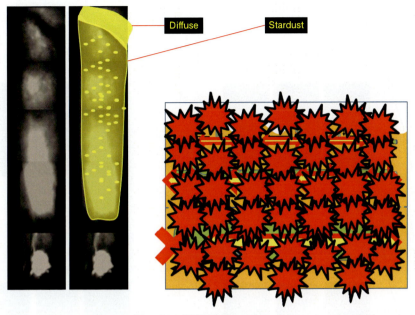

Fig. 4-3-9. Diffuse パターン部のリンパ循環動態　Lymphodynamics in a Diffuse region

であるのに対し、DB stage Ⅱでは自覚症状の有無にかかわらず保存療法抵抗性かつ進行性のため外科治療の適応である。DB stage Ⅰに関しては、約 1/3 が進行性であるが残り 2/3 は進行しないため、経過観察もしくは症例により予防的治療の適応となる。このように、従来 ISL 0 期と診断されていた病期は、DB stage により stage 0、stage Ⅰ、stage Ⅱという、予後の異なる 3 群に細分類されることになる。

Ⅲ. Characteristic ICG lymphography findings and DB stage

Plateau-phase observation in dynamic ICG lymphography reveals lymphodynamics of the targeted areas. Characteristic ICG lymphography findings in obstructive lymphedema are divided into 2 patterns ; normal Linear pattern and abnormal Dermal Backflow (DB) pattern. DB pattern is subdivided into 3 patterns ; Splash, Stardust, and Diffuse patterns. ICG lymphography finding changes from Linear to Splash, to Stardust, and finally to a Diffuse pattern (see **Fig. 4-2-6**). DB pattern can be seen in a transient phase as a Reticular pattern that is distinct from Splash/Stardust/Diffuse patterns. Since this Reticular pattern seen in transient phase changes to Splash or Stardust or Diffuse pattern in a plateau phase, DB pattern should not be evaluated in a transient phase (**Fig. 4-3-5**).

Linear pattern is seen in the normal condition, and represents lymph flows of lymphatic collectors (**Fig. 4-3-6**). Obstruction of lymph flow leads to dilation of lymphatic precollectors and capillaries that act as lymph collateral pathways, and is seen as Splash pattern on ICG lymphography (**Fig. 4-3-7**). When the collateral pathway is not enough to compensate lymph overload, lymph extravasation takes place, that is seen as spots on ICG lymphography ; Stardust pattern (**Fig. 4-3-8**). With progression of lymph extravasation, there are too many spots to identify each other, and a diffuse enhanced image is obtained on ICG lymphography ; Diffuse pattern (**Fig. 4-3-9**). Since these 4 ICG lymphography patterns represent different lymphatic vessel conditions, it is important to differentiate DB patterns to Splash/Stardust/Diffuse patterns.

Based on distribution of DB patterns in the plateau phase ICG lymphography findings, DB staging and pathophysiological severity, is determined. There are 4 DB stages ; arm DB (ADB) stage for arm

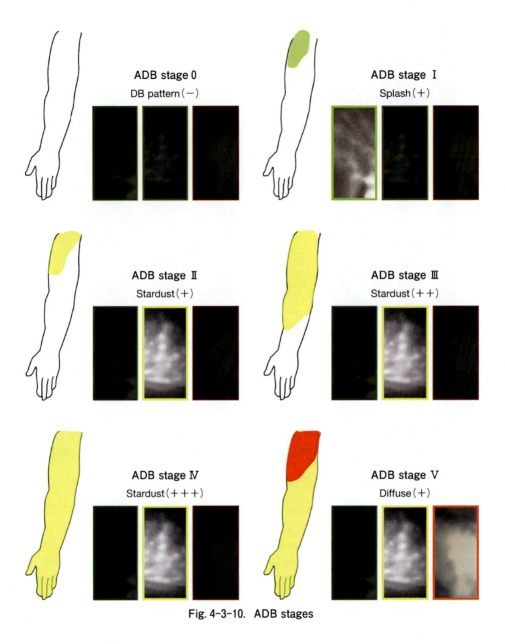

Fig. 4-3-10. ADB stages

lymphedema, leg DB (LDB) stage for leg lymphedema, genital DB (GDB) stage for genital lymphedema, and facial DB (FDB) stage for facial lymphedema (**Fig. 4-3-10 to 12**). In DB stage 0, there is only Linear pattern and no DB pattern. In DB stage Ⅰ, Splash pattern is seen around the obstruction site. From DB stage Ⅱ, Stardust pattern is seen and extends from obstruction site to the distal region with progression of lymphedema. In the advanced DB stage (DB stage Ⅳ/Ⅴ), Diffuse pattern is seen in the background of Stardust pattern (**Table 4-3-3**).

DB stage is very useful for lymphedema management, because prognosis of lymphedema can be predicted based on DB stage. ISL stage 0 can be further subdivided into 3 different stages ; DB stage 0, DB stage Ⅰ, and DB stage Ⅱ (**Fig. 4-3-13**). A patient with DB stage 0 has no lymphedema, and does not require treatment for lymphedema. DB stage Ⅱ lymphedema is a progressive condition refractory to conservative

4-3. ICGリンパ管造影による病態生理的重症度評価

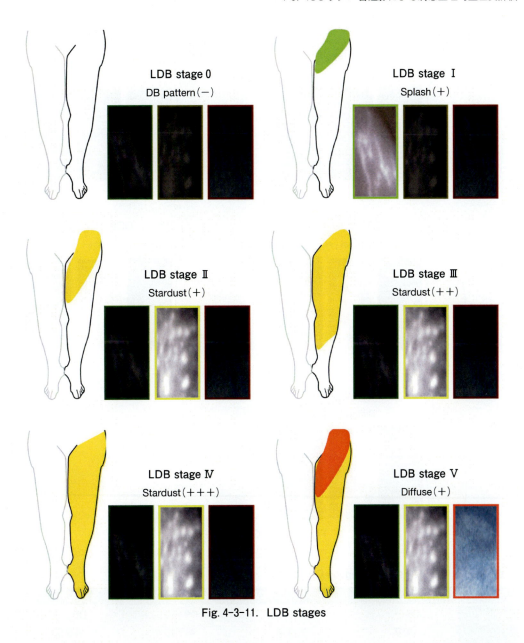

Fig. 4-3-11. LDB stages

treatments, and should be treated surgically regardless of subjective symptoms. Treatment strategy for DB stage I is controversial. Patients with DB stage I lymphedema are asymptomatic, but a 1/3 will develop symptomatic lymphedema and progressive lymphedema within 2 years ; 2/3 will not develop symptomatic lymphedema. Thus, either watchful waiting or prophylactic treatment can be indicated for DB stage I lymphedema.

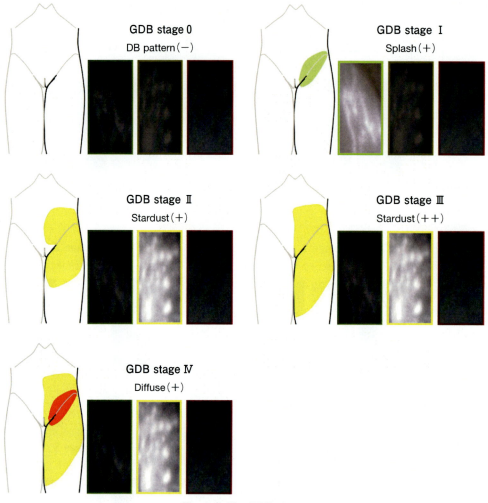

Fig. 4-3-12. GDB stage

Table 4-3-3. 各種 DB stage　Various DB stages

	ADB	LDB	FDB	GDB
Stage 0	DB(−)	DB(−)	DB(−)	DB(−)
Stage I	腋窩 Axilla **Splash**	鼠径部 Groin **Splash**	顎下部 Submandibular **Splash**	鼠径部 Groin **Splash**
Stage II	肘まで To elbows **Stardust(+)**	膝まで To knees **Stardust(+)**	顎下のみ Only submandibular **Stardust(+)**	下腹部のみ Only lower abdomen **Stardust(+)**
Stage III	肘より先も Beyond elbows **Stardust(++)**	膝より先も Beyond knees **Stardust(++)**	顔面も Face too **Stardust(++)**	陰部も Genital area too **Stardust(++)**
Stage IV	上肢全域 All upper extremities **Stardust(+++)**	下肢全域 All lower extremities **Stardust(+++)**	頭頸部全域 All head and neck **Stardust(+++)**	**Diffuse**
Stage V	**Diffuse**	**Diffuse**	**Diffuse**	—

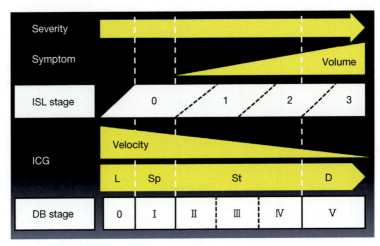

Fig. 4-3-13. ISL stage と DB stage　ISL stage and DB stage

Ⅳ　原発性リンパ浮腫の評価と ICG 分類

　原発性リンパ浮腫は二次性リンパ浮腫や他の浮腫性疾患の除外診断により診断される疾患で、さまざまな病態を含む疾患群である。近年、Milroy 病における *VEGFR3*、Meige 病における *GJC2*、Hennekam 症候群における *CCBE1* などさまざまな原因遺伝子が報告され、原発性リンパ浮腫の一部の病態が明らかになってきているが、大部分は孤発性かつ多因子による疾患で病態が明らかでない。毛細リンパ管からリンパ節などさまざまなレベル・部位での多様な奇形(形態異常のみならず機能障害を含めた広義の奇形)が原発性リンパ浮腫の成因と考えられているが、奇形の種類・程度・範囲により臨床象は多様である。分類法としては、先天性リンパ浮腫(congenital lymphedema：出生時発症)、早発性リンパ浮腫(lymphedema precox：35 歳までに発症)、遅発性リンパ浮腫(lymphedema tarda：35 歳以降に発症)と発症年齢による分類が一般的だが、病態を反映しておらず便宜上の分類と言わざるを得ない。二次性リンパ浮腫における知見をもとに、原発性リンパ浮腫を ICG リンパ管造影所見により分類することができる。

　原発性リンパ浮腫は ICG リンパ管造影により、proximal DB (PDB) パターン、distal DB (DDB) パターン、less enhancement (LE) パターン、no enhancement (NE) パターンの 4 群に分類される。PDB パターンは二次性リンパ浮腫同様に近位から遠位に DB パターンが拡大していくもので、中枢でのリンパ閉塞(リンパ管やリンパ節の低・無形成など)が原因と考えられる (**Fig. 4-3-14**)。悪性腫瘍が除外されていない場合は精査する必要がある。DDB パターンでは、下腿など末梢のみに DB パターンを認め中枢に DB パターンを認めないもので、同部に蜂窩織炎を頻発する例が多い (**Fig. 4-3-15**)。PDB パターン同様リンパ流の閉塞機転が病因と考えられる。LE パターンでは末梢のみに Linear パターンを認め中枢のリンパ節(鼠径リンパ節や腋窩リンパ節)が造影されない (**Fig. 4-3-16**)。病的な浮腫を認める前から"もともとむくみやすい"という例に多くみられ、浅リンパ系が低形成で深リンパ系が優位であることが多い。NE パターンではまったく造影されず Linear パターンも DB パターンもみられない (**Fig. 4-3-17**)。重度の低形成や無

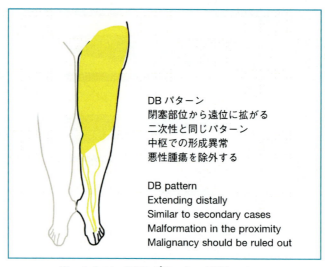

Fig. 4-3-14. PDB パターン　PDB pattern

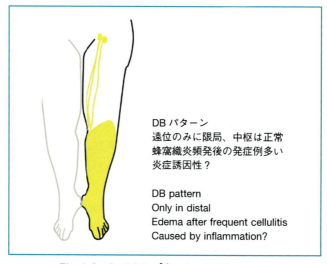

Fig. 4-3-15. DDB パターン　DDB pattern

形成もしくは吸収障害が原因と考えられるが、蜂窩織炎を併発することは少なく単一肢のみの障害であることが多い。

　ICG 分類を用いても病因を特定することはできないが、上述のとおりおおよその病態を予測することができ治療方針を検討するのに有用である（**Table 4-3-4**）。PDB パターン・DDB パターンでは閉塞機序があるため、うっ滞したリンパを減圧する LVA が効果的と考えられる。二次性の治療方針同様、リンパ管硬化が著しくバイパス効果が見込めない例・LVA で効果が不十分な例ではリンパ節移植が検討される。LE パターンでは閉塞機序が明らかでないため、通常厳格な圧迫療法が有効であることが多い。NE パターンではリンパ管自体を認めない可能性があり LVA の治療効果が見込み難く、リンパ節移植の方が有効と考えられる。

　原発性リンパ浮腫では深部のリンパ流評価が不可欠であり、ICG リンパ管造影のみでは評価が

4-3. ICG リンパ管造影による病態生理的重症度評価

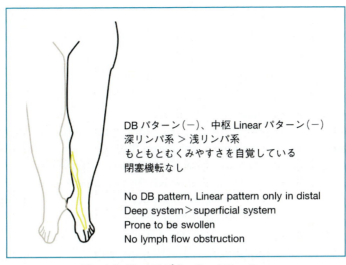

Fig. 4-3-16. LE パターン　LE pattern

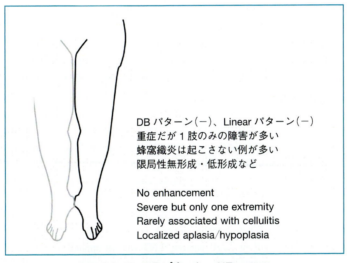

Fig. 4-3-17. NE パターン　NE pattern

Table 4-3-4. 原発性リンパ浮腫の ICG 分類　ICG classification for primary lymphedema

	PDB	DDB	LE	NE
想定される病態 Possible cause	中枢での閉塞 Obstruction (proximal)	末梢での閉塞 Obstruction (distal)	浅リンパ低形成 Superficial lymph hypoplasia	限局性無形成 Localized aplasia
臨床的特徴 Clinical characteristics	二次性と酷似 Similar to secondary cases	蜂窩織炎の後に発症 Manifestation after cellulitis	軽症でもともとむくみやすい Mild edema prone to be swollen	重症例多いが限局 蜂窩織炎少ない Severe, localized Cellulitis rare
治療方針 Treatments	1. LVA 2. LNT 3. LS	1. LVA 2. LNT	1. Strict compression 2. LVA	1. LNT（LVA） 2. LS

83

不十分である。MRI やリンパシンチグラフィ・SPECT/CT は深部評価に有用であるが、これらを用いた原発性リンパ浮腫の分類方法は確立されていない。ICG 分類はリンパ循環動態に基づいた初の分類方法であり、最適な治療方針の検討に役立つであろう。

(山本　匠)

IV. ICG classification for primary lymphedema

Primary lymphedema is diagnosed by excluding other edematous diseases such as venous edema and secondary lymphedema, and includes various pathologies. Some genetic mutations have recently been reported as causes of primary lymphedema such as *VEGFR3* gene for Milroy disease, *GJC2* gene for Meige disease, and *CCBE1* for Hennekam syndrome. However, the vast majority of primary lymphedemas are sporadic and multifactorial, and their pathogeneses are yet to be clarified. Various malformations are considered causes of primary lymphedema, and there are a wide variety of clinical manifestations according to severity, type, and distribution of malformation. Classification according to onset age (congenital lymphedema, lymphedema precox, and lymphedema tarda) is usually used for primary lymphedema, but does not address pathophysiology of the disease. Primary lymphedema can be classified based on abnormal lymph circulation using ICG lymphography.

Primary lymphedema is classified into 4 patterns based on ICG lymphography findings ; proximal DB (PDB) pattern, distal DB (DDB) pattern, less enhancement (LE) pattern, and no enhancement (NE) pattern. PDB pattern represents proximal lymph flow obstruction due to lymphatic vessel and/or lymph node malformation such as hypoplasia, and its image is similar to that seen in secondary lymphedema (**Fig. 4-3-14**). Malignancy should be ruled out when PDB pattern is seen. In DDB pattern, DB pattern is seen only in the distal region such as lower leg and not in the proximal region (**Fig. 4-3-15**). There is usually associated cellulitis that affects the pathophysiology. In LE pattern, Linear pattern is seen only in the distal region, and no enhanced image is seen in the proximal region (**Fig. 4-3-16**). Patients with LE pattern usually notice that their legs are likely to be swollen before manifestation of pathological lymphedema. In NE pattern, nothing is enhanced other than ICG injection site, and severe hypoplasia/aplasia and malabsorption are suspected (**Fig. 4-3-17**). Patients with NE pattern have usually only one affected limb, and rarely suffer from cellulitis.

ICG classification, cannot fully elucidate pathogenesis, clarify lymph circulation of primary lymphedema, suggest its pathophysiology and suitable treatment options (**Table 4-3-4**). In PDB pattern and DDB pattern, the obstructive mechanism plays an important role in the pathophysiology, and LVA is considered effective to decongest stagnated lymph. When lymphosclerosis is severe or LVA is not enough to improve lymphedema in patients with PDB or DDB pattern, LNT can be applied as a further treatment. Since obstructive mechanism is not apparent in LE pattern, rigorous compression therapy is usually effective. In NE pattern, lymphatic vessels suitable for LVA are rarely found, and LNT should be considered as a first-line surgical treatment.

Deep lymph flow evaluation is important for primary lymphedema, and ICG lymphography should be used in combination with MRI and/or lymphoscintigraphy that can visualize deep lymph flows. There is no classification using MRI or lymphoscintigraphy. ICG classification is the first one that distinguishes the staging of primary lymphedema based on lymph circulation. ICG classification can therefore be used to define the etiology and prognosis of primary lymphedema and to determine optimal management for primary lymphedema.

(*Takumi Yamamoto*)

1) International Society of Lymphology : The diagnosis and treatment of peripheral lymphedema ; 2013 Consensus Document of the International Society of Lymphology. Lymphology 46(1) : 1-11, 2013.

2) Yamamoto T, Yamamoto N, Yoshimatsu H, et al : Indocyanine green lymphography for evaluation of genital lymphedema in secondary lower extremity lymphedema patients. J Vasc Surg : Venous and Lym Dis 1(4) : 400-405, 2013.

3) Yamamoto T, Yamamoto N, Hara H, et al : Lower Extremity Lymphedema(LEL) Index ; A Simple Method for Severity Evaluation of Lower Extremity Lymphedema. Ann Plast Surg 70(1) : 47-49, 2013.

4) Yamamoto T, Yamamoto N, Hara H, et al : Upper Extremity Lymphedema(UEL) Index ; A Simple Method for Severity Evaluation of Upper Extremity Lymphedema. Ann Plast Surg 70(1) : 47-49, 2013.

5) Yamamoto N, Yamamoto T, Hayashi N, et al : Arm volumetry versus upper extremity lymphedema index ; validity of upper extremity lymphedema index for body-type corrected arm volume evaluation. Ann Plast Surg 76(6) : 697-699, 2016.

6) Yamamoto T, Yamamoto N, Hayashi N, et al : Practicality of lower extremity lymphedema index ; lymphedema index versus volumetry-based evaluations for body-type corrected lower extremity volume evaluation. Ann Plast Surg 77(1) : 115-118, 2016.

7) Yamamoto T, Yamamoto N, Yoshimatsu H, et al : LEC score ; A judgment tool for indication of indocyanine green lymphography. Ann Plast Surg 70(2) : 227-230, 2013.

8) Yamamoto T, Yamamoto N, Doi K, et al : Indocyanine green (ICG)-enhanced lymphography for upper extremity lymphedema ; a novel severity staging system using dermal backflow(DB) patterns. Plast Reconstr Surg 128(4) : 941-947, 2011.

9) Yamamoto T, Narushima M, Yoshimatsu H, et al : Indocyanine green velocity ; Lymph transportation capacity deterioration with progression of lymphedema. Ann Plast Surg 71(5) : 591-594, 2013.

10) Lee BB, Antignani PL, Baroncelli TA, et al : IUA-ISVI consensus for diagnosis guideline of chronic lymphedema of the limbs. Int Angiol 34(4) : 311-332, 2015.

11) Yamamoto T, Iida T, Matsuda N, et al : Indocyanine green (ICG)-enhanced lymphography for evaluation of facial lymphoedema. J Plast Reconstr Aesthet Surg 64(11) : 1541-1544, 2011.

12) Yamamoto T, Narushima M, Yoshimatsu H, et al : Dynamic indocyanine green(ICG) lymphography for breast cancer-related arm lymphedema. Ann Plast Surg 73(6) : 706-709, 2014.

13) Yamamoto T, Yoshimatsu H, Narushima M, et al : Indocyanine green lymphography findings in primary leg lymphedema. Eur J Vasc Endovasc Surg 49 : 95-102, 2015.

14) Yamamoto T, Koshima I : Subclinical lymphedema ; understanding is the clue to decision making. Plast Reconstr Surg 132(3) : 472e-473e, 2013.

15) Yamamoto T, Koshima I : Splash, stardust, or diffuse pattern ; differentiation of dermal backflow pattern is important in indocyanine green lymphography. Plast Reconstr Surg 133(6) : e887-e888, 2014.

16) Yamamoto T, Narushima M, Doi K, et al : Characteristic indocyanine green lymphography findings in lower extremity lymphedema ; the generation of a novel lymphedema severity staging system using dermal backflow patterns. Plast Reconstr Surg 127(5) : 1979-1986, 2011.

17) Yamamoto T, Yamamoto N, Narushima M, et al : Lymphaticovenular anastomosis with guidance of ICG lymphography. J Jpn Coll Angiol 52 : 327-331, 2012.

18) Yamamoto T, Narushima M, Yoshimatsu H, et al : Minimally invasive lymphatic supermicrosurgery (MILS) ; indocyanine green lymphography-guided simultaneous multi-site lymphaticovenular anastomoses via millimeter skin incisions. Ann Plast Surg 72(1) : 67-70, 2014.

19) Akita S, Mitsukawa N, Rikihisa N, et al : Early diagnosis and risk factors for lymphedema following lymph node dissection for gynecologic cancer. Plast Reconstr Surg 131(2) : 283-289, 2013.

20) Yamamoto T, Matsuda N, Doi K, et al : The earliest finding of indocyanine green (ICG) lymphography in asymptomatic limbs of lower extremity lymphedema patients secondary to cancer treatment ; the modified dermal backflow(DB) stage and concept of subclinical lymphedema. Plast Reconstr Surg 128(4) : 314e-321e, 2011.

21) Connell FC, Gordon K, Brice G, et al : The classification and diagnostic algorithm for primary lymphatic dysplasia ; an update from 2010 to include molecular findings. Clin Genet 84(4) : 303-314, 2013.

22) Lee BB, Villavicencio JL : Primary lymphoedema and lymphatic malformation ; are they the two sides of the same coin? Eur J Vasc Endovasc Surg 39(5) : 646-653, 2010.

Important Reference

■ 四肢リンパ浮腫患者の走査電子顕微鏡所見—リンパ管静脈吻合術で観察される皮下組織の微細構造的特徴

Scanning electron microscopy findings in patients with lower-and upper-extremity lymphedema : fine-structure characteristics of subcutaneous tissues observed during lymphaticovenous anastomosis

■はじめに

　近年、形成外科領域における超微小血管外科（supermicrosurgery）の技術とその手術器具の飛躍的な進歩に伴い、従来のリンパ浮腫に対する外科的療法よりも優れたリンパ管細静脈吻合術（lymphaticovenular anastomosis；LVA）が外科治療法として開発されてきた。特に、現在発展著しいインドシニアグリーン（ICG）蛍光造影法を LVA の術中ナビゲーションに応用できたことの臨床的意義は大きく、結果、LVA はリンパ浮腫の外科治療として目覚ましい進歩を遂げている。

　浮腫患者の LVA を多く経験する中で、術者は皮下リンパ管周囲の結合組織には規則的な構造変化が個体間で共通して出現することに気づく。また、LVA 術前に施行される ICG 蛍光造影で観察される Dermal Backflow、ICG の局所貯留、そしてリンパ迂回路の閉塞像なども、術中観察される線維性中隔との深い関係を容易に想起させる。したがって、浮腫発生メカニズムを理解する場合、生理学的因子の解析のみならず、皮下組織内に生じる種々の構造変化を電子顕微鏡的に詳細に明らかにすることも重要と考えられる。

　ここでは、術中よく観察される主に 7 つの浮腫固有の組織構造（**Fig. 1**）について走査電子顕微鏡（Hitachi, S-4800）を用いて観察した結果を症例ごとに供覧する。なお、検索組織は、SEM 試料作成に先立ってデジタルマイクロスコープ（KEYENCE, VH-5500）を用いてマクロ形態の特徴についても観察を行った。

　ここで使用した組織試料は、すべて術前に同意が得られた LVA を施行したリンパ浮腫患者（25 名）からの浮腫皮下組織（切除した余剰組織）を使用した。

■Introduction

　Lymphaticovenular anastomosis (LVA), which is superior to conventional lymphedema operative interventions, has been developed with the help of rapid advancement in techniques and devices in supermicrosurgery in recent years. Advances in indocyanine green (ICG) fluorescence imaging are particularly noticeable, and its role in navigation during LVA is of clinical significance. As a result, LVA has made significant advancement as a surgical procedure for lymphedema.

　During LVA, surgeons often notice common systematic changes in the connective

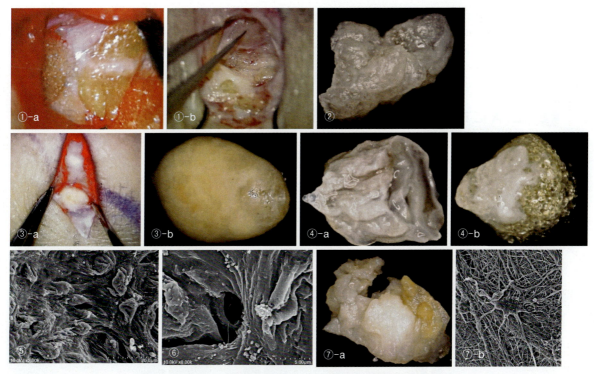

Fig. 1. LVA にて術中観察される皮下組織内の構造的特徴（7 つ）
Seven types of structural characteristics of lymphedema tissues observed during LVA surgery
①脂肪組織（被膜）(a)と細胞間物質の線維化（白色線維）(b)
  Excessive fibrosis of adipose tissue (capsule) (a) and intracellular matrix : white fibers (b).
②反復性蜂窩織炎に伴う白色結合組織
  White connective tissue accompanying recurrent cellulitis.
③皮下黄金顆粒（リンパ節様結節）
  Subcutaneous golden granules (lymph node-like nodules).
④リンパ管周囲の白色結合組織（肥厚線維束）
  White connective tissues (thick fiber bundles) around the lymphatic vessels (a : subcutaneous lymphatic vessels, b : white connective tissue).
⑤リンパ管内皮細胞の形態変化
  Fibrosis of the outer membrane of lymphatic vessels and morphological changes in endothelial cells.
⑥皮下前リンパ管通液路（SPLCs）の形態的特徴
  Morphological characteristics of subcutaneous prelymphatic channels (SPLCs) (endothelial gap).
⑦その他（線維芽細胞・放射線照射後の線維性瘢痕）
  Others (specific lymphedema accompanied by radiation ulcers, appearance of several fibroblasts) (a : scar tissue (fibrosis), b : fibroblast).

tissue surrounding subcutaneous lymphatic vessels. Also, findings of pre-LVA ICG fluorescence imaging, such as dermal backflow, local accumulation of ICG and bypass obstruction, can be strongly associated with fibrotic septa observed during surgery. Thus, in addition to analyzing physiological factors, close examination by electron microscopy to reveal various structural changes occurring in subcutaneous tissue is important to understanding the pathogenesis of chronic lymphedema.

In this chapter, seven types of structural characteristics of lymphedema tissues frequently observed during surgery, were introduced by scanning electron microscopy (SEM) findings in many clinical cases (**Fig. 1**). Prior to the preparation of SEM specimens, lymphedematous tissues were examined with a digital microscope (KEYENCE, VH-5500) to obtain their macroscopic morphological characteristics.

Tissue specimens included in this chapter were untouched by subcutaneous tissues recovered from lymphedema patients (n=25) who had underwent LVA. Consent was obtained from all patients before LVA surgery.

1　LVAにて術中観察される皮下組織内の構造的特徴（電顕所見）

1）脂肪組織と細胞間物質（基質）cellular substrates の過剰な線維化（白色線維）(Fig. 2〜10)

脂肪組織は、通常被膜の発達が悪く、肉眼的に脂肪組織表面において肥厚した白色線維は認められなかった。これは他の結合組織でも同じである。浮腫状態が続くと白色線維が広域で発達し、脂肪組織は線維性中隔を伴って段階的に肥厚した被膜によって完全に覆われるようになる。

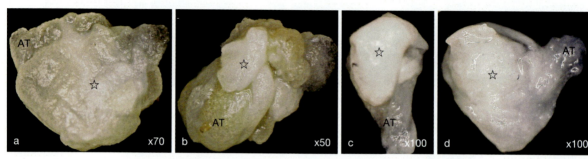

Fig. 2.　白色線維組織の所見（1）（a〜d：デジタルマイクロスコープ像）
Cases of white connective tissue (1) (a〜d : digital microscope images)

皮下リンパ管周囲の脂肪組織表層に形成される種々の白色線維組織（☆）。いずれもリンパ管に接する領域に局所的な線維化が生じた。しばしば脂肪組織の表面が光沢のある白色線維によって被覆された（d）（扁平線維芽細胞層との関連性）。
Various white fibrous tissues (☆) that form on the surface of the adipose tissue around subcutaneous lymphatic vessels. Fibroses occurred locally in every region contiguous with lymphatic vessels. The surface of the adipose tissue was often covered with shiny white fibers (d) (the relationship of flattened fibroblast layers).

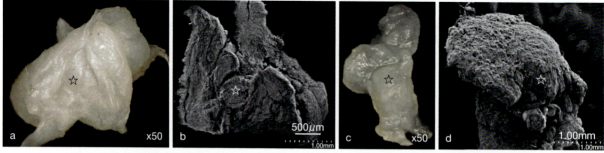

Fig. 3.　白色線維組織の症例（1）（a、c：デジタルマイクロスコープ像、b、d：走査電子顕微鏡像）
Cases of white connective tissue (1) (a, c : digital microscope images, b, d : SEM images)

79歳、女性、下腿。リンパ管から離れた間質に生じた白色線維組織（a、c：☆）。脂肪組織全体が白色線維で被覆された。白色線維は共に細い膠原線維の束から形成された（b、d：☆）。
A 79-year-old female, lower limb. White fibrous tissues (a, c : ☆) appeared on the subcutaneous matrix away from lymphatic vessels. The adipose tissue was completely covered with white fibers. Both of the white fibers were formed of thin collagenous fiber bundles (b, d : ☆).

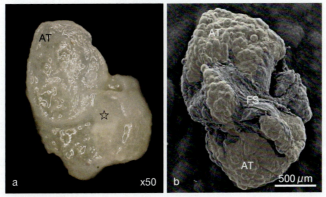

Fig. 4. 白色線維組織の症例 (2) (a：デジタルマイクロスコープ像、b：走査電子顕微鏡像)
A case of white connective tissue (2) (a：digital microscope image, b：SEM image)

75歳、女性、下腿。脂肪組織表面が白色線維 (a：☆) に被覆された。発達した線維性中隔 (FS) が脂肪組織 (AT：黄色着色) の間にクサビ状に進入した (b)。
A 75-year-old female, lower limb. The surface of the adipose tissue was covered with white fibers (a：☆). Wedge-shaped invasion of the fibrous septum (FS) was seen between the adipose tissue (AT：yellow-colored) (b).

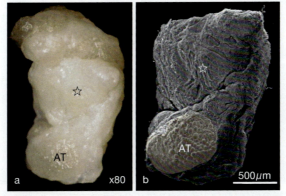

Fig. 5. 白色線維組織の所見 (2) (a：デジタルマイクロスコープ像、b：走査電子顕微鏡像)
Cases of white connective tissue (2) (a：digital microscope image, b：SEM image)

4歳、女児、前腕。通常の脂肪組織 (b：AT, 黄色着色) が光顕上観察された表層にも SEM 観察では線維性被膜の形成が認められた。
A 4-year-female child, forearm. Even on the surface of the normal adipose tissue (b：AT, yellow-colored) observed with an optical microscope, a formation of fibrous membrane was found with scanning electron microscope (SEM).

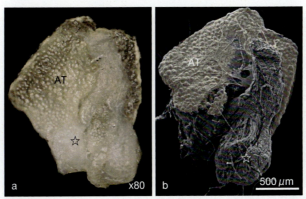

Fig. 6. 白色線維組織の所見 (3) (a：デジタルマイクロスコープ像、b：走査電子顕微鏡像)
Cases of white connective tissue (2) (a：digital microscope image, b：SEM image)

54歳、男性、下肢。両症例共にリンパ管周囲の脂肪組織には、表層 (a：☆) のみならず組織深部にも過度の線維化が認められた。
A 54-year-male, lower limb. Both cases had excess fibrosis not only on the surface of the adipose tissue (a：☆) around lymphatic vessels, but also in the deep portion of the adipose tissue.

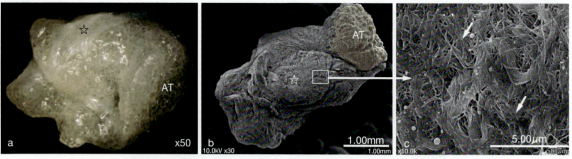

Fig. 7. 白色線維組織の症例(3)(a：デジタルマイクロスコープ像、b、c：走査電子顕微鏡像)
A case of white connective tissue (3) (a : digital microscope image, b, c : SEM images)

他の症例と比較して、脂肪組織(a：AT)は汚い色調の大きな脂肪細胞を多く含んでいた。脂肪組織表層の白色線維(b：☆)の発達は不均一であった。線維化が顕著な領域(b：white square)では、膠原線維(c：arrows)に密性網工が確認された。
The adipose tissue (a : AT) contained more large dirty-colored adipose cells than other cases. The development of white fibers (b : ☆) on the surface of the adipose tissue was inhomogeneous. A dense network of collagenous fibers (c : arrows) was recognized in regions with remarkable fibrosis (b : white square).

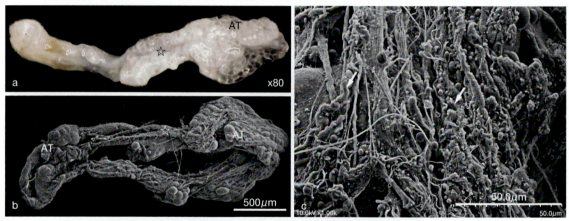

Fig. 8. 白色線維組織の症例(4)(a：デジタルマイクロスコープ像、b、c：走査電子顕微鏡像)
A case of white connective tissue (4) (a : digital microscope image, b, c : SEM images)

原発性リンパ浮腫・反復性蜂窩織炎：女性、下腿。特徴的な白色線維束(a：☆)がリンパ管を含む脂肪組織の間に進入した。SEM観察において、線維化が顕著な領域(b：☆)において蛇行する太い膠原線維束(c：arrows)が多数認められた。
Primary lymphedema・recurrent cellulitis：female, lower limb. Characteristic white fiber bundles (a : ☆) invaded areas between the adipose tissue, including lymphatic vessels. With scanning electron microscope (SEM) observation, many thick, tortuous, collagenous fiber bundles (c : arrows) were found in regions with remarkable fibrosis (b : ☆).

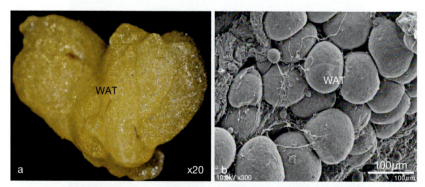

Fig. 9. 正常な白色脂肪組織(a：デジタルマイクロスコープ像、b：走査電子顕微鏡像)
Normal white adipose tissue without edema (a : digital microscope image, b : SEM image)

正常皮下組織内の白色脂肪組織(WAT)。通常、脂肪組織表層には白色線維被膜ならびに脂肪組織間に嵌入する発達した線維性中隔も認められなかった。
The white adipose tissue (WAT) in normal subcutaneous tissue. Commonly, the surface of the adipose tissue showed no white fibrous membrane or developed fibrous septum intruding between the adipose tissue.

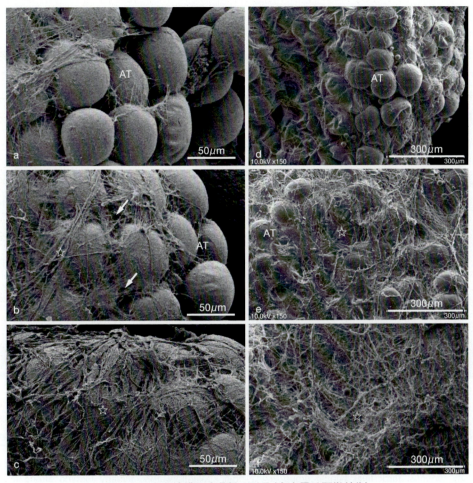

Fig. 10. 白色線維発達過程の所見（走査電子顕微鏡像）
Two cases of developmental process of white fibrosis (SEM images)
a〜c：脂肪組織（AT）表面に観察される強靭な線維性被覆（c）は、徐々に発達する膠原線維束が脂肪細胞間（b：large arrows）を充填するようにして広域に形成される。
d〜f：脂肪組織の表面ならびに脂肪細胞間に比較的細い膠原線維（e：☆）が浅深方向に多数交錯することで線維性被覆（c：☆）が形成される。
a〜c：A strong fibrous membrane (c) observed on the surface of the adipose tissue (AT) forms over a wide area, as if gradually developing collagenous fiber bundles form between adipose cells (b : large arrows).
d〜f：Many of the relatively thin collagenous fibers (e : ☆) mix in the shallow-deep direction on the surface of the adipose tissue as well as between adipose cells, which thereby leads to formation of the fibrous membrane (c : ☆).

2）反復性蜂窩織炎に伴う白色結合組織（Fig. 11〜13）

通常の浮腫組織と比較して、脂肪組織ならびに細胞間物質には過剰な線維化が認められた。出現する線維束は太く、やや蛇行するが相互に直交する特徴がみられた。細胞実質が壊死した領域（蜂窩）の周囲の線維化も顕著である。線維化の一部には扁平線維芽細胞による上皮様被膜化も認められた。

3）皮下黄金顆粒（リンパ節様結節）（Fig. 14〜18）

①皮下組織浅層には、浮腫患者のみ鮮やかな黄金色の結節様の顆粒が出現した。またそれに類

似した種々の顆粒(発達初期)も多数観察されたが、顆粒被膜の発達は黄金顆粒と比較して明らかに悪く、実質内に充満する脂肪細胞間の線維化も乏しかった。

　②顆粒被膜が特に肥厚した1症例(**Fig. 18**)において、実質内に隔離されたメチシリン耐性黄色ブドウ球菌(methicillin-resistant *Staphylococcus aureus*；MRSA)の菌巣が観察された。黄金顆粒の形成機序の1つとして、蜂窩織炎の起炎菌であるMRSAの皮下感染が関係する可能性が推測された。

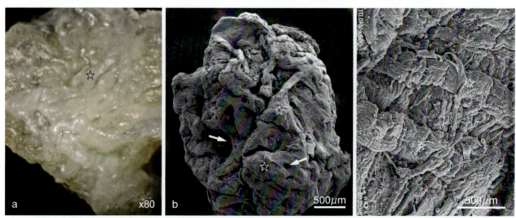

Fig. 11. 反復性蜂窩織炎の症例(1)(a：デジタルマイクロスコープ像、b、c：走査電子顕微鏡像)
A case of recurrent cellulitis(1)(a：digital microscope image, b, c：SEM images)

48歳、女性、大腿。反復性蜂窩織炎に罹患した皮下脂肪組織。不規則に蛇行する太い線維束群(a：☆)がそれぞれ直行することで強靭な線維被膜を形成された。SEM観察において、蛇行した肥厚線維束の間には多数の蜂巣状の小孔(b：arrows)も出現した。
A 48-year-female, lower limb. The subcutaneous adipose tissue in a patient with recurrent cellulitis. Each of the irregularly tortuous, thick fiber bundle group (a：☆) ran straightforwardly, thereby forming strong fibrous membranes. Scanning electron microscope(SEM) observation also showed many honeycomb pores(b：arrows) between the tortuous thickened fiber bundles.

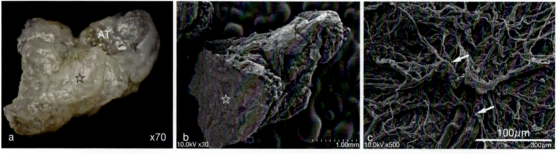

Fig. 12. 反復性蜂窩織炎の症例(2)(a：デジタルマイクロスコープ像、b、c：走査電子顕微鏡像)
A case of recurrent cellulitis(2)(a：digital microscope image, b, c：SEM images)

男性、大腿。光顕像観察にて、脂肪組織の表層には凹凸した大きな肥厚線維が認められた(a：☆)。試料断面をSEM観察すると、表層線維化の一部は組織内にも多数進入(b：☆)した。被膜形成には蛇行する多数の肥厚線維束(c：arrows)も形成に関係した。
A male, lower limb. With an optical microscope, uneven, large thickened fibers (a：☆) were noted on the surface of the adipose tissue. Scanning electron microscope(SEM) observation of the cross-section exhibited many invasions of a part of the surficial fibroses(b：☆). Many of tortuous and thickened fiber bundles(c：arrows) were also involved in the membrane formation.

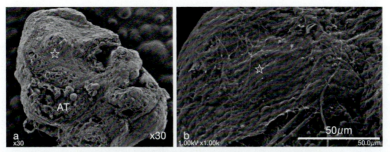

Fig. 13. 反復性蜂窩織炎の皮下所見（走査電子顕微鏡像）
Cases of recurrent cellulitis (SEM images)

脂肪組織（AT）には膠原線維の細胞間浸潤と表層線維化（a：☆）が明らかに認められた。線維被膜には局所的に上皮様のシート構造（b：☆）も出現した。
The adipose tissue (AT) obviously showed intercellular invasion and superficial fibrosis of collagenous fibers (a：☆). An epithelial-like sheet structure (b：☆) also locally appeared on the fibrous membrane.

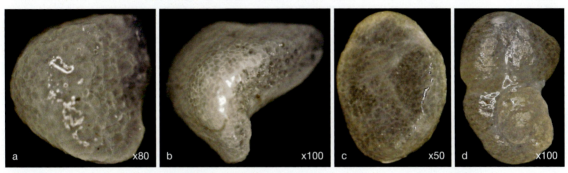

Fig. 14. 皮下黄金顆粒の光顕所見（1）（a〜d：デジタルマイクロスコープ像）
Cases of subcutaneous golden granules (1) (a〜d：digital microscope images)

皮下黄金顆粒（ScGG）には、被膜線維化の発達状況により種々の形成過程が観察された。黄金顆粒初期過程（a〜d）。
Subcutaneous golden granules (ScGG) showed various processes of their formation depending on the development conditions of the membrane fibrosis. The initial processes of ScGG (a〜d).

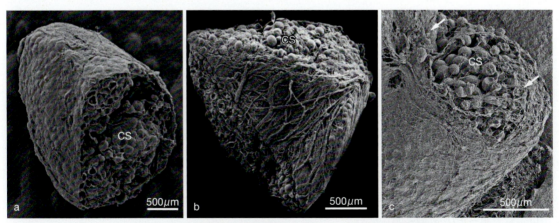

Fig. 15. 皮下黄金顆粒の電顕所見（2）（a〜c：走査電子顕微鏡像）
Cases of subcutaneous golden granules (1) (a〜c：SEM images)

皮下黄金顆粒（ScGG）断面（CS）の SEM 観察（a〜c）。ScGG は脂肪組織を実質主要素とするが、線維性被膜の発達状況に応じて独立した顆粒形態を形成（a、b）した。顆粒被膜の発達は顆粒内部の線維化（c：arrows）とも強く相関した。
Scanning electron microscope (SEM) images of the cross-sections (CS) of the subcutaneous golden granules (ScGG) (a〜c). The ScGG contain the adipose tissue as their matrix constituent but have granule morphology (a, b) depending on the development conditions of the fibrous membrane. The development of the granular membrane strongly correlated with fibrosis in the granules (c：arrows).

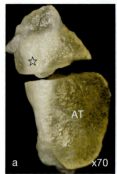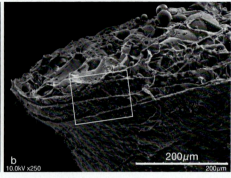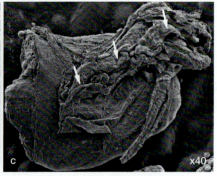

Fig. 16. 皮下黄金顆粒の症例(1)(a：デジタルマイクロスコープ像、b、c：走査電子顕微鏡像)
A case of subcutaneous golden granule(1) (a：digital microscope image, b, c：SEM images)

黄金顆粒の初期形成段階では、線維被膜(☆)の発達不全に伴い被膜下の脂肪細胞が透けて見えた(a：AT)。通常、顆粒被膜は重層化(b：white square)を呈した。顆粒表面には周囲の脂肪組織との間を連結する強靱な架橋線維束も発達した(c：arrows)。

In the initial stage of ScGG ormation, adipose cells under the membrane could be seen transparently (a：AT) because of the premature development of the fibrous membrane (☆). The granular membrane usually presents with stratification (b：white square). On the surface of granules, strong cross-linking fiber bundles developed to connect with the surrounding adipose tissue (c：arrows).

4) リンパ管周囲の白色結合組織(肥厚線維束)(Fig. 19, 20)

皮下リンパ管には脂肪組織が密着する。リンパ管に接する脂肪組織に局所的な線維化が生じることでリンパ管と結合組織が強く密着する。線維化が顕著な症例では、リンパ管の全周に肥厚した線維が発達する。リンパ管周囲の脂肪組織では特徴的な種々の線維化が観察された。

5) リンパ管外膜の線維化と内皮細胞の形態変化(Fig. 21〜23)

リンパ管線の線維化が顕著な症例では、内皮細胞の形態変化が生じた領域に内皮小孔の増加が認められた。またこの小孔下の結合組織層にも篩状斑様のいくつかの組織間隙が認められた。

6) 皮下前リンパ管通液路(prelymphatic channel；PLC)の形態的特徴(Fig. 24)

リンパ管の線維化が顕著な症例では、内皮細胞の形態変化が生じた領域に内皮小孔の増加が認められた。またこの小孔下の結合組織層にも篩状斑様のいくつかの組織間隙が認められた。

7) その他(線維芽細胞、放射線潰瘍を伴うリンパ浮腫)(Fig. 25〜29)

①リンパ浮腫組織では、線維化が顕著な領域においてしばしば活性化した線維芽細胞が認められた。また、反復性蜂窩織炎の症例を中心に、線維化表層に扁平線維芽細胞の被膜形成が認められた。扁平線維芽細胞で形成された被膜は肉眼的に光沢のある白色を呈した(Fig. 25, 26)。

②鼠径部リンパ浮腫領域に難治性の放射線潰瘍が認められたStewart-Treves症候群の疑いもある症例。脂肪組織の被膜のみならず、局所的に脂肪細胞間に進入する太い線維束が多数形成された。血管周囲の線維化の一部には石灰化も認められたが、試料内で観察できた血管内皮細胞は正常であった(Fig. 27〜29)。

1. Structural characteristics of subcutaneous tissues observed during LVA (electron microscopy findings)

1) **Excessive fibrosis of adipose tissue and intracellular matrix：white fibers** (Figs. 2 to 10)：
Adipose tissue usually has a poorly developed capsular membrane, and indeed, white-fiber thickening was macroscopically absent on the surface of adipose tissue. Findings obtained from examination of connective

Important Reference/四肢リンパ浮腫患者の走査電子顕微鏡所見

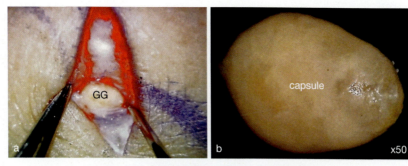

Fig. 17. 皮下黄金顆粒の症例(2)(手術所見)
A case of subcutaneous golden granule(2):LVA operative finding
黄金顆粒(GG)は LVA 術中、皮下浅層にしばしば出現した(a)。摘出した顆粒はリンパ節に似た独立した結節様構造を呈した(b)。
The ScGG (GG) frequently appeared in the subcutaneous superficial layers during lymphaticovenular anastomosis(a). The removed granules had an independent nodule-like structure resembling lymphatic vessels(b).

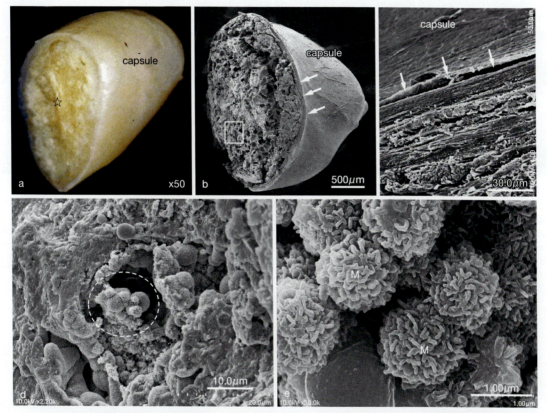

Fig. 18. 皮下黄金顆粒の発達症例(a:デジタルマイクロスコープ像、b〜e:走査電子顕微鏡像)
A case of developed golden granule(a:digital microscope image, b〜e:SEM images)
40 歳の女性下腿。黄金顆粒(ScGG)中央部を切断(a)。実質内部は通常の脂肪細胞のほか、粥状組織が広く分布した(a:☆、b:white square)。顆粒被膜は多層線維により顕著に肥厚した(b、c:arrows)。顆粒内部の粥状組織の一部(d:white dotted circle)には、MRSA の菌巣集簇が散在して認められた(e:M)。
A 40-year-female lower limb. The ScGG as cut at the central part(a). Wide distribution of normal adipose cells as well as atheromatous tissues was seen in the matrix(a:☆, b:white square). The granular membrane was markedly thickened due to multi-layer fibers(b, c:arrows). A part of the atheromatous tissue in granules(d:white dotted circle) sporadically showed aggregated fungal nests of MRSA(e:M).

95

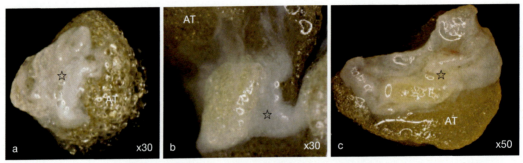

Fig. 19. リンパ管周囲の脂肪組織の白色線維化所見(a～c：デジタルマイクロスコープ像)
Cases of white connective tissue adjacent to the lymphatic vessels (a～c：digital microscope images)
皮下リンパ管周囲の脂肪組織(AT)には、リンパ管に隣接する領域に限局して発達した白色線維(☆)が出現した。
Well-developed white connective tissue(☆) appeared to the adipose tissue(AT) toward contact with subcutaneous lymphatic vessels preferentially.

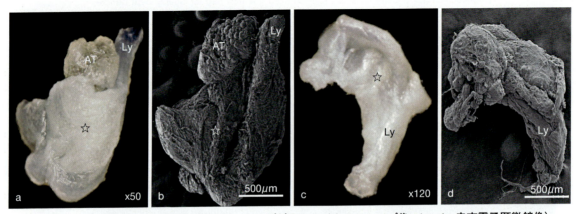

Fig. 20. リンパ管周囲の白色線維化症例(a、c：デジタルマイクロスコープ像、b、d：走査電子顕微鏡像)
Cases of white connective tissue around the lymphatic vessel (a, c：digital microscope images, b, d：SEM images)
58歳の女性下腿(a、b)と58歳の男性下腿(c、d)。両症例共にリンパ管(Ly)周囲に広く白色の肥厚線維(☆)が発達した。
A 58-year-female lower limb (a, b), A 58-year-male lower limb (c). In both cases, white thickened fibers (☆) developed extensively around lymphatic vessels (Ly).

tissue were similar. On the other hand, in sustained lymphedema, white fibers developed across a wide area, and eventually, adipose tissue became completely covered by a capsular membrane, which gradually thickened with development of fibrotic septa.

2) **White connective tissue accompanying recurrent cellulitis** (Figs. 11 to 13)：Excessive fibrosis was confirmed in adipose tissue and extracellular matrix, compared with ordinary (non-cellulitis) lymphedema tissue. Fiber bundles that developed were thick and crossed perpendicularly, albeit with slight tortuosity. Marked fibrosis was found around necrotic parenchymal areas (cellulitic areas). A capsular layer composed of activated fibroblasts was also found in parts of the fibrotic regions.

3) **Subcutaneous golden granules (lymph node-like nodules)** (Figs. 14 to 18)

①Bright golden nodule-like granules appeared in the superficial subcutaneous layer only in lymphedema patients. A large number of similar granules (early stage of development) were observed, but the development of a capsular layer was clearly poorer when these granules were present than when developing golden granules were present. Fibrosis between parenchymal adipose cells was less obvious in the former than in the latter cases.

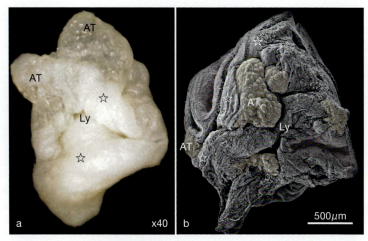

Fig. 21. リンパ管外膜の線維化症例(a：デジタルマイクロスコープ像、b：走査電子顕微鏡像)
A case of fibrosis of the outer membrane of lymphatic vessel (a：digital microscope image, b：SEM image)
58歳の女性下腿。皮下リンパ管(Ly)側面とその周囲に肥厚した白色線維(☆)が強く密着する所見。AT：脂肪組織
A 58-year-female lower limb. A finding of strong adhesion between the lateral side of subcutaneous lymphatic vessels and the surrounding thickened white fibers(☆). AT：fatty tissue

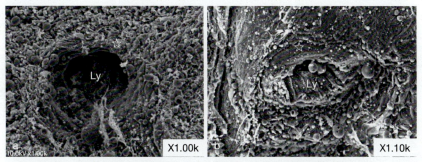

Fig. 22. リンパ管外膜の線維化(走査電子顕微鏡像)
Fibrosis of the adventitial tissue layer of lymphatic vessel (SEM images)
リンパ管(Ly)周囲には管壁に密着する厚い線維層(a、b：☆)の発達が認められた。
Around the lymphatic vessels, development of thick fibrous layers adhering to vessel walls was noted (a, b：☆).

②Isolated MRSA foci were observed in the tissue parenchyma in a patient with a particularly thickened capsular membrane of granules (**Fig. 18**). This suggests that subcutaneous MRSA infection, a causative agent of cellulitis, is possibly involved in the mechanism underlying the formation of these golden granules.

4) White connective tissues (thick fiber bundles) around lymphatic vessels (Figs. 19, 20)：
Adipose tissue is tightly attached to subcutaneous lymphatic vessels. Local fibrosis in such adipose tissue resulted in tight attachment of connective tissue to lymphatic vessels. Circumferential thick fiber formation was found in patients with severe fibrosis. Characteristic fibrosis in various forms was found in adipose tissues around lymphatic vessels.

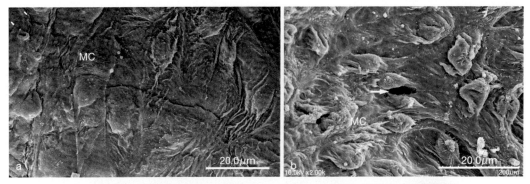

Fig. 23. リンパ管内皮細胞の形態変化（a：正常、b：異常）（走査電子顕微鏡像）
Morphological changes in endothelial cells (a : normal, b : abnormal) (SEM images)

通常、リンパ管内皮細胞 (MC) は敷石状に整然と配列 (a) するが、発達した線維化領域ではリンパ管内皮細胞の一部に萎縮・膨化などの形態変化が認められた。また endothelial gaps (large arrow) も散在して出現が認められた (b)。
Lymphatic endothelial cells (MC) are generally arranged methodically like cobblestones (a). However, lymphatic endothelial cells partly had morphological changes such as atrophy or swelling in the regions with developed fibrosis. Endothelial gaps (large arrow) were also sporadically seen (b).

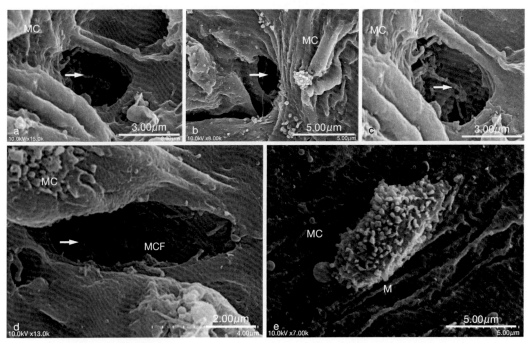

Fig. 24. 皮下前リンパ管通液路（a〜d：リンパ管内皮小孔）とリンパ管内皮細胞の形態変化（e：マクロファージ）（走査電子顕微鏡像）
Subcutaneus prelymphatic channels (a〜d : lymphatic endothelial gaps) and Morphological changes in endothelial cells (e : Macrophage) (SEM images)

リンパ管内皮細胞 (MC) 間に出現する内皮小孔 (a〜d：large arrow) と基底膜下に macula cribriformis (MCF) の存在も認められた (d)。リンパ管内皮 (e：MC) 小孔周囲にはしばしばマクロファージ (e：M) の存在が確認された。
The existence of MCF was also found in endothelial gaps (a〜d : large arrow) between lymphatic endothelial cells and beneath the basement membrane (d). The presence of macrophages (e : M) was often noted around the pores on the lymphatic endothelium (e : MC).

Important Reference/四肢リンパ浮腫患者の走査電子顕微鏡所見

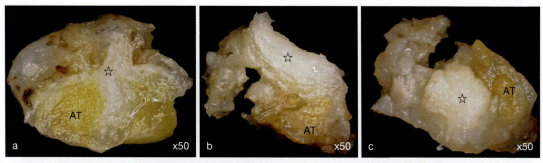

Fig. 25. 放射線放射後の瘢痕線維(1) (a～c：デジタルマイクロスコープ像)
Specific fibrosis accompanied by radiation ulcers(1) (a～c：digital microscope images)

76歳の女性鼠径部。難治性潰瘍生検組織。リンパ管周囲の脂肪組織(AT)に、不規則に走行する石灰化を伴う強靭な膠原線維束(☆)が発達した。ただし脂肪組織全体を被覆する肥厚線維束の形成は認められなかった。
A 76-year-female groin region. The biopsy tissues of refractory ulcer. On the adipose tissue around lymphatic vessels (AT), a strong collagenous fiber bundle(☆) running irregularly and associated with calcification appeared. However, there was no formation of thickened fiber bundles covering the whole adipose tissue.

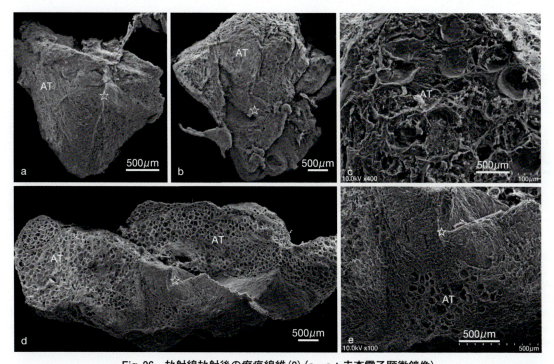

Fig. 26. 放射線放射後の瘢痕線維(2) (a～e：走査電子顕微鏡像)
Specific fibrosis accompanied by radiation ulcers(2) (a～e：SEM images)

光顕観察において線維化(☆)が乏しい脂肪組織では、比較的発達した線維被膜(AT)の形成された(a、b)。線維化が顕著な脂肪組織の断面観察では、密性の膠原線維束の進入(d、e：☆)も認められた。また、試料組織断面に進入する脂肪細胞間の線維性中隔の発達も顕著であった(c、e)。
In the adipose tissue found to have poor fibrosis(☆) by observation with an optical microscope, relatively developed fibrous membrane was formed(AT) (a, b). Observation of the cross-section of the adipose tissue with noticeable fibrosis demonstrated invasion of dense collagenous fiber bundles(d, e：☆). Additionally, remarkable development was also noted in septal fibers between the adipose tissue that invades sections of sample tissues(c, e).

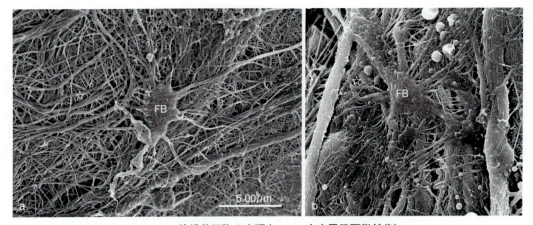

Fig. 27. 線維芽細胞の出現 (a、b：走査電子顕微鏡像)
Appearance of normal fibroblasts (a, b : SEM images)

脂肪組織の被膜 (☆)。被膜表層の線維化が顕著な領域において、散在して活性化線維芽細胞 (FB) (a、b：青色着色) の出現も認められた。

The membrane of the adipose tissue (☆). Sporadically activated fibroblasts (FB) (a, b : blue-colored) also appeared in the regions with marked fibrosis on the surface of the membranes.

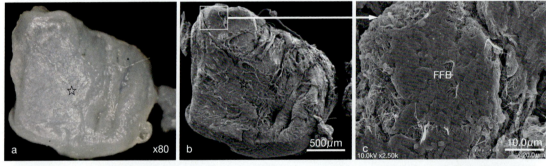

Fig. 28. シート様扁平線維芽細胞の出現 (1) (a：デジタルマイクロスコープ像、b、c：走査電子顕微鏡像)
Appearance of sheet like-flatter fibroblasts (1) (a : digital microscope image, b, c : SEM images)

慢性浮腫組織ではしばしば鮮やかな白色を呈する線維性被膜 (a：☆) が観察された。SEM 観察では白色領域は線維性被膜 (b：☆) で形成されていたが、光沢のある表層は上皮シート様の扁平線維芽細胞 (FFB) によって覆われていた (c)。c は b 内に示した square の拡大。

The fibrous membranes (a : ☆) frequently presenting with bright white color in tissues of chronic edema were found. Scanning electron microscope (SEM) observation showed that white areas were formed by fibrous membrane (b : ☆), but the glossy surface was covered with epithelial sheet-like flattened fibroblasts (FFB) (c). c is the magnification of the square shown in b.

5) **Fibrosis of the adventitial tissue layer of lymphatic vessels and morphological changes in endothelial cells** (**Figs. 21 to 23**)：Patients with severe fibrosis of adventitia of lymphatic vessels showed increases in the number of small holes in the area containing morphologically altered endothelial cells. In addition, gaps in a cribriform pattern were observed in the connective tissue layer below these small holes.

6) **Morphological characteristics of prelymphatic channels (PLCs)** (**Fig. 24**)：Patients with severe fibrosis of the adventitia of lymph vessels showed increases in the number of small gaps in the area with morphologically altered endothelial cells. In addition, gaps in a macula cribriform pattern were observed in the connective tissue layer below these small holes.

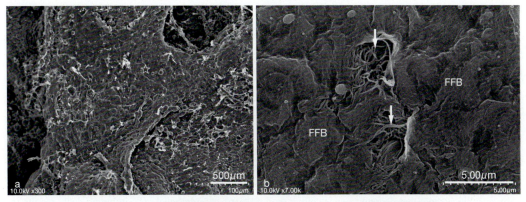

Fig. 29. シート様扁平線維芽細胞の出現(2)(a、b：走査電子顕微鏡像)
Appearance of sheet like-flatter fibroblasts(2)(a, b：SEM images)

シート様の扁平線維芽細胞(FFB)(a：☆)が存在する領域を拡大すると、単層扁平上皮様に変化した扁平線維芽細胞(b)の特殊形態が確認できた。FFB の間隙(b：large arrows)からその直下に位置する発達した膠原線維が存在した。
Magnification of the region with the sheet-like flattened fibroblasts(FFB)(a：☆) allowed identification of FFB(b：large arrows) that had changed to have a particular morphology of simple squamous epithelium-like FFB. From the gap(b) between the FFB, developed collagenous fibers could be seen immediately below FFB.

7) Others(fibroblasts, lymphedema accompanied by radiation ulcers)(Figs. 25 to 29)

①Activated fibroblasts were confirmed in obviously fibrotic areas in lymphedema tissues. Also, a layer composed of fibroblasts was confirmed on the surface of the fibrotic region, especially in patients with recurrent cellulitis. Macroscopic characteristics of the outer layer composed of fibroblasts giving its glossy-white appearance(Figs. 25, 26).

②A case of a refractory radiation ulcer developed in a lymphedema-affected site of the groin in a patient with suspected Stewart-Treves syndrome. Local formation of a large number of thick fiber bundles that inserted into the spaces between adipocytes, as well as the formation of a capsular layer enclosing adipose tissues were observed. Calcification was found in fibrotic parts around blood vessels, but examination of the specimens revealed normal vascular endothelial cells(Figs. 27 to 29).

2 まとめ

LVA の術中によく観察される皮下組織内の種々の構造変化について、それぞれ SEM を用いて微細構造的特徴を観察した。リンパ浮腫にかかわる皮下組織内の構造変化の特徴は以下のとおりである。皮下組織には、他の器官系と同じように prelymphatic channel(PLC)に類似した結合組織間隙(篩状斑)およびリンパ管内皮細胞隙の存在が観察された。またリンパ管内皮細胞が変性(膨化・縮小)することで内皮細胞間隙の異常な増加または弁変性が生じ、リンパ管の輸送機能が低下することが推測された。浮腫発生メカニズムには、PLC 関連構造の線維化(①肥厚線維化・②脂肪線維被膜ならびに結合組織間線維中隔の形成、③線維層板の発達を伴う黄金顆粒など)とリンパ管内皮細胞の膨化などの変性、そしてリンパ管外膜とリンパ管密着脂肪組織(含む adipose-derived stem cell ADSC)の局所的な線維化がそれぞれ深く関係することが示唆された。

他方、反復性蜂窩織炎を伴うリンパ浮腫症例では、脂肪組織被膜に発達したシート状の扁平線維芽細胞、そして線維化の主部には交錯した太い線維束の重層形成が特徴的に出現した。さらに

MRSAに感染した皮下浅層内では、線維性中隔ならびに発達した被膜を呈する黄金顆粒などの形成がその特徴と考えられた。これらの構造的特徴は、リンパ循環不全を引き起こす責任構造因子であると考えられる。なお、抗がん剤使用や放射線照射の影響が懸念されるリンパ浮腫患者では、皮下組織に局所的な強い線維性瘢痕が多数認められた。

（三浦真弘、濱田裕一）

2. Summary

Structural changes in subcutaneous tissues, frequently observed during LVA, were examined using SEM to obtain microstructure characteristics of lymphedema. There were PLC-like cribriform gaps between the connective tissue and gaps in the endothelium of lymph vessels in subcutaneous tissues as seen in other organs. We assume that degeneration (swelling or shrinkage) of endothelial cells in lymph ducts results in abnormal increases in gaps in the endothelium or valvular degeneration, thereby reducing lymphatic transport function. We suggested that mechanisms in lymphedema pathogenesis strongly involve fibrosis of PLC-associated structure (fibrous thickening ; formation of fibrotic capsules enclosing adipose tissue and fibrotic septum between connective tissues ; and golden granules associated with fibrotic layers), endothelial degeneration (*e.g.*, swelling) in lymph vessels, and local fibrosis in the adventitial tissue layer of lymph vessels and in adipose tissues closely attached to lymph vessels.

On the other hand, formation of a fibroblast sheet on the surface of adipose tissues, and formation of layers of intersecting thick fiber bundles in the focal part of the fibrotic regions are characteristics observed in patients with lymphedema accompanied by recurrent cellulitis. Furthermore, formation of fibrotic septa and subcutaneous golden granules with a well-developed outer membrane were characteristics of the MRSA-infected, superficial, subcutaneous layer. It is likely that such structural characteristics are causative structural factors triggering failure in lymph circulation. Also, local formation of a large number of severe fibrotic scars was found in the subcutaneous tissue of lymphedema patients, which may have been caused by anticancer drugs and radiation exposure.

（*Masahiro Miura, Yuichi Hamada*）

Important Reference

■ 遺伝子変異マウスの胎児浮腫とリンパ管形成異常

Embryonic edema and defective lymphatic vascular development in gene mutant mice

■はじめに

胎児浮腫は心奇形やリンパ管形成異常などが原因で、胎児の末梢組織中に水分が異常に貯留した状態である。ここでは、胎生期のリンパ管形成機構とその異常が原因で生じる浮腫を中心に概説する。

■Introduction

Embryonic edema is an abnormal accumulation of water in the peripheral tissues, and its causes include heart malformations and dysplasia of the lymphatic vessels. In this manuscript, both the mechanism of embryonic lymphatic vessel formation, and resultant edema due to abnormalities in this process will be reviewed.

1 胎児浮腫

1）ヒトの症例

ヒト妊娠中に実施される胎児の超音波検査で項部浮腫（首の後ろのむくみ）が見つかることがあり、NT（Nuchal Translucency）肥厚と呼ばれている。正確な判定には、①妊娠 11 週 0 日〜13 週 6 日での測定、②超音波画像の拡大率が十分であり、胎児上半身が大きく描出されていること、③矢状断面で計測されていること、の 3 点に留意して測定された NT 値が重要である。NT 値の 95 パーセンタイル値は頭臀長（Crown-Rump Length；CRL）に応じて異なるが、これを超えた胎児の約 10%程度に羊水検査で胎児染色体異常（13 トリソミー、18 トリソミー、21 トリソミーなど）が見つかる。一方で、妊娠週数にかかわらず 99 パーセンタイル値は 3.5 mm であるが、NT 値がこれを超えても染色体正常で出生に至った児においては、90%強の無病生存が期待できるとされている[1]。

2）マウスの場合

遺伝子突然変異マウスやノックアウトマウスを用いた発生遺伝学研究で、胎児が項部浮腫をきたす例が数多く報告されている。概ね胎生 13.5 日目から 15.5 日目にかけて顕著であるが、妊娠後期においては水分の貯留による皮膚の張りが抑えられてやや不明瞭になる傾向がある。マウスの項部浮腫を判定するための標準的測定法は定められていないが、われわれは胎児の透過領域の面積を CRL の 2 乗で割った値を Edema index として、遺伝子型ごとの比較解析に用いている。

1. Embryonic edema

1) In humans : Edema in the nuchal region (swelling in the rear of the neck), called nuchal translucency (NT), is sometimes found in fetal ultrasounds taken during pregnancy in humans. An understanding of the following three points are important in making an accurate assessment through the measurement of NT values : (I) that the measurement is made between 11 weeks and 13 weeks 6 days of the pregnancy, (II) that the ultrasound images are of a sufficient magnification and provide a large view of the fetus' upper body, and (III) that measurements are made in the sagittal plane. While the 95th percentile of the NT values differ depending on the crown-rump length (CRL), about 10% of fetuses with a value greater than this are found to have chromosomal abnormalities (trisomy 13, trisomy 18, trisomy 21, etc.) by amniotic diagnosis. In contrast, while the 99th percentile is 3.5 mm regardless of the week of the pregnancy, even with an NT value higher than this, disease-free survival can be expected in more than 90% of those children born with normal chromosomes.

2) In mice : In developmental genetic research, there have been a large number of reports on cases of induced nuchal edema in embryos using gene mutant mice and knockout mice. Generally, while most prominent between 13.5 and 15.5 days of gestation, the extension of the skin due to the accumulation of water is suppressed and tends to become indistinct in late pregnancy. There is not a standard measurement method for assessing nuchal edema in mice ; however, we take the area of the translucent region of the embryo divided by the square of the CRL as an edema index for analytical comparison of different genotypes.

2 リンパ管の発生

1）リンパ管の構造

リンパ管系は開放循環系であり、末梢組織で盲端から始まり組織間液・蛋白・脂質・免疫細胞・異物などを取り込む毛細リンパ管（起始リンパ管とも呼ぶ）と、リンパ液の運搬路となり心臓近くの静脈に開口する集合リンパ管からなる。毛細リンパ管の内皮細胞は特徴的な柏の葉状の輪郭を示し、内皮細胞間接着はボタン様結合（button-like junction）であり、広く開いた細胞間隙から大型物質を取り込むのに適している。集合リンパ管の内皮細胞間接着は密であり、ジッパー様結合（zipper-like junction）と呼ばれている。集合リンパ管には逆流を防ぐ弁が備わり、径の大きなものには平滑筋細胞が集積してそれらの収縮がリンパ流をつくるのに役立っている。2つの弁の間で平滑筋を備える領域は lymphangion と呼ばれ、集合リンパ管の機能単位と考えられている。

2）リンパ管内皮細胞の由来

静脈を構成する血管内皮細胞から分化するという遠心説（centrifugal theory）と、静脈周囲の間葉系細胞から分化するという求心説（centripetal theory）という2つの有力な説が提唱されている。近年のゼブラフィッシュを用いたリアルタイム解析は静脈内皮細胞が分化・出芽してリンパ管が形成される様子を捉えており、遠心説を支持している。一方、トリを用いた移植実験は静脈内皮細胞以外の系譜からリンパ管内皮細胞が発生することを示しており、求心説を支持している。マウスの遺伝学的手法を用いた細胞系譜解析では、両方の由来が存在することが示唆されている。

3）リンパ管の形態形成機構

a．分化・遊走・融合

　マウス胚では胎生 10 日目頃に、頸部静脈を構成する内皮細胞の一部に転写制御因子 Sox18、Prox1 が順次発現し、リンパ管内皮細胞へ分化する。分化誘導因子として、レチノイン酸や Wnt5b が示されている。静脈特異的に発現する核内受容体 COUP-TFII が Prox1 の発現誘導と維持に必要であり、Sox18 は *Prox1* 遺伝子の転写を促進する。Prox1 はリンパ管内皮細胞の分化に必須であり、受容体型チロシンキナーゼ（vascular endothelial growth factor receptor 3；VEGFR3）や糖蛋白質（Podoplanin；Pdpn）などのリンパ管内皮細胞マーカーの発現に中心的な役割を果たしている。分化したリンパ管内皮細胞は VEGFR3 を強く発現し、そのリガンドである血管内皮増殖因子 VEGF-C を産生する近傍の間葉組織に向かって遊走する。VEGF-C は前駆体として産生され、細胞外基質蛋白 Ccbe1 依存的にプロセシングされて成熟型蛋白となることで活性型となる。

　ゼブラフィッシュのリアルタイム解析において、静脈に由来するリンパ管内皮細胞が節状に分布し、それらがお互いに融合して胸管形成が進行する像が捉えられている。マウスの頸部静脈から分化したリンパ管内皮細胞は、その近傍で互いに接着して初期リンパ嚢を形成し、それらがお互いに融合して管腔形成しながら伸長すると考えられている。一方で、頸部静脈に由来するリンパ管内皮細胞の一部は体表まで遊走して皮膚のリンパ管形成に貢献する。このような移動の際には先に形成されている血管とりわけ動脈の上を移動することが知られている。

b．リモデリング（弁形成・平滑筋被覆）

　原始リンパ管叢が形成された後に、弁を備え平滑筋で被覆された集合リンパ管が構築されていく。弁形成には、フォークヘッド転写因子 FoxC2 が Prox1 および機械刺激（ずり応力）と協調して作用する。発現誘導される Cx37（Connexin37）が弁形成領域で内皮細胞のリング状凝集に、活性化される Calcineurin-NFAT シグナルが境界形成に必要である。平面内細胞極性制御因子 Celsr1 と Vangl2 が VE-cadherin による接着結合の安定化を遅らせて、弁を構成する内皮細胞の再配向を制御することも必要である。Integrin α9 とそのリガンドである細胞外基質 Fibronectin EIIIA 領域の相互作用が弁尖の伸長に必要である。さらに、Semaphorin 3 A が Neuropilin-1 と PlexinA1 からなる受容体シグナルを介して平滑筋細胞に対して反発作用を及ぼすことで、集合リンパ管の弁領域に平滑筋が集積することを妨げている。一方で、平滑筋細胞の集合リンパ管への正常な集積には、Akt/Protein kinase B シグナルや分泌性糖蛋白 Reelin が必要である。

c．血管との分離

　リンパ管は心臓近くの生理的開口部位（通常は静脈角と呼ばれる内頸静脈と鎖骨下静脈の合流部位）以外では、通常血管と吻合しない。胎生期において、転写因子 Meis1 依存的に発生する巨核球に由来する血小板が、リンパ管と血管の分離を保障していることが明らかになっている。リンパ管内皮細胞特異的に発現する Pdpn が血小板上の受容体 CLEC-2 に結合して、Syk-Slp76-Plcg2（Phospholipase Cγ2）シグナル経路依存的に血小板を活性化させることが重要である。本来リンパ管内に存在しない血小板がどこでどのようにリンパ管内皮細胞と接触するのかなど、作用機序の詳細には不明な点が残されている。

2. Development of the lymphatic vessels

1) Structure of the lymphatic vessels : The lymphatic system is an open circulatory system that is made up of lymphatic capillaries (also known as the initial lymphatics), which start at blind ends in the peripheral tissue and take up interstitial fluid, protein, lipids, immune cells, and foreign bodies ; and the collecting lymphatics, which comprise the lymph transport route and open into the veins near the heart. The endothelial cells of the lymphatic capillaries have a characteristic appearance, with a profile similar to that of an oak leaf. The endothelial cells are connected via button-like junctions, and the large openings between the cells are well adapted for the uptake of macromolecules. The endothelial cells of the collecting lymphatics are closely adherent by what are called zipper-like junctions. The collecting lymphatics are equipped with valves to prevent backflow of lymph and those with a large diameter accumulate smooth muscles, the contraction of which is instrumental in creating the lymphatic flow. The functional unit of the collecting lymphatic vessels is considered to be the region with smooth muscle between two valves, and is called a lymphangion.

2) Derivation of the lymphatic endothelial cells : Two plausible theories have been proposed, centrifugal theory, which surmises that the cells are differentiated from the vascular endothelial cells that comprise the veins ; and the centripetal theory, which surmises that the cells are differentiated from mesenchymal cells surrounding the veins. Recent real-time analysis using zebrafish captured the differentiation and budding of venous endothelial cells to form lymphatic vessels, supporting the centrifugal theory. In contrast, transplant experiments using birds showed that lymphatic endothelial cells developed from cell lineages other than that of venous endothelial cells, supporting the centripetal theory. Genetic lineage tracing analysis in mice suggests both derivations exists.

3) Mechanism of lymphatic vessel formation

a. Differentiation, migration, and fusion : In mouse embryos, at around 10 days of gestation, a proportion of the endothelial cells of the cervical vein sequentially express the transcriptional regulators Sox18 and Prox1, and differentiate into lymphatic vessel endothelial cells. Retinoic acid and Wnt5b have shown to be differentiation-inducing factors. The nuclear receptor COUP-TFII, which is expressed specifically in the veins, is necessary for the maintenance and induction of the expression of Prox1, and Sox18 promotes the transcription of the Prox1 gene. Prox1 is necessary for the differentiation of lymphatic endothelial cells, and plays a central role in the expression of lymphatic endothelial cell markers such as the receptor tyrosine kinase, vascular endothelial growth factor receptor 3 (VEGFR3), and the glycoprotein podoplanin (Pdpn). Differentiated lymphatic endothelial cells express VEGFR3 strongly and migrate toward the neighboring mesenchymal tissue, which produces its ligand, VEGF-C. VEGF-C is produced as a precursor and its processing, which is dependent upon the extracellular substrate protein Ccbe1, that leads to the matured, active form of the protein.

In real-time analysis of zebrafish, images showed that lymphatic endothelial cells derived from veins that had a segmented distribution that fused together, leading to the formation of the thoracic duct. Lymphatic endothelial cells differentiated from the cervical vein in mice form early lymph sacs by adhering to other lymphatic endothelial cells in their vicinity, and are thought to fuse together and elongate to form the lumen. Meanwhile, a portion of cervical vein-derived lymphatic endothelial cells migrates to the body surface to participate in the formation of the lymphatic vessels in the skin. Such migration is known to occur via the blood vessels, especially the arteries, which are formed earlier.

b. Remodeling (valve formation, and investment with smooth muscle cells) : After the formation of the early lymphatic plexus, construction of the lymphatic vessels includes the provision of valves and their integration with smooth muscle cells. In valve formation, the forkhead box transcription factor FoxC2 acts alongside Prox1 and mechanical stimuli (shear stress). The induction of the expression of Connexin-37 (Cx37) and the activation of calcineurin-NFAT are required for the ring-shaped aggregation of endothelial cells in the region of the forming valve, and a defined boundary formation, respectively. The planar cell polarity regulators Celsr 1 and Vangl 2 postpone the stabilization of VE-cadherin-mediated cell-cell adhesion, and are necessary for the regulation of the reorientation of endothelial cells that comprise the valve. Interaction between integrin α9 and its ligand, the extracellular substrate Fibronectin EIIIA domain, is necessary for the extension of the valve cusp. Additionally, Semaphorin 3A, acts to repel smooth muscle cells via a receptor signal comprised of Neuropilin-1 and PlexinA1, and in doing so prevents the accumulation of smooth muscle cells in the valve region of the collecting lymphatic vessels. Meanwhile, Akt/Protein kinase B signaling and the secretory glycoprotein Reelin are necessary for the normal accumulation of smooth muscle cells on collecting lymphatic vessels.

c. Separation from the blood vessels：Other than the physiological opening close to the heart (usually the region where the internal jugular vein and subclavian vein converge, called the venous angle), the lymphatic vessels do not ordinarily open onto the blood vessels. It has been found that, in the embryo, the separation of the lymphatic and blood vessels is ensured by the Meis1 transcription factor-dependent production of megakaryocyte-derived platelets. This requires that Pdpn, expressed specifically by lymphatic endothelial cells binds to the receptor CLEC-2 on the platelets, and activates the platelets in a Syk-Slp76-Plcg2 (Phospholipase Cγ2) signaling pathway-dependent manner. A number of details regarding the mechanism of how and where the platelets, which do not originally exist in the lymphatic vessels, contact the lymphatic endothelial cells remain unclear.

❸　リンパ管形成異常をきたす遺伝子変異

ヒト遺伝性リンパ浮腫の原因遺伝子を **Table 1** に示す。また、リンパ管形成異常をきたす遺伝子変異マウスモデルのうち、胎児浮腫が報告されているものを中心に **Table 2** に示す。

3.　Mutations resulting in abnormalities of lymphatic vessel formation

Genes responsible for hereditary lymphedema in humans are shown in **Table 1**. Additionally, **Table 2** focuses on those gene-mutant mouse models resulting in lymphatic vessel malformation that were reported to cause embryonic edema.

Table 1. ヒト遺伝性リンパ浮腫の原因遺伝子　Responsible genes of human hereditary lymphedema

遺伝子 Gene	遺伝形式 Inheritance	病名 Disease
CCBE1	AR	Hennekam 症候群 Hennekam syndrome
FLT4（VEGFR3）	AD	Milroy 病 Milroy disease
FOXC2	AD	リンパ水腫-睫毛重生症候群 Lymphatic hydrops-biciliate syndrome
GATA2	AD	Emberger 症候群 Emberger symdrome
GJC1（CX43）	AD	眼歯牙骨異形成症-リンパ浮腫 Oculodentoosseous dysplasia-lymphedema
GJC2（CX47）	AD	遺伝性リンパ浮腫 Congenital hereditary lymphedema
IKBKG（NEMO）	XR	無汗性外胚葉形成不全-免疫不全-骨大理石症-リンパ浮腫 Anhidrotic ectodermal dysplasia-immunodeficiency-osteopetrosis-lymphedema
ITGA9	AR	先天性乳び胸 congenital chylothorax
KIF11（EG5）	AD	リンパ浮腫-小頭症-網脈絡膜症症候群 Lymphedema-microcephaly-chorioretinopathy syndrome
PTPN11（SHP2）	AD	Noonan 症候群 Noonan syndrome
PTPN14	AR	リンパ浮腫-後鼻孔閉鎖症候群 Lymphedema-choanal atresia syndrome
SOX18	AD	貧毛症-リンパ浮腫-毛細血管拡張症候群 Hypotrichosis-lymphedema-trichangiectasia syndrome

AD：常染色体優性遺伝　autosomal dominant inheritance
AR：常染色体劣性遺伝　autosomal recessive inheritance
XR：伴性劣性　X-linked recessive inheritance

Table 2. リンパ管形成異常をきたす遺伝子変異マウス　Gene mutant mice developing defective lymphatic vessels

遺伝子 Gene	表現型 Phenotype
1．染色体異常　Chromosomal abnormality	
Trisomy 16（Ts16）	ヒト 21 番染色体の相同遺伝子の多くは、マウスにおいて 16 番染色体遠位部に位置しており、ヒト 21 トリソミー（ダウン症候群）のモデルマウスとして解析されてきた。心奇形や頸部リンパ嚢形成異常を伴う胎児浮腫をきたし、胎生後期に致死となる。 It was analyzed as human trisomy 21（Down syndrome）model mice since a large part of homologous genes of human chromosome 21 exists at the distal portion of chromosome 16 in mice. It will be lethal at the latter term of embryonic stage due to the embryonic edema with cardiac malformation or cervical lymph sac malformation.

Important Reference/遺伝子変異マウスの胎児浮腫とリンパ管形成異常

Table 2. 続き　Continued

遺伝子 Gene	表現型 Phenotype
2．優性変異　Dominant mutation	
Prox1	ヘテロ欠損マウスはリンパ管形成異常による胎児浮腫をきたす。特に生理的リンパ管血管吻合弁の形成異常があり、リンパ管内に血球細胞が流入する。遺伝子背景によって生存率は著しく異なるが、成体の Prox1 ヘテロ欠損マウスではリンパ管からの漏出が起こって乳び腹水が貯留し、肥満や炎症の病態を呈する。ホモ欠損マウスではリンパ管内皮細胞が分化せず、胎児浮腫をきたして致死となる。 Heterozygous mice develop embryonic edema due to the malformation of lymphatics. There is a particular malformation of lymphovenous valve and it induces influx of blood cells to the lymphatic vessels. Although survival rates significantly vary depending on the genetic background, adult Prox1 heterozygous mice reveals obesity and inflammatory conditions due to the chylous ascites that transudate from the lymphatic vessels. Homozygous mice show the embryonic edema and lethality due to the lack of lymphatic endothelial cell differentiation.
VEGFR3	遺伝子突然変異により誘導された VEGFR3 キナーゼ欠損型のヘテロ変異である Chy マウスは、新生仔期に乳び腹水を伴うリンパ浮腫をきたす。ハイポモルフ変異体も、ヘテロ接合型でリンパ管低形成を伴う胎児浮腫をきたす。ホモ欠損マウスでは血管形成が異常となり、リンパ管発生期以前に致死となる。 Chy mice, heterozygosity of the VEGFR3 kinase deficiency induced by ENU-mediated gene mutation, develops lymphedema with chylous ascites in the neonatal period. Heterozygosity of the hypomorphic variant develops embryonic edema with lymphatic hypoplasia. Homozygous deficient mice are embryonic lethal before lymphatic vessel formation because of the defective blood vessel formation.
VEGF-C	ヘテロ欠損マウスは皮膚リンパ管が低形成となり新生仔期に乳び腹水をきたす。第8染色体の一部を欠失する Chy-3 マウスは VEGF-C がヘテロ欠損しており、同様の表現型をきたす。ホモ欠損マウスでは頸部静脈から分化したリンパ管内皮細胞が遊走せず、リンパ管形成不全による胎児浮腫をきたして致死となる。 Heterozygous mice develop hypoplasia of the skin lymphatic vessels and it will be the cause of chylous ascites in the neonatal period. Chy-3 mice, heterozygous deletion of a part of chromosome 8 including the VEGF-C gene shows the same phenotype. Homozygous mice show embryonic edema and lithality with malformation of lymphatics since lymphatic endothelial cell differentiated from the jugular vein cannot migrate.
Vezf1	転写制御因子。ヘテロ欠損マウスは頸部リンパ管の過形成を伴う胎児浮腫をきたす。ホモ欠損マウスは血管形成異常で出血をきたし致死となる。 Heterozygous mice of the transcriptional regulator show embryonic edema accompanied by hyperplasia of cervical lymphatics. Homozygous mice are lethal accompanied by bleeding vascular dysplasia.
3．劣性変異　Recessive mutation	
a．分化・遊走・融合の異常　Defective differentiation, migration, or fusion	
Sox18	Prox1 の発現が欠失して、リンパ管形成不全による胎児浮腫をきたして致死となる。 Lack of Prox1 expression results in embryonic edema and lethality accompanied by lymphatic dysplasia.
Ccbe1	VEGF-C のプロセシングによる成熟化が障害されて、リンパ管形成不全による胎児浮腫をきたして致死となる。 Impaired processing and maturation of VEGF-C protein results in embryonic edema and lethality accompanied by lymphatic dysplasia.
Neuropilin-2	VEGF-C および Semaphorin の受容体。小径のリンパ管が減少する。 Receptor for VEGF-C and Semaphorins. Decrease in small lymphatic vessels.
Wnt5a	胎児皮膚に小径のリンパ管が減少し巨大なリンパ管がみられる。 Large lymphatic vessels are seen in embryonic skin.

109

Table 2. 続き　Continued

遺伝子 Gene	表現型 Phenotype
AM (Adrenomedullin)	生理活性ペプチド。頸部リンパ嚢の低形成による胎児浮腫をきたし致死となる。 Bioactive peptide. Embryonic edema and lethality accompanied by hypoplasia of cervical lymph sacs.
Ramp2, Calcrl	AM受容体。いずれにおいても、頸部リンパ嚢の低形成による胎児浮腫をきたし致死となる。 AM receptor. Embryonic edema and lethality accompanied by hypoplasia of cervical lymph sacs.
Cxcr7	7回膜貫通型受容体。AM活性が亢進して血球細胞を含んで拡張したリンパ嚢を伴う胎児浮腫をきたす。 Seven-transmembrane receptor. Enhanced AM activity. Embryonic edema accompanied by expanded lymph sacs which contain blood cells.
Cyp26b1	レチノイン酸分解酵素。血球細胞を含んで拡張したリンパ嚢を伴う胎児浮腫をきたす。 Retinoic acid degrading enzyme. Embryonic edema accompanied by expanded lymph sacs which contain blood cells.
Aspp1	リンパ管ネットワーク形成が遅延して胎児浮腫をきたす。 Embryonic edema accompanied by delayed lymphatic vascular network formation.
Pkd1, Pkd2	いずれにおいても、リンパ管内皮細胞の平面内細胞極性が異常で遊走方向が乱れて、リンパ管形成異常による胎児浮腫をきたす。Pkd2ホモ欠損マウスにおいては、リンパ管内に血球細胞がみられる。 Disorganized planar cell polarity and migration of lymphatic endothelial cells results in embryonic edema accompanied by defective lymphatic vessel formation. Blood cells are seen in lymphatic vessels of Pkd2-homozygous mice.
b．リモデリング(弁形成・平滑筋被覆)の異常 Defective remodeling (valve formation or investment with smooth muscle cells)	
FoxC2	弁形成不全および毛細リンパ管に基底膜蛋白と平滑筋細胞の異所性集積がみられる。胎生14.5日目頃までリンパ管形成は正常であるが、他の心血管系異常が原因で浮腫をきたす。 Valve dysplasia and ectopic accumulation of basament membrane proteins and investment of smooth muscle cells on lymphatic capillaries. Lymphatic vessel formation is not affected by E14.5 but cardiovascular abnormality causes embryonic edema.
Cx37, Cx43	二重欠損マウスでは弁形成不全および血球細胞を含むリンパ管がみられる。顕著な胎児浮腫をきたし、先天性乳び胸により致死となる。 Doubly-deficient mice show valve dysplasia and lymphatic vessels which contain blood cells. Severe embryonic edema and neonatal lethality caused by congenital chylothorax.
Integrin α9	弁形成不全となり、先天性乳び胸により致死となる。 Valve dysplasia and neonatal lethality caused by congenital chylothorax.
Angiopoietin-2	弁形成異常や平滑筋細胞の異常な被覆などのリンパ管リモデリング異常を呈し、新生仔期に乳び腹水を伴うリンパ浮腫をきたす。毛細リンパ管がボタン様結合に成熟しないため、組織間液吸収不全となる。一方で、集合リンパ管のジッパー様結合も傷害され、リンパ液が管外に漏れ出す。 Remodeling disorders of valve dysplasia and ectopic investment of smooth muscle cells. Lymphedema with chylous ascites in the neonatal period. Impaired maturation of zipper-like endothelial cell-cell junctions in lymphatic capillaries results in defective absorption of interstitial fluid. Impaired zipper-like endothelial cell-cell junctions in collecting lymphatic vessels is also seen, which causes leakage of the lymph fluid.
Tie1	出血をきたさず生存したものは、リンパ管形成異常を伴う胎児浮腫をきたす。ハイポモルフ変異体も同様の表現型をきたす。 Embryonic edema accompanied by defective lymphatic vessel formation, if mouse embryos survive without bleeding. Hypomorphic mutation results in the same phenotype.
Net/Elk3	転写制御因子。ハイポモルフ変異マウスは先天性乳び胸により致死となる。 Transcriptional regulator. Hypomorpic mutation results in neonatal lethality accompanied by congenital chylothorax.

Table 2. 続き　Continued

遺伝子 Gene	表現型 Phenotype
c．血管との分離の異常　Defective separation from the blood vessels	
CLEC-2, Syk, Slp76, Plcg2	いずれにおいても血小板活性化障害があり、リンパ管内に血球細胞がみられる軽度の胎児浮腫をきたす。 Defective platelet activation. Mild embryonic edema accompanied by lymphatic vessels which contain blood cells.
Pdpn	リンパ管内に血球細胞がみられる軽度の胎児浮腫をきたす。 Mild embryonic edema accompanied by lymphatic vessels which contain blood cells.
C1galt1	糖転移酵素。Pdpn 蛋白の糖鎖修飾が起こらず、Pdpn 欠損マウスと同様の異常をきたす。 Glycosyltransferase. Loss of O-glycosylation of Pdpn protein causes the same phenotype as Pdpn-deficient mice.
Spred1, Spred2	Ras/ERK 経路に対する負の調節因子。二重欠損マウスは、リンパ管内に血球細胞がみられる胎児浮腫をきたす。 Negative regulatory factor to Ras/ERK pathway. Doubly-deficient mice show embryonic edema accompanied by lymphatic vessels which contain blood cells.
Angiopoietin-like protein 4	腸管のリンパ管に血液が流入して生後3週以内に致死となる。 Intestinal lymphatic vessels contain blood cells. Lethal within 3 weeks of birth.

■おわりに

　ヒトの胎児浮腫が超音波検査で見つかるようになってからの歴史はまだ浅く、原因・病態・予後・疾患発症リスクなどに関して十分に理解されていない。ヒト遺伝性リンパ浮腫の多くは遺伝子変異マウスモデルで再現されており、胎児浮腫についてもマウスモデルを用いた今後の研究推進が期待される。

（平島正則）

■Conclusion

　There is little history to draw from since it has became possible to identify embryonic edema in humans via ultrasound, and we still do not have a sufficient understanding of the causes, pathology, prognoses, or the risk of disease onset. Many human hereditary lymphedemas have been reproduced in gene mutant mouse models, and it is hoped that further research using these genetic mouse models will make a great contribution for gaining insights into embryonic edema.

(*Masanori Hirashima*)

1) 日本産科婦人科学会, 日本産科婦人科医会（編・監）：NT（nuchal translucency）肥厚が認められた時の対応は？　産婦人科診療ガイドライン；産科編 2014, pp89-93, 日本産科婦人科学会, 東京, 2014.

CHAPTER 5

術前評価
Preoperative evaluation
1. CT・MRI

CT・MRI

■はじめに

リンパ浮腫の画像診断としては、CT、MRI、リンパシンチグラフィ、インドシアニングリーン蛍光リンパ管造影法（ICG 検査）などが用いられる。リンパ浮腫と呼ばれる状態の中には、さまざまな病態や重症度のものが含まれており、種々の検査を組み合わせて個々の病態を把握することが必要である。

■Introduction

For diagnostic imaging of lymphedema, CT, MRI, lymphoscintigraphy, indocyanine green fluorescent lymphangiography (ICG examination) and the like are used. Lymphedema can include several disease states of variable severity, and it is necessary to investigate individual disease states by combining various examinations.

I　CT

まず、患肢の CT では「そこに浮腫がある」ことが診断できる（**Fig. 5-1-1**）。リンパ浮腫なのか静

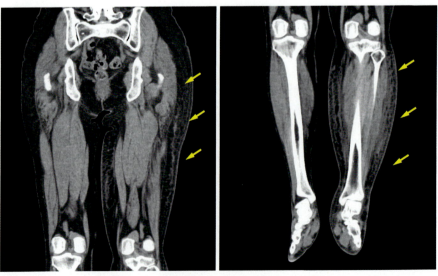

Fig. 5-1-1. 左下肢リンパ浮腫患者の CT 像　CT image of left lower extremity lymphedema patients
左が大腿で、右が下腿。黄色矢印の部位に浮腫を認める。
The thigh is imaged on the left and the lower leg on the right. Edema is noted at the sites indicated by the yellow arrows.

脈性浮腫なのか、または内科的疾患による浮腫なのかを判別するのは難しいことが多いが、静脈血栓を除外することが可能である。骨盤〜胸部 CT では、骨盤内や縦隔内に、リンパ流を妨げるような占拠性病変がないかを診断する。下肢リンパ浮腫を発症した際は、骨盤内〜胸部の癌初発または再発が原因となっていることもあり、その検索は必須である。

婦人科癌術後では、骨盤内にリンパ嚢胞が形成されることがある(**Fig. 5-1-2-左**)。骨盤内リンパ嚢胞は、下肢から上行してきたリンパ管が手術操作によって骨盤内に開放され、リンパ液が持続的に骨盤内に流入するために生じる。つまり、骨盤内リンパ嚢胞がある場合、下肢リンパ管から胸管に至る途中のリンパ管に損傷があることを意味し、他覚的に下肢浮腫を認めない場合でも下肢にリンパ還流障害が生じていることが多い。そのため、後に下肢リンパ浮腫を発症することもあり、骨盤内リンパ嚢胞を有する患者は下肢リンパ浮腫の高リスク群といえる。下肢でリンパ管細静脈吻合術(LVA)を行うことで、骨盤内に流入するリンパ液の量を減少させることができるため、LVA 術後には骨盤内リンパ嚢胞が消失することがある(**Fig. 5-1-2-右**)。

そのほかにも、治療前後の下肢 CT でボリューム測定を行うことで、リンパ浮腫治療の効果判定を行うことも可能である。

I. CT

First of all, CT of the affected limb can diagnose "the presence of edema"(**Fig. 5-1-1**). It is often difficult to distinguish whether it is lymphedema, venous edema or edema secondary to a medical disorder. However it is possible to exclude venous thrombosis. In a pelvic to chest CT, we can diagnose whether there is an obstructive lesion in the pelvis or mediastinum that interferes with lymph flow. When lower extremity lymphedema develops, it is sometimes caused by the initial incidence or recurrence of cancer in the pelvis〜chest.

After gynecologic cancer surgery, lymphatic cysts may form in the pelvis(**Fig. 5-1-2-L**). Pelvic lymphatic cysts arise because the lymph ducts ascending from the lower limb are severed secondary to surgical intervention and lymph fluid flows permanently into the pelvis. In other words, the presence of pelvic lymphatic cysts, means that lymph ducts draining the lower limb are damaged along their route to the thoracic duct. Even in cases where objective lower limb edema is not initially identified, a lymph circulation

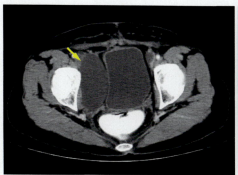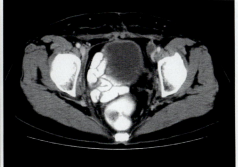

Fig. 5-1-2. 骨盤内リンパ嚢胞の CT 像　CT image of a pelvic lymphatic cyst
左が LVA 術前、右が LVA 術後。LVA 術前には中央の膀胱の右側にリンパ嚢胞を認めるが(黄色矢印)、術後にはリンパ嚢胞は消失している。
Left image before LVA operation, right is after LVA operation. Prior to LVA surgery, lymphatic cysts are found on the right side of the central bladder(yellow arrow), but the lymphatic cyst disappears after surgery.

disorder of the lower limb exists in many cases. Therefore, clinical lymphedema can develop in the future. Patients with pelvic lymphatic cysts are considered at high-risk for developing lower limb lymphedema. By performing lymph venous anastomosis (LVA) on the lower limbs, the amount of free lymph flowing into the pelvis can be reduced and pelvic lymphatic cyst may disappear after LVA surgery (**Fig. 5-1-2-R**).

Moreover, the outcome of lymphedema treatment can be evaluated by measuring the pre- and post-treatment lower limb volume with CT.

II MRI

一般的な下肢単純 MRI では、CT と同様、「そこに浮腫がある」ことが診断できる (**Fig. 5-1-3**)。それ以外にも、リンパ浮腫診療において MRI は多彩に応用されている。

1. 造影剤を用いた MR リンパ管造影法 (MRL)

造影剤を皮下注射することで造影剤がリンパ管に取り込まれる。正常では細いリンパ管が描出され、リンパ液還流障害がある場合は拡張したリンパ管が描出されたり、皮膚への逆流がみられたりする。原発性リンパ浮腫では、リンパ管の低形成や過形成が存在することがあり、MR リンパ管造影法 (Magnetic Resonance Lymphography；MRL) を用いてその診断が可能である。

造影剤の皮下注射には強い疼痛が伴うため、先に 1％キシロカインなどの局所麻酔薬を両側の全指間部（または趾間部）に注射しておく方が、患者の精神的負担が軽減される。その後、同部位に Gd-DTPA（マグネビスト®）などの造影剤を約 1 mL ずつ皮下注射する。造影剤と局所麻酔薬を混和して用いる方法もある。一定時間経過後、MRI を撮影する。撮影には 1.5〜3 T の MRI を

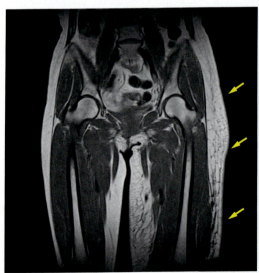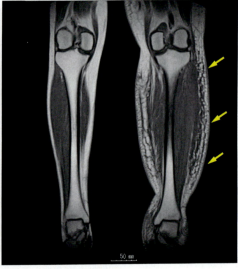

Fig. 5-1-3. 左下肢リンパ浮腫患者の単純 MRI 像
Simple MRI image of left lower extremity lymphedema patients
左は大腿、右は下腿。黄色矢印の部位に浮腫を認める。
The thigh on the left and the lower leg on the right. Edema is noted at the sites indicated by the yellow arrows.

用いる。撮影条件については諸々の報告がある[1]-[3]。

　造影剤を用いて MRL を撮影する場合、造影剤がリンパ管内を上行する速度と、撮影タイミングの関係が問題となる。タイミングが早過ぎる場合には、リンパ管が十分に描出されない。また、遅過ぎる場合には、造影剤が通り過ぎてしまい薄くなったり、体循環に入った造影剤により静脈が描出されてしまい、リンパ管との鑑別が困難になったりする。Lohrmann らは、撮影タイミングと下腿、大腿のリンパ管の描出について調査を行い、下腿は注射後 25 分、大腿は注射後 55 分に最もよくリンパ管が描出されたと報告している。

　現在、日本では MRI の造影剤の皮下注射は禁忌とされている。造影剤を皮下注射して MRI 撮影を行うことについては、動物実験および臨床応用について既に多数の報告があるが、造影剤の皮下注射によって明らかな炎症反応や皮膚壊死などの合併症が生じたという報告は今のところない。投与量については、通常 MRI の造影剤は 0.2 mL/kg の投与量で経静脈的に投与されており、MRL における投与量は許容範囲と考えられる。

　MRL においては、リンパ管と静脈の鑑別が問題となる。リンパ管と静脈は比較的類似した走行をするためである。静脈は滑らかで比較的まっすぐな形状をしている一方、リンパ管は数珠玉状の形状をしていることが多く、形態による鑑別を行うことが多い。しかし、形態以外に確実に両者を鑑別する基準はなく、現在でも議論の的となっている。

　造影剤を用いた MRL は、MRI の造影剤アレルギーの患者、ペースメーカー使用中の患者、体内に金属の埋入がある患者、閉所恐怖症の患者などには施行できない。また、特に上肢リンパ浮腫の患者では、乳房再建の過程でティシューエキスパンダーを使用している期間も、エキスパンダーに金属が含まれている場合は施行できないので注意が必要である。

2. 造影剤を用いない MRL

　フランスの Lionel Arrivé は、下肢リンパ浮腫患者において造影剤を用いない MRL でリンパ管を撮影したことを報告している[4]。解像度や明瞭さは造影剤を用いた MRL と比較してさほど遜色ない印象である。造影剤を用いた MRL では、造影剤の広がる速度と撮影タイミングを合わせる必要があるが、造影剤を用いない MRL ではそのタイミングを考慮する必要がない。また、日本においては MRI の造影剤の皮下注射は禁忌とされており、その点では造影剤を用いないMRL の方が施行にあたっての障壁は少ないともいえる。さらに、造影剤アレルギーの患者にも行うことが可能である。造影剤を用いた MRL と同様、静脈とリンパ管の鑑別が課題であるが、今後の発展が望まれる検査法である。

3. MR 胸管撮影法(MRTD)

　筆者らは、MR 胆膵管撮影(Magnetic Resonance Thoracic Ductography；MRCP)のプロトコールを縦隔に応用し、胸管を撮影している[5]。撮影は呼吸に同期して行い、造影剤は使用しない。健常人でははっきりとした胸管像が得られるが、原発性リンパ浮腫の患者では、胸管像の欠損や著しい蛇行を認めることがある(**Fig. 5-1-4, 5**)。この所見は、特に若年で発症した原発性リンパ浮腫患者で多くみられる。若年で発症した原発性リンパ浮腫患者においては、胸管の形態異

115

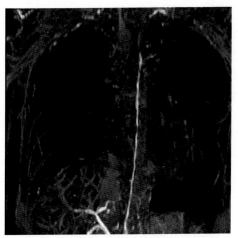

Fig. 5-1-4. MRIによる、健常人の胸管像
Magnetic resonance thoracic ductography of a healthy person by MRI
拡張、蛇行、途絶などのない胸管が左静脈角まで描出されている。
A normal thoracic duct without any dilation, tortiousness, disruption etc. is illustrated extending the left vein horn.

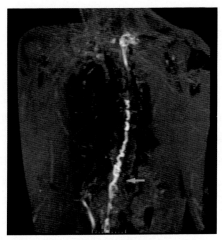

Fig. 5-1-5. MRIによる、原発性リンパ浮腫患者の胸管像
MRI resonance thoracic ductography of patients with primary lymphedema
腹部で蛇行した胸管を認める。
Note a tortuous thoracic duct in the abdomen.

常だけでなく、浮腫の部位以外にリンパ管奇形が存在したり、乳び尿、乳び胸水、乳び腹水などをきたしたりすることも多い[6]。リンパ浮腫とリンパ管奇形は紙一重の病態であり、共にリンパ管の形態異常、機能異常の現れであると考えられる。実際、原発性リンパ浮腫とリンパ管奇形はしばしば合併する。リンパ管不全の進展範囲は患者ごとにさまざまなモザイク型を呈し、足関節より末梢のごく一部のみに限局した浮腫が生じることもあれば、両上下肢のリンパ浮腫、乳び胸腹水を合併するような広範囲リンパ管機能不全が存在する場合もある。若年で発症したリンパ浮腫患者では、リンパ管機能不全が高度で、同時に身体の広範囲に及んでいる傾向にあると、筆者は考えている。特に10歳以下で発症した原発性リンパ浮腫の場合にはこれらのことに留意し、胸腹部のMRI検査も含め、精査を検討する必要がある。

（原　尚子）

II. MRI

In general terms a standard MRI, like CT, can help to diagnose the presence of edema (**Fig. 5-1-3**). However more specific MRI investigations are widely applied in lymphedema diagnosis.

1. **Magnetic Resonance Lymphography (MRL) with contrast agent**：The contrast medium is injected subcutaneously and is taken up by the lymphatic ducts, highlighting the flow pattern, which can be traced on the skin. When a lymphatic reflux deficit is present, the dilated lymphatic duct is depicted by a dermal backflow pattern.

In primary lymphedema, there may be hypoplasia or hyperplasia of lymphatic vessels, which can also be diagnosed with MRL.

Subcutaneous injection of the contrast agent is painful. Therefore it is advisable to inject local anesthetic such as 1% xylocaine in the interdigital spaces on both sides to reduce patient discomfort. Thereafter 1 ml of a contrast medium such as Gd-DTPA (Magnevist) is injected subcutaneously into the same site. It is also possible to inject a mixture of the contrast agent and a local anesthetic. After a period of time, MRI images can be taken. MRI of 1.5 to 3 T is used for photography. There are various reports relating to the interpretation of these MRI images[1)-3)].

When using a contrast again in MRL imaging, the time interval for imaging following contrast injection is very critical. Baring in mind that lymph flow through an edematous extremity is slower than unaffected limbs. If imaging is performed too early after contrast injection, the lymphatic vessels will not be fully visible. Conversely, if imaging is performed late after injection and contrast material has already passed into the venous system, highlighting the vein and making it difficult to distinguish from the lymph duct. Lohrmann and colleagues investigated imaging timing and visualization of the lymph vessels of the lower leg and thigh, and reported that the lymphatic vessels were best visualized at the lower leg 25 minutes after injection and the thigh at 55 minutes after injection.

At the present time, MRI imaging with subcutaneously injected contrast medium is contraindicated in Japan despite the existence of many reports from animal experiments and clinical applications. To date there are no reported complications in the literature such as obvious inflammatory reactions or skin necrosis secondary to subcutaneous injection of the contrast agent. Regarding the dosage, usually MRI contrast medium is administered intravenously at a dose of 0.2 mL/kg, and this is considered to be an acceptable range for MRL.

In MRL, the distinction between lymph vessels and veins can be problematic, because the course of both vessels is similar. However, veins are smooth and relatively linear while lymphatics often have a bead-like appearance, helping the distinguish them apart. This point remains controversal, as there is no other reliable standard to distinguish between them.

MRL using contrast agent cannot be performed to patients with MRI contrast agent allergy, patients with pacemakers, patients with metal implants, patients with claustrophobia, etc. This may also be contraindicated in patients with upper limb lymphedema and breast reconstruction with tissue expander, if the expander contains metal.

2. MRL without using contrast agent : Lionel Arrivé of France reported that lymph ducts were imaged with MRL without contrast medium in lower limb lymphedema[4)]. The resolution and clarity are not much inferior to MRL using contrast medium. In the MRL using contrast agent, it is necessary to synchronize the flow rate of the contrast agent with the timing of imaging, but this considersation is not necessary to when performing MRL without contrast medium. In Japan, subcutaneous injection of contrast medium with MRI is prohibited, and therefore MRLs that do not use contrast media pose less restrictions. Furthermore, it can be applied to patients with contrast agent allergy. In MRL using contrast agent, the difficulty to distiguish between veins and lymph vessels is problematic, therefore further development is necessary.

3. Magnetic Resonance Thoracic Ductography (MRTD) : The authors photographed the thoracic duct by applying the protocol of MR biliary pancreatic duct (MRCP) to the mediastinum[5)]. The imaging is performed in synchronization with respiration and no contrast medium is used. A clear thoracic image can be obtained in healthy subjects, but in patients with primary lymphedema, there is usually no clear image of the thoracic duct, and significant morphologic abnormality may be observed (**Fig. 5-1-4, 5**). This finding is more common in patients with primary lymphedema, especially in young patients. Patients with primary lymphedema who developed the disease at a young age, showed not only morphological abnormalities of the thoracic duct but also lymphatic malformations at separate sites other than the locations of clinical oedema, often leading to milky urine and watery breast discharge that is also milky in appearance, etc[6)]. Lymphedema and lymphatic malformations are pathological conditions, both of which display morphological and functional abnormalities of lymphatic vessels. Indeed, it is often difficult to distinguish primary lymphedema and lymphatic malformations. The spectrum of lymphatic insufficiency depends on the various mosaic subgroups : edema may be confined distally to only involve the ankle, it can involve both upper and lower limbs, or substantial chylous ascites. In some cases extensive lymphatic vessel dysfunction may exist. Patients who develop lymphedema at a young age, tend to have extensive lymphatic dysfunction that is found at multiple locations throughout the body. Particularly cases of primary lymphedema that develop at the age of 10 years or less, it is necessary to pay attention to these points and thoroughly screen distant locations including MRI investigations of the thorax and abdomen.

(Hisako Hara)

1) Lohrmann C, Foeldi E, Langer M : Indirect magnetic resonance lymphangiography in patients with lymphedema preliminary results in humans. Eur J Radiol 59(3) : 401-406, 2006.
2) Lu Q, Delproposto Z, Hu A, et al : MR lymphography of lymphatic vessels in lower extremity with gynecologic oncology-related lymphedema. PLoS One 7(11) : e50319, 2012.
3) 佐久間 恒 : 下肢リンパ浮腫に対する MR Lymphangiography. PEPARS 22 : 23-28, 2008.
   Sakuma H : MR Lymphangiography in lower extremity lymphedema. PEPARS 22 : 23-28, 2008.
4) Arrivé L, Derhy S, El Mouhadi S, et al : Noncontrast Magnetic Resonance Lymphography. J Reconstr Microsurg 32(1) : 80-86, 2015.
5) Hara H, Mihara M, Okuda I, et al : Presence of thoracic duct abnormalities in patients with primary lymphoedema of the extremities. J Plast Reconstr Aesthet Surg 65(11) : e305-e310, 2012.
6) Hara H, Mihara M, Ohtsu H, et al : Indication of lymphaticovenous anastomosis for primary lower limb lymphedema. Plast Reconstr Surg 136(4) : 883-893, 2015.

CHAPTER **5**

術前評価
Preoperative evaluation

2. リンパシンチグラフィ・SPECT-CT

Lymphoscintigraphy and SPECT-CT

■はじめに

リンパ浮腫の患者ではリンパ管機能が次第に低下していくことが知られている。リンパ浮腫診療においては、患肢の外見やボリュームだけでなく、その患者のリンパ管の機能がどの程度保たれているかを把握することが治療成功の鍵となる。リンパ管機能を評価するための検査方法として、リンパシンチグラフィは古くから行われている比較的低侵襲な方法である。その後、インドシアニングリーン蛍光リンパ管造影法（ICG 検査）が広く行われるようになった。最近では MRリンパ管造影法、SPECT-CT なども行われ、国内外で報告がなされるようになっている。

本章では、リンパシンチグラフィ、SPECT-CT について述べる。

■Introduction

It is known that lymphatic function gradually decreases in patients with lymphedema. In lymphedema diagnosis, evaluating both the appearance and volume of the affected limbs in addition to the internal function of the lymphatic system is key to the successful treatment of these patients. Lymphoscintigraphy is a relatively minimally invasive investigation that has existed for a long time to evaluate lymphatic vessel function. Indocyanine green fluorescent lymphangiography (ICG examination) is a newer technology that has become widely used to visualize lymphatics. More recently, MR lymphangiography and SPECT-CT etc. are also reported both domestically and abroad.

This section describes lymphoscintigraphy and SPECT-CT.

I リンパシンチグラフィ

リンパシンチグラフィは、放射性同位元素で標識されたコロイドを患肢に皮下注射し、リンパ管機能を評価する方法である。リンパ管機能が良好な部位では、リンパ管がはっきりとした線状に、所属リンパ節が数珠玉状に描出される（**Fig. 5-2-1**）。一方、リンパ管閉塞などによりリンパ液のうっ滞がある部位では、集合リンパ管から皮膚へリンパ液が逆流する所見が、ぼんやりとした影のようにみられる。さらにリンパ管機能が著しく低下している場合は、注射した放射性同位体がまったくリンパ管に取り込まれず、線状のリンパ管も皮膚への逆流もみられなくなる。

済生会川口総合病院における下肢リンパ浮腫に対する具体的な方法は以下のとおりである。仰臥位で、両足の第 1 趾間部に 1% キシロカイン®を皮下注射する。^{99m}Tc の皮下注射には強い疼痛が伴うため、局所麻酔薬注射を先行させた方が患者の精神的負担は小さくなる。その後、同部位にそれぞれ 0.3 mL（222 MBq）の ^{99m}Tc を皮下注射し、シンチカメラで撮影を行う。撮影のタイミングは施設によって異なるが、同病院では注射後 15 分、30 分、60 分、90 分で撮影を行っている。4 回の撮影が困難な場合は注射後 60 分のみでもよいが、できれば注射後早期像（15 分）と遅延像

(60分)の両方を撮影することが望ましい。早期像が必要な理由は、早期像で鼠径部まで線状のリンパ管が描出される場合と、膝下までしか描出されない場合では、リンパ管機能に違いがあるためである。また、皮膚への逆流所見を認めるようになるには60分程度の時間が必要であるため遅延像も重要である。90分では、トレーサーが通り過ぎてしまい、集合リンパ管や皮膚への逆流が薄くなることがある。注射後、安静臥床の場合はトレーサーが上行するのに時間がかかる。注射部のマッサージや、関節運動などにより、撮影までの時間を短縮させることができる。

上肢の場合は第2指間部に下肢と同量の^{99m}Tcを皮下注射する。

リンパシンチグラフィを用いた重症度分類としては前川分類が一般的である[1]。以下に、前川分類に基づいてリンパシンチグラフィの画像を供覧する。

1. 正　常

大伏在静脈に沿ったリンパ管が描出されている(**Fig. 5-2-1**)。前後像と後前像が得られるため、写っているリンパ管が腹側、背側のいずれに近いのかが判別できる。左右差はほとんどなく、皮膚への逆流も認めない。注射後15分で既に左静脈角までトレーサーが到達している。非常に良好なリンパ管機能である。

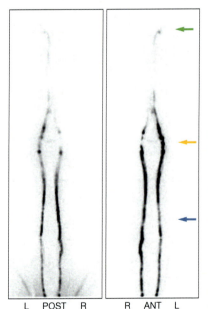

Fig 5-2-1. 健常人におけるリンパシンチグラフィ画像
Lymphoscintigraphic image in a healthy person
左が後 → 前像、右が前 → 後像。注射後15分で、線状の下肢リンパ管と数珠玉状の鼠径リンパ節が描出されている。また、既に左静脈角も描出されている。
青矢印：リンパ管、黄色矢印：鼠径リンパ節、緑矢印：左静脈角。
The left is the posteroanterior image, the right is the anteroposterior image. Linear lower limb lymphatic vessels and beaded groin lymph nodes are depicted 15 minutes after the injection. In addition, the left vein horn is already evident. Blue arrow：lymph vessel, yellow arrow：inguinal lymph node, green arrow：left venous horn.

2. 前川分類タイプ I

タイプ I では、皮膚への逆流は認めないが、拡張したリンパ管を認めたり、描出される所属リンパ節の個数が減少したりする。**Fig. 5-2-2** は両側ともタイプ I である。皮膚への逆流は認めないが、両下腿および右大腿に拡張した多数の側副リンパ管を認める。右鼠径リンパ節の個数が減少している。

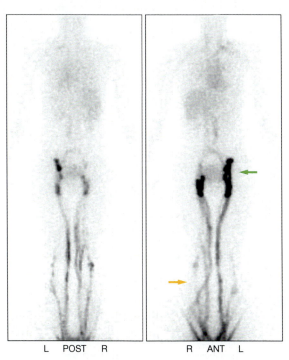

Fig. 5-2-2. タイプ I のリンパシンチグラフィ画像
Type I lymphoscintigraphic images
注射後60分。左が後→前像、右が前→後像。両下肢に線状のリンパ管を認めるが、両下肢とも側副リンパ路が発達しており、蛇行している。鼠径リンパ節の描出は右側で減少している。
黄色矢印：発達した側副リンパ路、緑矢印：鼠径リンパ節。
60 minutes after injection. The left is the posteroanterior image, the right is the anteroposterior image. Linear lymphatic vessels are found in both lower limbs, but collateral lymphatic pathways in both lower limbs are evident and tortuous. The view of the inguinal lymph node is diminished on the right side.
Yellow arrow: developing collateral lymphatic pathway, green arrow: inguinal lymph node.

3. 前川分類タイプ II

タイプ II の下肢では、大腿部に皮膚への逆流を認めるが、下腿には認めない。上肢では、上腕のみに皮膚への逆流を認め、前腕に認めない。**Fig. 5-2-3** は右下肢がタイプ II である。

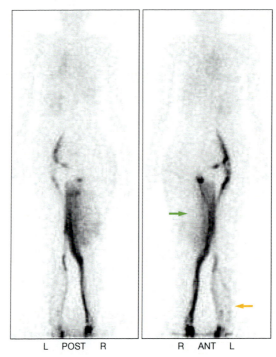

Fig. 5-2-3. タイプⅡのリンパシンチグラフィ画像
Type Ⅱ lymphoscintigraphic images

注射後60分。左が後→前像、右が前→後像。右大腿部に皮膚への逆流現象を認め、タイプⅡである。左下肢では発達した側副リンパ路を認め、タイプⅠである。
黄色矢印：発達した側副リンパ路、緑矢印：皮膚への逆流現象。
60 minutes after injection. The left is the posteroanterior image, the right is the anteroposterior image. Backflow to the skin on the right thigh is evident, type Ⅱ. In the left lower limb, expansion of the collateral lymphatic path is detected, and it is Type Ⅰ.
Yellow arrow：developed collateral lymphatic pathway, green arrow：backflow to the skin.

4. 前川分類タイプⅢ

　タイプⅢの下肢では、大腿、下腿部に皮膚への逆流を認める。上肢では、上腕、前腕に皮膚への逆流を認める。**Fig. 5-2-4** は右下肢がタイプⅢである。

5. 前川分類タイプⅣ

　タイプⅣの下肢では、下腿のみに皮膚への逆流を認める。上肢では前腕のみに皮膚への逆流を認める。大腿や上腕のリンパ管機能が著しく障害されている場合、浮腫が極めて重度のためリンパ液がほとんど輸送されない場合がある。また、下腿や前腕のみに皮膚への逆流を認め、大腿や上腕には線状のリンパ管が描出されることもあり、これは原発性リンパ浮腫に多くみられる。**Fig. 5-2-5** は右下肢がタイプⅣである。

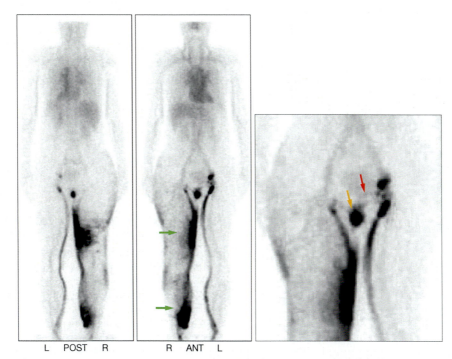

Fig. 5-2-4. タイプⅢのリンパシンチグラフィ画像　Type III lymphoscintigraphic image
注射後60分。左が後→前像、中が前→後像、右が陰部拡大像。右大腿、下腿に皮膚への逆流現象を認め、タイプⅢである。両鼠径リンパ節から陰部へ向かう側副リンパ路が形成されており、陰部にトレーサーの貯留を認める。このような所見を認めるときは、リンパ小胞が形成されていることが多い。
緑矢印：皮膚への逆流現象、赤矢印：鼠径リンパ節から陰部へ向かう側副リンパ路、黄色矢印：陰部に貯留したトレーサー。
60 minutes after injection. Left is posteroanterior image, middle is anteroposterior image, right is an enlarged image of the genital area. Reflux to the skin on right thigh and lower leg illustrated, type III. Collateral lymphatic channels are formed from both inguinal lymph nodes to the genital area, and tracer retention is present in the genital area. When such findings are observed, lymphoid follicles are often also formed.
Green arrow: reflux to the skin, red arrow: collateral lymphatic pathway from the inguinal lymph node to the genital area, yellow arrow: tracer reserved in the pudenda.

6. 前川分類タイプⅤ

タイプⅤの下肢では足から足関節に皮膚への逆流（またはハレーション）を認め、それより近位には何も描出されない。上肢では手から手関節に皮膚への逆流（またはハレーション）を認め、それより近位には何も描出されない。リンパ管機能がほとんど失われた状態である。**Fig. 5-2-6** は右下肢がタイプⅤである。

7. 陰部リンパ浮腫

Fig. 5-2-4 では、鼠径リンパ節を経由したトレーサーが陰部皮膚に向かって逆流している様子がみられる。このような場合、陰部浮腫やリンパ小胞が形成される。病理学的には真皮乳頭に異

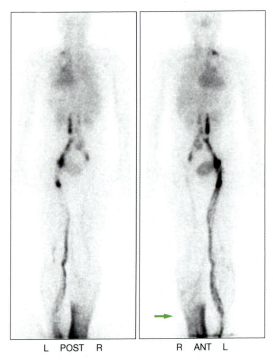

Fig. 5-2-5. タイプIVのリンパシンチグラフィ画像
Type IV lymphoscintigraphic images
注射後60分。左が後→前像、右が前→後像。右大腿部に皮膚への逆流所見を認める。
緑矢印：皮膚への逆流現象。
60 minutes after injection. The left is the posteroanterior image, the right is the anteroposterior image. Reflux to the skin on the right thigh is observed. Green arrow：reverse flow phenomenon to the skin.

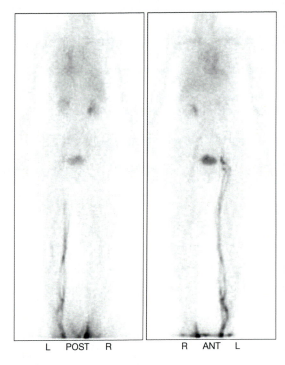

Fig. 5-2-6. タイプVのリンパシンチグラフィ画像
Lymphoscintigraphic image of type V
注射後60分。左が後→前像、右が前→後像。右下肢では足から足関節に皮膚への逆流（またはハレーション）を認め、それより近位には何も描出されていない。
60 minutes after injection. The left is the posteroanterior image, the right is the anteroposterior image. In the right lower limb, there is a reflux (or halation) from the foot to the ankle, with nothing else evident in its proximity.

5-2. リンパシンチグラフィ・SPECT-CT

常に拡張したリンパ管が認められる[2]。これは非常に浅い層であるため、下着がこすれるなどの軽微な刺激で破綻し、そこからリンパ液が持続的に流出することになる。

I. Lymphoscintigraphy

Lymphoscintigraphy is a method of evaluating lymphatic function by subcutaneously injecting radioisotope-labeled colloid into the affected limb. At the site of good lymph duct function, the regional lymph nodes are beaded and linear (**Fig. 5-2-1**). On the other hand, at sites of lymphatic stasis due to lymph duct obstruction, the lymph fluid back flow from the collecting lymph duct to the skin is seen as a blurred shadow. In addition, if the lymphatic vessel function is significantly decreased, the injected radioactive isotope will not be taken into the lymph vessel at all and therefore, no lymphatic roadmap will be visualized.

Specific methods for lower extremity lymphedema imaging in Saiseikai Kawaguchi General Hospital are as follows. In the supine position, 1% xylocaine is injected subcutaneously into the first interdigital space of both feet. Because subcutaneous injection of ^{99m}Tc is accompanied by intense pain, patient discomfort is reduced by prior injection of local anesthetic. Subsequently, 0.3 mL (222 MBq) of ^{99m}Tc is injected subcutaneously into the same site, and imaging is performed with a cinch camera. The timing of imaging depends on the facility, in Saiseikai Kawaguchi General Hospital, imaging is done at 15 minutes, 30 minutes, 60 minutes and 90 minutes after injection. If it is difficult to photograph four times, it can be done only 60 minutes after injection, but it is preferable to photograph both the early image after injection (15 minutes) and the delayed image (60 minutes), if possible. An early image is necessary because it helps to elucidate the extent of lymphatic vessel function ranging from early detectable linear lymphatic vessels visible to the inguinal region or only to the level of the knee. A delayed image is also important because it takes about 60 minutes to observe dermal backflow to the skin. At 90 minutes, the tracer advances through the system, which may reduce the backflow to the collecting lymph vessels and the skin. Timing of the imaging can be shortened by massaging the site of injection.

When Imaging the upper limb, ^{99m}Tc of the same amount as the lower limb is injected subcutaneously into the second web space.

Maegawa's classification is a common classification using lymphoscintigraphy[1]. The images of lymphoscintigraphy are listed below based on Maegawa's classification.

1. Normal：A lymph duct along the large saphenous vein is illustrated (**Fig. 5-2-1**). Since the antero-posterior and the posterior-anterior images are obtained, it can be determined whether the visualized lymphatic vessels are close to the ventral side or the dorsal side. There is little difference between left and right, with no evidence of backflow to the skin. The tracer has already reached the left vein angle at 15 minutes after injection. Indicating very good lymphatic vessel function.

2. Maegawa classification type I：Type I, there is no backflow to the skin, but the dilated lymphatic vessels are evident, and the number of highlighted regional lymph nodes is reduced. **Fig. 5-2-2** shows type I on both sides. There is no reflux to the skin, but there are numerous collateral enlarged lymphatic vessels in both the left and right thighs. The number of highlighted right inguinal lymph nodes is reduced.

3. Maegawa classification type II：In the lower limb of type II, reflux to the skin is observed in the thigh, but not in the lower leg. In upper limb, reflux to the skin is only seen in the upper arm, but not in the forearm. In **Fig. 5-2-3**, the right lower limb is type II.

4. Maegawa classification type III：In the lower limb of type III, back flow to the skin is observed in the thigh and lower leg. In the upper limbs, reflux to the skin is observed in both the upper arm and forearm. In **Fig. 5-2-4**, the right lower limb is type II.

5. Maegawa classification type IV：In the lower limbs of type IV, the back flow to the skin is seen only in the lower leg. In the upper limbs, reflux to the skin is seen only in the forearms. In cases where the lymphatic function of the thigh or upper arm is severely impaired, almost no lymph fluid is transported due to extremely severe edema. In addition, there is a reflux to the skin only in the lower leg and forearm. Linear lymphatic vessels are sometimes evident on the thigh and upper arm, which is commonly seen in primary lymphedema. In **Fig. 5-2-5**, the right lower limb is type Ⅳ.

6. Maegawa classification type Ⅴ：In the lower limb of type Ⅴ, there is a reflux (or halation) from the foot to the ankle to the skin, nothing is highlighted closer to it. In the upper limb, reflux (or halation) from the hand to the wrist joint is recognized, and nothing is seen more proximally. Lymph vessel function is almost lost. In **Fig. 5-2-6**, the right lower limb is type Ⅴ.

7. Pubic lymphedema：In **Fig. 5-2-4**, the tracer can be observed flowing back toward the skin of the genital region via the inguinal lymph node. In such cases, pudendal edema and lymphoid vesicles are formed. Pathologic, abnormally dilated lymphatic vessels are found in the dermal papilla. 2 Since this is a very superficial layer, it will collapse with even minor stimulus such as underwear friction, causing the lymph fluid to continuously flow out.

Ⅱ　SPECT-CT

リンパ浮腫におけるリンパシンチグラフィは、一般的に前後像だけの2次元画像で評価されることが多いが、これはリンパ管の3次元的な局在を評価できないというデメリットをもっており、リンパ管静脈吻合術などの術前検査としては限界があった。頭頸部癌、悪性黒色腫、乳癌などのセンチネルリンパ節の評価を行う際や胸管の評価に、リンパシンチと SPECT-CT の併用の有用性が報告されており、この手法をリンパ浮腫に対するリンパシンチに応用すると、3次元的なリンパ管の局在を評価することができる[3]。

下肢に対する方法は以下のとおりである。400 MBq の[99m]Tc で標識したアルブミンを両側の第1趾間部に皮下注射する。注射後 15 分に両下肢全体の SPECT-CT を撮影する。SPECT は収集マトリックス 128×128、エネルギーウィンドウ 140-keV、360 度収集、5 度ステップで 1 view 12 秒収集としている。ピクセルサイズは 4.8 mm としている。コリメータは低エネルギー高分解能コリメータを使用する。SPECT、CT の画像を水平断、冠状断、矢状断でフュージョンさせ、評価を行う。

これにより、**Fig. 5-2-7** のような像を得ることができる。リンパシンチグラフィでは右大腿に皮膚への逆流所見を認め、タイプⅡである。右では総腸骨動脈に沿うリンパ管の高さで途絶しているようにみえる。SPECT-CT では、右大腿リンパ管を通るトレーサーの量が左大腿より少なく、リンパ管機能が左大腿よりも右下肢で低いことがうかがえる。また、右大腿部では皮膚への逆流を認める。両大腿で、リンパ管は皮下組織内を走行している。

Ⅱ. SPECT-CT

Lymphoscintigraphy imaging in lymphedema is usually evaluated with a two-dimensional image of only the anterior-posterior image, but this has the disadvantage that the three-dimensional location of lymphatic vessels cannot be evaluated, and this poses a limitation as a postoperative examination of lymphatic venous anastomosis. The combined use of lymphatic cystic and SPECT-CT has been reported in evaluating sentinel lymph nodes in head and neck cancer, malignant melanoma, breast cancer and the thoracic duct. When applied, it is possible to evaluate the location of three-dimensional lymphatic vessels[3].

The method for the lower limb is as follows. Albumin labeled with 400 MBq of ^{99m}Tc is injected subcutaneously into the first interdigital space on both sides. A SPECT-CT of both lower limbs is taken 15 minutes after injection. SPECT collects matrix 128×128, energy window 140-keV, collects 360 degrees,

5-2. リンパシンチグラフィ・SPECT-CT

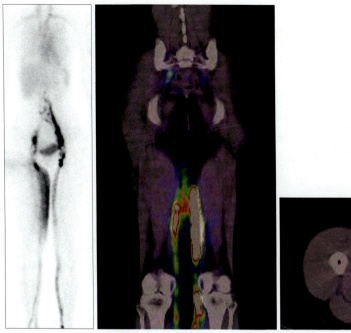

Fig. 5-2-7. SPECT-CT リンパシンチグラフィ画像　SPECT-CT lymphoscintigraphic image
左がリンパシンチグラフィ画像、中が SPECT-CT の coronal 像、右が SPECT-CT の axial 像。リンパシンチグラフィでは右大腿に皮膚への逆流所見を認め、タイプⅡである。SPECT-CT では、リンパ管機能が左大腿よりも右下肢で低いことがうかがえる。また、右大腿部では皮膚への逆流を認める。
Left is a lymphoscintigraphic image, inside is a coronal image of SPECT-CT, right is the axial image of SPECT-CT. Lymphoscintigraphy revealed reflux to the skin on the right thigh, type Ⅱ. SPECT-CT shows that the lymphatic function is lesser in the right lower limb compared to the left thigh. In addition, at the right thigh, reflux to the skin is evident.

collects 1 view for 12 seconds in 5 degree steps. The pixel size is set to 4.8 mm. The collimator uses a low energy high resolution collimator. SPECT, CT images are fused with horizontal cut, coronal disconnection, sagittal breakdown, and evaluated.

In this way, an image as shown in **Fig. 5-2-7** can be obtained. Lymphoscintigraphy revealed backflow to the skin on the right thigh, typeⅡ. On the right it appears to be disrupted by the height of the lymph duct along the common iliac artery. SPECT-CT shows that the amount of tracer passing through the right femoral lymph duct is less than that of the left thigh, and the lymphatic function is less in the right lower limb than in the left thigh. Also, reflux to the skin is evident in the right thigh. In both thighs, lymphatic vessels are traveling through the subcutaneous tissue.

Ⅲ　種々の画像診断の比較

本章では、主にリンパシンチグラフィと SPECT-CT について述べた。
　リンパシンチグラフィは放射線被曝というデメリットをもつものの、深部のリンパ管機能まで評価できるという点で有用な、比較的低侵襲な検査である。しかし、手術中にリアルタイムで検査を行うことは不可能である。さらに、リンパ管静脈吻合術などの際に正確にリンパ管の位置を

同定するためにはICG検査の方が有用である。一方でICG検査は深さ1〜2cmまでしかリンパ管を観察することができず、その点ではリンパシンチグラフィの方が勝っている。

リンパシンチグラフィは前後像しか得られないため、リンパ管の位置の深さ診断が困難であった。そのデメリットを克服するのがSPECT-CTである。やはり放射線被曝というデメリットはあるが、断層像でリンパ管の局在を診断でき、筋層内を走行するリンパ管まで描出することが可能である。今後、リンパ浮腫の病態解明においても期待される検査法である。

リンパ浮腫の診療においては、それぞれの検査の特性を活かし、複数の検査法を組み合わせてリンパ浮腫の評価を行うことが必要であろう。

（原　尚子、三原　誠）

III. Comparison of various diagnostic images

This section mainly described lymphoscintigraphy and SPECT-CT.

Although lymphoscintigraphy has the disadvantage of radiation exposure, it is a relatively minimal invasive and useful examination, because it helps to evaluate deep lymphatic function. However, it is impossible to conduct the examination in real time during surgery. On the other hand, ICG examination is more useful for accurately identifying the location of lymphatic vessels during lymph venous anastomosis. Yet, ICG examination can only observe lymph vessels 1 to 2 cm in depth, in this regard spect lymphoscintigraphy is superior.

Only Anterior and Posterior images are possible with lymphoscintigraphy, making it difficult to diagnose the depth of lymphatic vessel position. This drawback can be overcome by performing SPECT-CT. Despite the drawback of radiation exposure, it is possible to determine the position of lymphatic vessels with a tomographic image and also to visualize lymph vessels traveling within the muscles. In the future, a better understanding of the pathology of lymphedema will be invaluable to its management.

In the diagnosis and evaluation of lymphedema, it is necessary to combine multiple diagnostic modalities incorporating the diverse characteristics of each examination in order to obtain a complete picture of the underlying condition.

(*Hisako Hara, Makoto Mihara*)

1) Maegawa J, Mikami T, Yamamoto Y, et al：Types of lymphoscintigraphy and indications for lymphaticovenous anastomosis. Microsurgery 30(6)：437-442, 2010.
2) Hara H, Mihara M, Hayashi A, et al：Therapeutic strategy for lower limb lymphedema and lymphatic fistula after resection of a malignant tumor in the hip joint region；a case report. Microsurgery 34(3)：224-228, 2014.
3) Pecking AP, Wartski M, Cluzan RV, et al：SPECT-CT fusion imaging radionuclide lymphoscintigraphy；potential for limb lymphedema assessment and sentinel node detection in breast cancer. Cancer Treat Res 135：79-84, 2007.

CHAPTER 5	術前評価 Preoperative evaluation

3. エコーによるリンパ管の同定とリンパ浮腫の評価

Identification of the lymphatic vessels and evaluation of lymphedema using ultrasound

■はじめに

保存療法に対し抵抗性のある軽症から中等症の二次性リンパ浮腫に対しては、早い段階で手術を行えばリンパ管細静脈吻合術（LVA）をはじめとする外科手術の効果が著明に出ることが多い。限られた時間の中で、より効率的・効果的な手術を行うには、術前のリンパ管同定や吻合に最適な細静脈・リンパ管の選択が重要となってくる。

現在広く使われるようになった ICG リンパ管造影においては、浮腫があまり出現していない Linear 領域でリンパ管の位置同定が ICG に沿って造影されたライン上で可能である。しかし浮腫が認められる部位に多くみられる Dermal Backflow 領域では、病期の進行に伴いリンパ管の同定は困難となり、術中のリンパ管同定における確実性は低下する。近年エコーの進歩に伴い、これまでエコーでは捉えられなかったリンパ管が捉えられるようになったことが報告されている。これにより、ICG リンパ管造影上 Dermal Backflow を示す領域や ICG リンパ管造影が行えない症例においてもリンパ管の同定ができるようになり、LVA をはじめとするリンパ浮腫外科治療の術前評価に活用され始めている。

また、これまでリンパ浮腫の重症度評価には、リンパ管シンチグラフィや ICG リンパ管造影を用いることが主であったが、近年エコーを用いた機能の１つである elastography を用いリンパ浮腫の重症度を評価できることが報告されている。

■Introduction

There has been well-known, positive surgical effect of performing the lymphatico-venous anastomoses (LVA), mainly in treating early stage of mild-to-moderate secondary lymphedema resistant to conservative therapy. The optimal choice of venules and the lymphatic vessels and the way how to perform the most efficient and time effective anastomosis is influenced by the preoperative lymphatic vessels imaging studies.

The most commonly used method has been Indocyanine Green Fluorescent Lymphography/lymphangiography (ICG) proved to be very usefull tool for identification of the lymphatic vessels, and for evaluation of the dynamic lymphatic status especially in early stages of lymphedema with many patent lymphatic vessels with linear pattern of perfusion. However, the identification of the lymphatic vessel becomes more difficult with progression of the stage of lymphedema with severe dermal backflow in worst afected parts of lymphedema.

Despite the invaluable importance of the lymphatic vessel scintigraphy and ICG lymphangiography in staging of severity of lymphedema, the introduction and progression of the new imaging and diagnostic utilities like sonography (Echo) and elastography has recently been reported. They proved to be more superior in detecting the lymphatic vessel in comparison with ICG lymphangiography, even in cases with severe dermal backflow. Thereby this imaging tool begins to be utilized more commonly in preoperative evaluation of the lymphedema.

I エコーによるリンパ管の同定と手術への応用

身体の表在・浅層組織を観察するのに適した15〜18MHzのリニア型プローブを用い、カラードプラモードでリンパ管を注意深く観察すると(**Fig. 5-3-1**)、3つの特徴的な所見を認める(①homogeneous、②hypoechoic、③spicular misshapen image)(**Fig. 5-3-2**)。これらの特徴的所見は、エコーの3D再構築像やソナゾイドによるリンパ管造影からもリンパ管であることが証明され、LVAなどのリンパ浮腫外科手術における術中所見の結果と比較しても、高い感度と特異度を示している。0.4mm以上のリンパ管であれば、エコーにより高い同定率でリンパ管を検出でき、細静脈や皮神経との鑑別も十分に可能である(**Fig. 5-3-3**)。術前にエコーを用いリンパ管と細静脈の位置を同定することにより、ICGリンパ管造影上Dermal Backflowを示す領域(**Fig. 5-3-4**)やICGリンパ管造影が行えない症例においても、より小さな皮切において短時間で正確なLVAをはじめとするリンパ浮腫の外科治療が可能となり始めている(**Fig. 5-3-5**)。

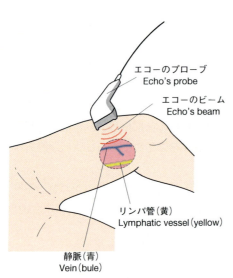

Fig. 5-3-1. 超音波によるリンパ管の同定
Ultrasound visualization of lymphatic vessels

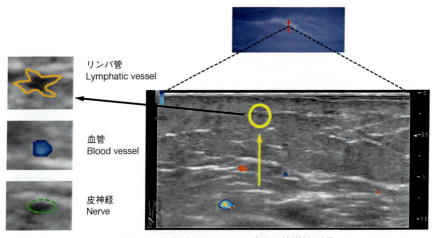

Fig. 5-3-2. 超音波によるリンパ管の特徴的所見
Characteristic ultrasonographic finding of lymphatic vessels

	Shape	Echogenic texture	Color Doppler mode
リンパ管 Lymphatic vessel 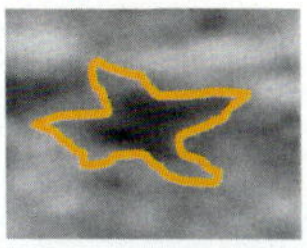	spicular missshapen	hypoechoic	−
血管 Blood vessel 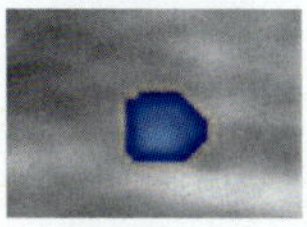	round	hypoechoic	+/−
皮神経 Nerve 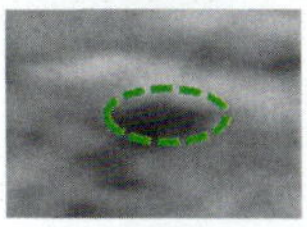	honey comb oval (superficial N.)	bright echogenic texture with hypoechoic fascicle one hypoechoic fascicle (superficial N.)	−

Fig. 5-3-3. 超音波所見におけるリンパ管、細静脈、皮神経の鑑別
Differentation of lymphatic vessel, blood vessel and nerve in ultrasound

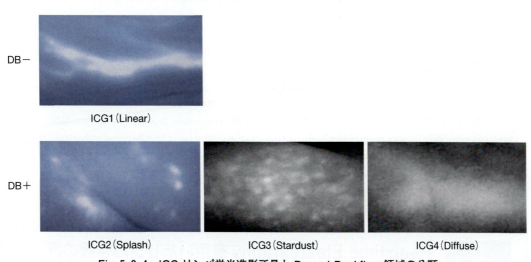

Fig. 5-3-4. ICG リンパ蛍光造影所見と Dermal Backflow 領域の分類
Classification of Dermal Backflow area in ICG lymphography

I. For the identification of the lymphatic vessel by the ultrasound and application to surgery

We use a linear type probe of 15-18 MHz for observation of the superficial tissue layers of the body (**Fig. 5-3-1**), and color Doppler mode that typically shows three characteristic views of the lymphatic vessel (①homogeneous, ②hypoechoic, ③spicular misshapen image) (**Fig. 5-3-2**). Based on the comparisons of the

131

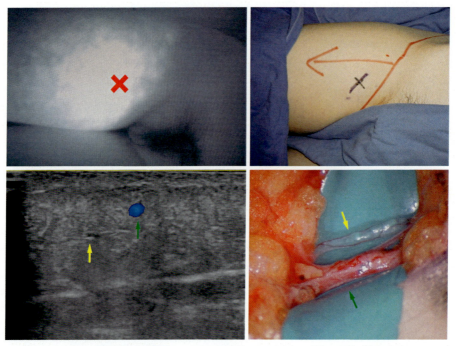

Fig. 5-3-5. Dermal Backflow 領域における超音波によるリンパ管の同定（黄色矢印：リンパ管、緑矢印：静脈）
Identification of lymphatic vessel in Dermal Backflow area using ultrasound (yellow arrow : lymphatic vessel, green arrow : venule)

3D reconstruction lymphangiography and the ultrasound of the echo device in identification of the lymphatic vessels, with the intraoperative views during LVA procedures we found these new modalities to have high sensitivity and specificity. It was found to be able to detect lymphatic vessels with a diameter as small as 0.4 mm with high s degree of reliability and also to distinguish the lymfatics from venules and cutaneous sensitive nerves. degree of reliability (**Fig. 5-3-3**). However, the identification of the lymphatic vessel becomes more difficult with progression In case of the more severe stage of lymphedema with severe dermal backflow on ICG lymphangiography (**Fig. 5-3-4**) preoperative echo imaging modality (**Fig. 5-3-5**) is very helpful in identifying position of both venular and lymphatic vessels thus making surgery shorter with possibility of smaller skin incision needed.

II　Real-time Elastography を用いたリンパ浮腫の評価

　Elastography は 1990 年代に初めて報告された、超音波を用いて組織のゆがみやひずみを評価する新しい技術の 1 つであり、これまで乳癌、前立腺癌、肝臓・膵臓・リンパ節の悪性腫瘍などの精査に使用されてきた。リンパ浮腫の症例において、液体貯留部、つまりひずみの大きい領域は Elastgraphy 上赤色に示される（**Fig. 5-3-6**）。この赤色の面積に応じ分類したものが Elastography Stage（0：0%、1：1〜25%、2：26〜50%、3：51〜75%、4：76〜100%）であり、これは ICG リンパ管造影を用いた重症度と相関し、ICG 所見が重症になるにつれリンパ液の貯留が増大する傾向にあることが報告されている（**Fig. 5-3-7**）。ただし Elastography は絶対評価では

5-3. エコーによるリンパ管の同定とリンパ浮腫の評価

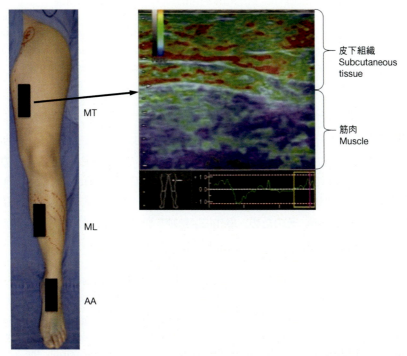

Fig. 5-3-6. Elastography による超音波所見（MT：大腿内側、ML：下腿内側、AA：足前面）
Elastographic finding of lower limb lymphedema (MT：medial thigh, ML：medial leg, AA：anterior ankle)

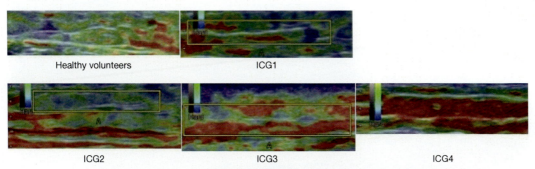

Fig. 5-3-7. ICG リンパ管造影の重症度と比較した Elastography 像
Elastographic image compared with the severity of ICG lymphography

なく相対評価であることや、皮下組織が厚い場合は超音波が深部まで届かないため正確に評価できない場合があることに注意しなければならない。

II. Evaluation of lymphedema using Real-time Elastography

Elastography has been one of the new techniques to evaluate a softiness and a distortion of the tissue using a supersonic waves. It was first reported in the 1990s. It has been widely used in the oncological fields, such as breast cancer, prostate cancer, the malignant tumor of liver, pancreas, the lymph node. In the case of lymphedema, the liquid storage area is demonstrated in red in Elastgraphy (**Fig. 5-3-6**). This that the thing which we classified according to this red area is Elastography Stage (0：0％, 1：1-25％, 2：26-50％, 3：51-

133

75%, 4：76-100%). There is direct correlation between the disease severity as seen on the ICG lymphangiogram (Fig. 5-3-7) and the degree of the lymph fluid retention. However, it is important to say that Elastography has its negatives, looses its reliability and precision with the higher degree of thickness of subcutaneous tissue, as it is harder for supersonic waves to penetrate the deeper tissues.

■おわりに

リンパ管シンチグラフィや ICG リンパ管造影検査が行えない施設においても、より一般的に普及しているエコーだけで、リンパ浮腫の重症度評価やリンパ管の同定が可能な時代が到来してきている。エコーを用いることで、リンパ管の特定が困難な Dermal Backflow 領域や解剖学的にリンパ管の数が少ない部位、アレルギーなどで ICG を用いることができない症例においてもリンパ管の位置を把握できる。そのため、操作には熟練を要するが、リンパ浮腫外科治療の領域においてエコーは今後ますます必須のツールとなることが予測される。

（林　明辰、林　伸子）

■Conclusion

In the institutions without lymphatic vessel scintigraphy or ICG lymphangiography facilities, the very useful tool in assessing the stage of lymphedema disease and the identification of the lymphatic vessel would be using the echo/ultrasound. By using an ultrasound we can predict more reliably the location of the lymphatic vessel in high degree lymphedema cases with severe dermal backflow than by ICG lymphangiography method, secondly as an option in contrast allergy cases. The echo preoperative imagine modality in the lymphedema surgical treatment is predicted to be reliable and valuable diagnostic tools in future.

(*Akitatsu Hayashi, Nobuko Hayashi*)

CHAPTER 5

術前評価
Preoperative evaluation

4. ICGリンパ管造影を用いた術前評価
Preoperative evaluation using ICG lymphography

I ICGリンパ管造影所見の評価

　Chapter 4-3「ICGリンパ管造影による病態生理的重症度評価」で述べられているとおり、ICGリンパ管造影所見はリンパ浮腫の病態生理を反映している（**Fig. 5-4-1**）。すなわち、集合リンパ管を流れているリンパ流はLinearパターン、浅い部位の毛細リンパ管などが拡張したリンパ側副路はSplashパターン、軽度から中等度のリンパ漏出はStardustパターン、重度のリンパ漏出はDiffuseパターンとして造影される。リンパシンチグラフィではDermal Backflow（DB）と表現される異常所見が、ICGリンパ管造影ではSplash・Stardust・Diffuseと3つの所見に細分類される。Splashは可逆的なリンパ流の変化に対しStardust・Diffuseは不可逆的な変化であり、Splash・Stardust領域ではリンパ管細静脈吻合術（LVA）が可能なリンパ管が見つけられる率が高いのに対し、Diffuse領域ではLVAに適したリンパ管を見つけることが困難など、DBパターンの所見の違いは臨床的に大きな意味をもつ。

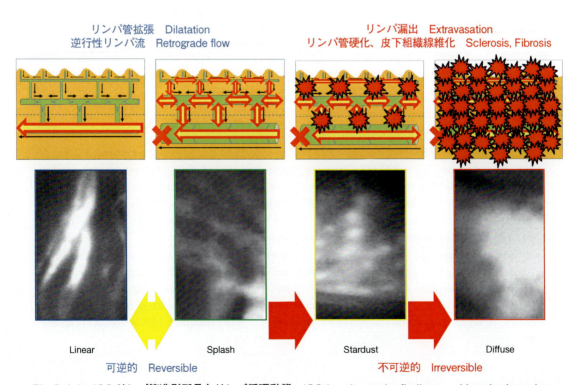

Fig. 5-4-1. ICGリンパ管造影所見とリンパ循環動態　ICG lymphography findings and lymphodynamics

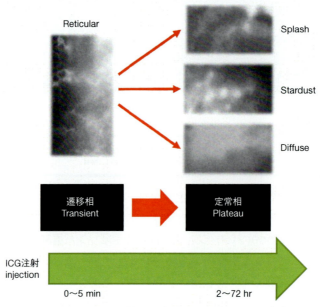

Fig. 5-4-2. ICG 注射経過時間と DB パターンの変化
DB pattern change with elapsed time after ICG injection

　手術直前の ICG 注射では遷移相のみの評価となり、Linear パターンの走行と DB の分布しかわからない。DB パターンの区別(Splash か Stardust か Diffuse か)が可能なのは注射後 2～72 時間のため、手術前日での注射が望ましい(**Fig. 5-4-2**)。手術前日に ICG を注射し遷移相における評価を行い(ICG velocity の評価と Linear パターンのマッピング)、手術直前(手術室で創部の消毒前)に定常相における評価を行う(DB の種類と分布のマッピング)。LVA においても血管柄付きリンパ節移植術(LNT)においても、ICG リンパ管造影を用いたマッピングをもとに手術部位を決めると効率的なリンパドレナージが図れる(**Fig. 5-4-3**)。

I. Evaluation of ICG lymphography findings

　ICG lymphography findings demonstrate lymphedema pathophysiology as mentioned in Chap. 4-3 (**Fig. 5-4-1**). DB pattern detected with lymphoscintigraphy can be divided into 3 distinct patterns : Splash, Stardust, and Diffuse. Splash represents a reversible lymph flow change whereas Stardust and Diffuse represent irreversible lymph flow changes. Lymphatic vessels suitable for LVA can be usually found in Splash or Stardust regions, but finding suitable lymphatic vessels for LVA is difficult in Diffuse patterns. Thus, the differentiation of DB pattern is very important for lymphedema management.

　There is no diagnostic value in ICG injection immediately before lymphatic surgery, because only a transient phase can be evaluated and not a plateau phase. On average, it takes 2-72 hours after ICG injection to achieve a plateau phase. As such, ICG should be injected the day before surgery (**Fig. 5-4-2**). This allows for measurements of ICG velocities, determining a Linear pattern and evaluation of the plateau phase in order to determine DB pattern. The pattern will guide the appropriate treatment : LVA and or LNT (**Fig. 5-4-3**).

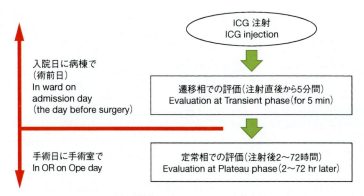

Fig. 5-4-3. LVA 術前のダイナミック ICG リンパ管造影
Preoperative dynamic ICG lymphography before LVA

II 造影所見による術中所見予測

リンパ浮腫外科治療の基本は LVA となるが、LVA においてはリンパ流量が豊富なリンパ管を確実につなぐことが求められる。いかなる吻合においてもそうであるように、リンパ管吻合においても開存率は経時的に低下していく。したがって、吻合リンパ管が開存し続けバイパス効果を持続させるためになるべく多くの吻合を作成することが肝要である。吻合数に相関しバイパス量も増えるため、術後の減量効果も高い (**Fig. 5-4-4**)。限られた手術時間で多くのバイパスを作成するには無駄なく吻合に適したリンパ管を探し吻合しなければならないが、ICG リンパ管造影によりリンパ管の状態を予測し適切な手術部位を選択できる。

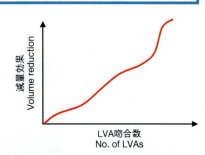

Fig. 5-4-4. LVA 吻合数と減量効果
Relation between the number of LVAs and volume reduction

吻合に用いられるリンパ管は、大伏在静脈や頭側皮静脈といった主要な皮静脈に沿った領域に多くあるが、リンパ浮腫肢ではその部位(末梢側か中枢側か)によってリンパ管の性状が大きく異なる。Linear 領域や Splash 領域ではリンパ管硬化はほとんどないが、Stardust 領域ではリンパ管硬化を認めるようになり、Diffuse 領域ではリンパ管硬化が著しくリンパ管径も細いことが多い (**Fig. 5-4-5**)。LVA 215 吻合における ICG リンパ管造影所見と術中所見を比較したデータでは、Linear 領域・Splash 領域・Stardust 領域ではリンパ管発見率は 90% 以上でリンパ管径は平均 0.45 mm 程度であったが、Diffuse 領域では吻合に適したリンパ管発見率は 45% でリンパ管径は平均 0.26 mm でありリンパ管硬化が著しかった。ICG リンパ管造影所見に応じて手術部位や術者配置を検討し、最も効率的にバイパスが作成できるようにすべきである (**Fig. 5-4-6**)。DB パターンの細分化により術中リンパ管所見の予測ができることがリンパシンチグラフィではできない ICG リンパ管造影の強みの 1 つである。

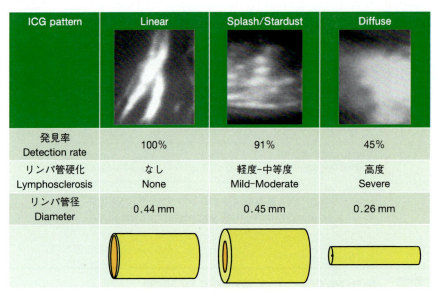

Fig. 5-4-5. ICG リンパ管造影所見とリンパ管の性状
Lymphatic vessels' conditions according to ICG lymphography pattern

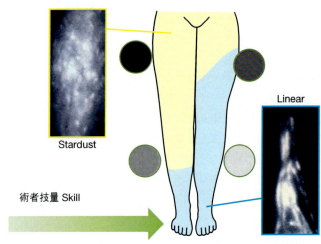

Fig. 5-4-6. 複数術者による LVA における術者の配置
Operators' positioning for simultaneous multisite LVAs by multiple surgeons

II. Prediction of lymphatic architecture based on ICG lymphography findings

LVA requires secure anastomosis of lymphatic vessels allowing for abundant lymph flow. Similar to other vascular anastomoses, lymphatic anastomosis patency also decreases with time. Consequently, it is important to anastomose as many lymphatic vessels as possible to maintain overall lymphatic reduction. The more anastomoses that are created, the more volume reduction can be obtained post-operatively (**Fig. 5-4-4**). By utilizing ICG lymphography, the surgeon is able to identify key regions where LVA should be performed in an effective and efficient manner.

Lymphatic vessels selected for LVA are usually found, running along major subcutaneous veins. However these vessels will vary in location depending on where the pathology is. Lymphosclerosis, or narrowing of the lymphatic vessel due to fibrosis is none to mild in Linear or Splash patterns, whereas lymphosclerosis is moderate in Stardust patterns. In Diffuse patterns of lymphedema, lymphosclerosis is severe and lymphatic vessels are significantly smaller than that seen in other ICG patterns (**Fig. 5-4-5**). For example, according to study of over 200 LVAs performed comparing ICG lymphography patterns and lymphatic vessel diameters, there was a significant difference between the different DB patterns. In Linear, Splash and Stardust patterns, detecting suitable lymphatic vessels was over 90% with the average vessel diameter of 0.45 mm. In Diffuse patterns the detecting a suitable vessel dropped by half to 45% with a vessel diameter of 0.26 mm. This highlights the importance of ICG lymphography in creating a roadmap of select lymphatic vessels to perform LVA on (**Fig. 5-4-6**).

It is one of the most useful strengths in ICG lymphography to predict intraoperative lymphatic vessels' conditions by differentiating DB patterns, which cannot be done with lymphoscintigraphy.

III 術前評価における Linear パターンの意義

ICG リンパ管造影で Linear パターンを認めた場合、その部位には浅い位置にリンパ集合管があり、LVA においても確実にリンパ管を発見できる（**Fig. 5-4-7**）。しかし、リンパ外科の経験豊富な術者であれば、Linear パターンを認めない部位でも容易にリンパ管を発見できるため、Linear パターンの臨床的な意義は"可及的に小さい皮切で LVA を行える"ことにある。もちろん"術前ガイダンス"としては有用で、初心者でも安心して確実にリンパ管を探し出せるが、Linear 領域での LVA で重要なことは 1 cm 程度の最小切開で低侵襲に整容面にも十分に配慮された手術をすることにある（**Fig. 5-4-8**）。Linear 領域を狙い短時間・小切開で最も低侵襲に LVA ができる（最小侵襲リンパ超微小外科 Minimally Invasive Lymphatic Supermicrosurgery；MILS）。

Linear パターンが見えない部位でも吻合に適したリンパ管はあるため、Linear パターンがあ

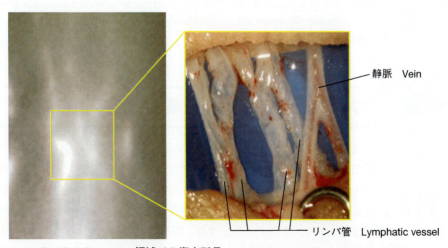

Fig. 5-4-7. Linear 領域での術中所見　Lymphatic vessels in Linear region

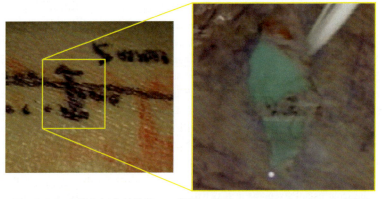

Fig. 5-4-8. MILSにおける数mm切開　Millimeter skin incision in MILS

る部位に固執してLVAを行ってはならない。特にStardust領域はある程度リンパうっ滞による負荷がかかっており、Linear領域より豊富なリンパ流をもち拡張したリンパ管を認めることが多い。前述のとおり、遷移相でLinearパターンであった領域が定常相でStardustパターンとなることがあるため、遷移相にLinearパターンをマッピングしておき、定常相でStardust領域となった領域を狙うと、初心者でも流量が豊富なリンパ管を確実に吻合することができる。

III. Meaning of linear pattern in preoperative evaluation

When a Linear pattern is seen on ICG lymphography, a surgeon can usually identify a lymphatic vessel relatively close (<2 cm) from the skin (**Fig. 5-4-7**). This allows for a small skin incision in which even a novice surgeon can localize the lymphatic vessel through. For aesthetic purposes, surgeons should be attentive in minimizing skin incision lengths (<1 cm) (**Fig. 5-4-8**). For a skilled surgeon performing multiple minimally invasive lymphatic supermicrosurgery (MILS), LVAs done in a region with Linear patterns can be performed in a short time (<2 hr) and small incisions (<10 mm); expore lymphatic supermicrosurgeon can complate 1 LVA within 30 min.

However, surgeons should not always opt to perform LVAs in regions showing Linear patterns. As stated earlier, a Linear pattern seen during the transient phase could very well evolve into a Splash or Stardust pattern. Lymphatic vessels seen in the latter two patterns are dilated due to higher intralymphatic pressures. Therefore at times it can be technically easier and physiologically advantageous to perform LVA in a region of Splash or Stardust patterns.

IV　ICGリンパ管造影所見に基づいた手術戦略

　ICGリンパ管造影所見はLVA・LNT・減量術いずれのリンパ外科手術においても有用である。LVAではうっ滞したリンパ流を減圧することが目的であるため、ある程度リンパ負荷のかかっており、かつ、リンパ管硬化も中等度まででリンパ管径も細くないStardust領域におけるLVAが効果的である。Stardust領域では逆行性のリンパ流を生じているため、リンパ管末梢端のEE吻合だけでなく、中枢端もバイパスするよう心がける。最も優先して吻合を行うのはStardust領域であり、その次がLinear領域となる。Linear領域では確実にリンパ管が見つかるため短い

5-4. ICGリンパ管造影を用いた術前評価

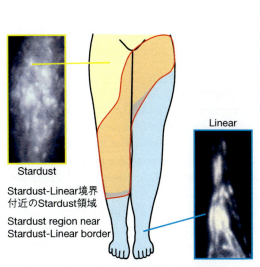

Fig. 5-4-9. LVAをすべき優先部位（赤線内）
Priority sites for LVA（red circle）

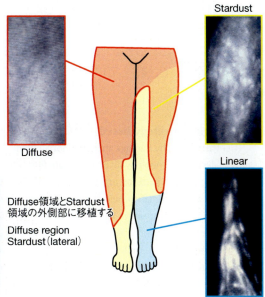

Fig. 5-4-10. LNTをすべき優先部位（赤線内）
Priority sites for LNT（red circle）

皮切と手術時間で吻合するよう心がける。もともとのリンパ流を途絶えさせないようSE吻合・SS吻合を行った方がよい。Diffuse領域では効果的なLVAを行える可能性は低いので避けるべきである（**Fig. 5-4-9**）。複数人でLVAを同時に行う際は、経験豊富な術者がStardust領域を優先し、経験が少ない術者がLinear領域でLVAを行うとよい。

　LNTはリンパ管硬化が強くLVAだけでは治療効果が不十分な症例に行われるが、当科では通常LNTをLVAと同時に行っている。LVAで効果が得られにくいDiffuseパターンを認める症例でも、Stardust領域がありLVAの治療効果が見込める部位も存在するからである。したがって、LNTを行う部位はLVAが効きにくい部位となり、Diffuse領域に優先的に移植するとよい（**Fig. 5-4-10**）。Diffuse領域がなければStardust

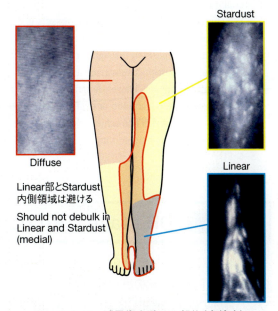

Fig. 5-4-11. 減量術を避ける部位（赤線内）
Untouchable sites in debulking surgery（lymph preserving lipectomy）（red circle）

領域のうちLVAの効きにくい大腿中枢や大腿・下腿外側に移植するとLVAでは得られない効果が得られやすい。

　減量術は、長期間のリンパ漏出で脂肪沈着によりnon-pitting edemaとして増大した皮下脂肪を除去する外科治療である。皮下脂肪とその部位にあるリンパ管が除去されるため、減量術後

141

には同部のリンパ流は途絶えてしまう。したがって減量術は原則的に Diffuse 領域などリンパ機能が廃絶した部位・症例で行われるが、LVA・LNT と併用してリンパ循環改善と沈着脂肪除去の両方を目的に行うこともある。減量術の際は ICG リンパ管造影で通常 Linear パターンを認める部位を避けることで、残存しているリンパ機能を障害することなく皮下脂肪を除去できる（**Fig. 5-4-11**）。

IV. Surgical strategy based on ICG lymphography findings

ICG lymphography findings are useful for all lymphatic surgeries including LVA, LNT, and debulking. LVA aims to decongest lymph by diverting lymph flow into the venous circulation. Stated previously, regions with Splash or Stardust patterns are good surgical sites to perform LVA on account of the larger lymphatic diameters with minimal to mild lymphosclerosis SE or SS anastomosis is preferable in regions of Linear patterns in order to preserve native lymph flow. In a Stardust pattern, lymphatic flow is both antegrade and retrograde. Consequently a surgeon should bypass antegrade flow using an EE anastomosis and retrograde flow using a double EE, lambda (EE + ES), SE, and SS anastomoses. LVA should not be performed in regions of Diffuse patterns, because the possibility to create an effective bypass is low (**Fig. 5-4-9**). When multiple surgeons simultaneously perform LVAs, an experienced surgeon should focus in on regions with Splash and Stardust patterns whereas a less experienced surgeon should focus in on regions with Linear patterns.

LNT is indicated in refractory lymphedema cases or in cases in which there is partial improvement with LVA but continued edema due to severe lymphosclerosis. LNT when performed with LVA can augment the overall therapeutic response, although additional scan (s) is (are) left. Additionally LNT should be considered in regions where identifying lymphatic vessels is difficult such as the lateral aspect of limbs (**Fig. 5-4-10**).

Debulking surgery with resection and liposuction, is performed in cases with non-pitting edema representing fat deposition through chronic protein-rich lymph retention in the interstitial space. Debulking surgery typically removes subcutaneous fat with lymphatic vessels and as such lymph flow is obstructed in these debulked regions. Therefore debulking surgery should be performed in cases where the lymphatic system is completely disrupted or dysfunctional such as in Diffuse patterns. Debulking surgery may also be performed with LVA/LNT to achieve decongestion of lymph and removal of fat deposition simultaneously. In Linear patterns, Lymph preserving lipectomy can be performed to maintain the lymphatic architecture (**Fig. 5-4-11**).

Ⅴ　DB stage に応じた治療戦略

ICG リンパ管造影所見を用いた DB stage はリンパ循環動態に基づいた病態生理的重症度評価で stage 0〜Ⅴ（陰部のみ stage Ⅳまで）の 6 つの stage からなる（**Table 4-3-3**、80 頁参照）。リンパ浮腫の臨床病期は DB stage により予後の異なる 4 つに分けられる。DB stage 0 はリンパ循環異常がなくリンパ浮腫は発症していないため治療適応はない。DB stage Ⅰ は自覚的にも他覚的にも浮腫は認めない不顕性リンパ浮腫（subclinical lymphedema）で、リンパ循環異常を認めるが可逆的な変化であり治療方針には議論の余地がある。DB stage Ⅱ は早期リンパ浮腫（early lymphedema）で、不可逆的なリンパ循環異常を伴い保存療法にても軽快せず、自覚症状がない例においても 2 年以内にほぼ全例が進行性のリンパ浮腫を発症するため外科治療の適応である。DB stage Ⅲ 以降は進行リンパ浮腫（progressed lymphedema）で、合併外科治療を含め積極的に外科治療を行うべきである（**Table 5-4-1**）。

Table 5-4-1. ICGリンパ管造影による重症度分類と各種外科治療の適応
Indication of each lymphatic surgery according to ICG lymphography severity staging

	臨床病期 Clinical condition	治療方針 Management
Stage 0	リンパ浮腫(−) Lymphedema(−)	治療不要 No treatment
Stage Ⅰ	不顕性リンパ浮腫 Subclinical	経過観察 or 予防 Follow or Prophylaxis
Stage Ⅱ	早期リンパ浮腫 Early	低侵襲治療 LVA
Stage Ⅲ～	進行リンパ浮腫 Progressed	積極的外科治療 LVA＋LNT±LS

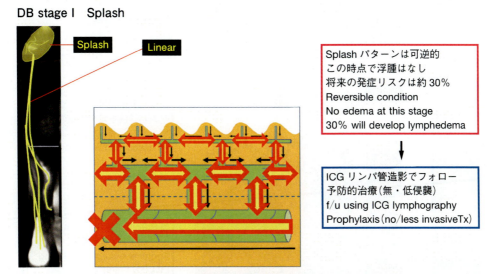

Fig. 5-4-12. DB stage Ⅰに対する治療方針　Management for DB stage Ⅰ

　DB stage 0 では DB パターンを認めずリンパ循環動態に異常を認めない。広範囲のリンパ節郭清と放射線照射はがん治療後リンパ浮腫のリスクを高めるが、いかにハイリスクとされる場合であっても DB stage 0 の例に対してはリンパ浮腫の治療適応はない。自覚的もしくは他覚的浮腫があったとしてもリンパ循環異常を伴わないため、深部静脈血栓や全身性浮腫など他の浮腫性疾患の鑑別をすべきで、リンパ浮腫に対する治療は不要である。

　DB stage Ⅰでは Splash パターンを認めるが、これは浅い部位におけるリンパ側副路を示しており可逆的な変化である。DB stage Ⅰではリンパ漏出はないため自覚的・他覚的浮腫は認めず、自覚症状もない場合がほとんどである。自覚症状がある場合は"張り""重い"感覚を訴えることが多い。DB stage Ⅰの約 1/3 は進行するが残りは進行しない（**Fig. 5-4-12**）。予防的にリンパドレナージを行い側副路の発達を補助することは有用かも知れないが、侵襲を伴う外科治療には慎重でなければならない。外科治療を行う場合は十分に低侵襲かつ短時間で施行可能な mini-

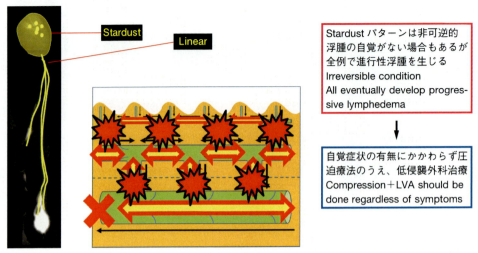

Fig. 5-4-13. DB stage Ⅱに対する治療方針　Treatment for DB stage Ⅱ

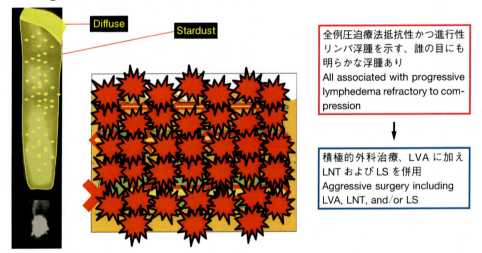

Fig. 5-4-14. DB stage Ⅲ以降に対する治療方針　Treatments for DB stage Ⅲ〜

mally invasive lymphatic supermicrosurgery(MILS)や efferent lymphatic vessel-to-venous anastomosis(ELVA)が好ましい。経過観察する場合は、ICGリンパ管造影を用いて慎重にフォローする必要があり、Stardustパターンの出現を認めた場合は速やかに治療開始すべきである。

　DB stage Ⅱでは不可逆的な変化であるStardustパターンを認め、保存療法を行ってもDB stage Ⅰもしくは DB stage 0 に改善することはなく進行性のため、外科治療の適応となる(**Fig. 5-4-13**)。保存療法により見た目の浮腫はコントロールできることもあるが、長期経過ではStardustパターンの領域が広がり、いずれ保存療法抵抗性のリンパ浮腫として悪化していくこととなる。浮腫は軽度なこともあり、なるべく侵襲の少ない治療が好ましくLVAが第一選択と

なる。ICG velocity が比較的保たれている例に十分なバイパスを作成することができれば治癒、すなわち浮腫は消失し圧迫療法も不要となり DB stage 0 にリンパ循環が改善することができる。下肢リンパ浮腫例では主に大腿部に Stardust パターンを認めるため、大腿部で吻合することが望ましい。

DB stage Ⅲ以降では中等症以上のリンパ浮腫を認め、多くの症例では保存療法抵抗性の進行性リンパ浮腫としてリンパ外科治療を求めて来院する。DB stage Ⅲでは DB stage Ⅱ同様に流量の豊富なリンパ管を認め LVA で改善する例も多いが、治癒まで改善することは容易ではない（特に下肢リンパ浮腫）。DB stage Ⅳおよび stage Ⅴでは LVA により改善することもあれば、効果が乏しいこともあり、リンパ循環改善に LNT を要することも多い。特に Diffuse パターンが広がっている DB stage Ⅴの症例では LVA による改善は見込み難く LNT を治療の基本とすべきである（**Fig. 5-4-14**）。DB stage Ⅲ以降では少なからず脂肪沈着を認めるので、LVA やLNT によるリンパ循環を改善しても患肢の容積は完全には戻らない。さらなる整容面の改善には減量術を行う必要がある。

（山本　匠）

V. Therapeutic strategy according to DB stage

Based on ICG lymphography and DB stages, a clinical staging system is utilized in lymphedema cases. There are 6 clinical stages (genital lymphedema has 5 stages) (see **Table 4-3-3**). In stage 0, there is no abnormal lymph circulation, and no lymphedema treatment is indicated. In stage Ⅰ, reversible lymph circulatory changes are seen (Splash pattern) without subjective or objective edema. This is otherwise known as "subclinical lymphedema" and prophylactic intervention is currently unclear and controversial. In stage Ⅱ, irreversible lymph circulatory changes are seen (Stardust pattern) and all these patients will likely result in symptomatic and progressive lymphedema refractory to conservative treatments within 2 years. Surgery is indicated for this "early lymphedema". Stage Ⅲ through Ⅴ represent "progressive lymphedema" and require aggressive surgical interventions sometimes even combined lymphatic surgery (**Table 5-4-1**).

No abnormal lymph circulation is detected in stage 0 and as such, should not be surgically treated. Should a patient with stage 0 complain of edema or other related symptoms such as tension and hardness, other pathological sources should be evaluated as a cause of the edema.

Splash pattern as seen in stage Ⅰ represents reversible changes of superficial lymphatic collateral pathways. As no lymph extravasation occurs in stage Ⅰ, edema is not seen but there can be subjective symptoms such as a feeling of heaviness, tension, or firmness of the affected extremity. One third of stage Ⅰ patients progress to develop symptomatic and progressive lymphedema, whereas the remaining two thirds do not develop symptomatic lymphedema (**Fig. 5-4-12**). Prophylactic LVA may be useful to facilitate further development of collateral lymphatic pathways, but the degree of invasiveness should be considered. If performed, surgical treatment should be minimally invasive with short operation times. A good method is to utilize ICG lymphography to follow patients with stage and intervene surgically when a Stardust pattern is seen.

Stardust pattern as seen in stage Ⅱ represents irreversible lymph flow changes. Clinically this is considered "early lymphedema." Conservative treatment will rarely improve pre-existing lymphatic flow and therefore surgical treatment is indicated (**Fig. 5-4-13**). Symptomatic edema can be temporarily improved by conservative treatments, but due to progressive lymphedema, all conservative treatments will become refractory with time. The surgical treatment for stage Ⅱ is LVA. LVA can cure stage Ⅱ patients by correcting abnormal lymphatic circulation especially when enough bypasses are performed. It is important to anastomose lymphatic vessels in the thigh for leg lymphedema, because the thigh usually shows Stardust pattern on ICG lymphography.

In stage III and higher, lymphedema is clinically apparent and is refractory to conservative treatments. Patients with stage III are usually improved with LVA, but are the success for complete cure is much less than that of stage II. For patients with stage IV/V, LVA is effective to reduce volume and to improve lymphatic circulation, but LNT is required to further improve lymphedema. In patients with stage V exhibiting a Diffuse pattern, LNT should be the first line therapy with/without LVA, because lymphatic vessels are likely to be severely sclerotic (**Fig. 5-4-14**). Starting from stage III, both LVA and LNT cannot completely reduce an affected limbs' volume despite significant improvement seen with lymph circulation. The reason for this is that the remaining volume is due to chronic fat deposition. Therefore to completely reduce the volume in order to match the contralateral extremity, debulking surgery (usually liposuction) is required to achieve an improved aesthetic result.

(Takumi Yamamoto)

1) Yamamoto T, Yamamoto N, et al : Indocyanine green (ICG)-enhanced lymphography for upper extremity lymphedema ; a novel severity staging system using dermal backflow (DB) patterns. Plast Reconstr Surg 128(4) : 941-947, 2011.
2) Yamamoto T, Narushima M, Yoshimatsu H, et al : Indocyanine green velocity ; Lymph transportation capacity deterioration with progression of lymphedema. Ann Plast Surg 71(5) : 591-594, 2013.
3) Yamamoto T, Yamamoto N, Yoshimatsu H, et al : Indocyanine green lymphography for evaluation of genital lymphedema in secondary lower extremity lymphedema patients. J Vasc Surg : Venous and Lym Dis 1(4) : 400-405, 2013.
4) Yamamoto T, Iida T, et al : Indocyanine green (ICG)-enhanced lymphography for evaluation of facial lymphoedema. J Plast Reconstr Aesthet Surg 64(11) : 1541-1544, 2011.
5) Yamamoto T, Narushima M, Yoshimatsu H, et al : Dynamic indocyanine green (ICG) lymphography for breast cancer-related arm lymphedema. Ann Plast Surg 73(6) : 706-709, 2014.
6) Yamamoto T, Yoshimatsu H, et al : Indocyanine green lymphography findings in primary leg lymphedema. Eur J Vasc Endovasc Surg 49 : 95-102, 2015.
7) Yamamoto T, Koshima I : Subclinical lymphedema ; understanding is the clue to decision making. Plast Reconstr Surg 132(3) : 472e-473e, 2013.
8) Yamamoto T, Koshima I : Splash, stardust, or diffuse pattern ; differentiation of dermal backflow pattern is important in indocyanine green lymphography. Plast Reconstr Surg 133(6) : e887-e888, 2014.
9) Yamamoto T, Matsuda N, Doi K, et al : The earliest finding of indocyanine green (ICG) lymphography in asymptomatic limbs of lower extremity lymphedema patients secondary to cancer treatment ; the modified dermal backflow (DB) stage and concept of subclinical lymphedema. Plast Reconstr Surg 128(4) : 314e-321e, 2011.
10) Yamamoto T, Yamamoto N, Narushima M, et al : Lymphaticovenular anastomosis with guidance of ICG lymphography. J Jpn Coll Angiol 52 : 327-331, 2012.
11) Yamamoto T, Narushima M, et al : Minimally invasive lymphatic supermicrosurgery (MILS) ; indocyanine green lymphography-guided simultaneous multi-site lymphaticovenular anastomoses via millimeter skin incisions. Ann Plast Surg 72(1) : 67-70, 2014.
12) Yamamoto T, Narushima M, et al : Less invasive supermicrosurgical treatment for lymphedema. Jpn J Phlebol 25 : 355-359, 2014.
13) Yamamoto T, Narushima M, et al : Evaluation of lower abdominal and genital lymphedema using ICG lymphography. Jpn J Phlebol 25 : 43-47, 2014.
14) Yamamoto T, Narushima M, et al : Characteristic indocyanine green lymphography findings in lower extremity lymphedema ; the generation of a novel lymphedema severity staging system using

dermal backflow patterns. Plast Reconstr Surg 127(5)：1979-1986, 2011.

15) Yamamoto T, Narushima M, et al：Lambda-shaped anastomosis with intravascular stenting method for safe and effective lymphaticovenular anastomosis. Plast Reconstr Surg 127(5)：1987-1992, 2011.

16) Yamamoto T, Yoshimatsu H, et al：Split intravascular stents for side-to-end lymphaticovenular anastomosis. Ann Plast Surg 71(5)：538-540, 2013.

17) Yamamoto T, Chen WF, Yamamoto N, et al：Technical simplification of the supermicrosurgical side-to-end lymphaticovenular anastomosis using the parachute technique. Microsurgery 35(2)：129-134, 2015.

18) Yamamoto T, Kikuchi K, et al：Ladder-shaped lymphaticovenular anastomosis using multiple side-to-side lymphatic anastomoses for a leg lymphedema patient. Microsurgery 34(5)：404-408, 2014.

19) Yamamoto T, Yamamoto N, Hayashi A, et al：Supermicrosurgical deep lymphatic vessel-to-venous anastomosis for a breast cancer-related arm lymphedema with severe sclerosis of superficial lymphatic vessels. Microsurgery 37(2)：156-159, 2017.

20) Yamamoto T, Yoshimatsu H, et al：Sequential anastomosis for lymphatic supermicrosurgery；multiple lymphaticovenular anastomoses on one venule. Ann Plast Surg 73(1)：46-49, 2014.

21) Yamamoto T, Hayashi N, et al：Pathophysiological approach to obstructive lymphedema. Jpn J Lymphol 37(2)：2014.

22) Yamamoto T, Yamamoto N, Yamashita M, et al：Efferent lymphatic vessel anastomosis(ELVA)；supermicrosurgical efferent lymphatic vessel-to-venous anastomosis for the prophylactic treatment of subclinical lymphedema. Ann Plast Surg 76(4)：424-427, 2016.

23) Yamamoto T, Yoshimatsu H, et al：A modified side-to-end lymphaticovenular anastomosis. Microsurgery 33(2)：130-133, 2013.

24) Yamamoto T, Yamamoto N, et al：Evaluation of peripheral lymphedema using ICG lymphography. Jpn J Phlebol 24：57-62, 2013.

25) Yamamoto T：Supermicrosurgical reconstruction of lymphatic system. Jpn J Microsurg 28(3)：89-96, 2015.

26) Yamamoto T, Narushima M, et al：Dynamic indocyanine green lymphography for breast cancer-related arm lymphedema. Ann Plast Surg 73(6)：706-709, 2014.

27) Yamamoto T, Yamashita M, et al：Lymph preserving lipectomy under indocyanine green lymphography navigation. J Plast Reconstr Aesthet Surg 68(1)：136-137, 2015.

術前評価
Preoperative evaluation

5. 早期診断
Early diagnosis

I 早期診断

　リンパ浮腫は一度発症すると治療法のない不治の病と考えられてきた。保存的療法を行っても徐々に進行する。中には血管肉腫（Stewart-Treves 症候群）を発症し、死に至る場合もある。しかし、最近はリンパ管静脈吻合術の発達により、早期治療にて完治する（弾性ストッキングなどによる圧迫が不要となる）例が出てきている。けれども、リンパ浮腫の診断基準はいまだ確立しておらず、どの時点からリンパ浮腫が発症しているかという明確な判断は困難である。これまでのように症状の有無や周径測定での変化が認められる時点では、病期が進みリンパ管や組織は不可逆的に変化してしまっている。そのため、未症状や症状がごく軽度のうち（ISL 分類ステージ 0〜1期）にリンパ浮腫が発症と確定診断できる方法の確立が必要である。ここでは、リンパ浮腫の早期診断について、Indocyanine green（ICG）蛍光リンパ管造影法を用いたわれわれの方法を紹介する。

1. 病期

　リンパ浮腫の病期分類は種々あり、ここでは International Society of Lymphology（ISL）の病期分類（**Table 4-3-1**、71 頁参照）を用いる。早期とは 0〜1 期である。特に無症状である 0 期のうちに、今後進行していく可能性が高いものを見つけ、治療を行っていく必要がある。

2. 対象

　リンパ浮腫発症の高リスク群（乳癌、子宮癌、前立腺癌などでリンパ節郭清を伴う腫瘍摘出術を施行された人）に対して行う。

3. 検査方法

　ICG 蛍光リンパ管造影法を用いて、ICG 注射後 4 時間のリンパ流を撮影する。術後 1 週間、術後 1 ヵ月、以降 1 ヵ月ごとの撮影を行う。術後半年からは 3 ヵ月ごと、術後 1 年からは半年ごとに検査を行う。リンパ浮腫は早ければ術後 6 ヵ月以内に発症し、術後 1 年以内の発症が最も多いからである（**Fig. 5-5-1**）。

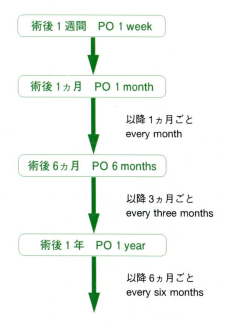

Fig. 5-5-1. ICG蛍光リンパ管造影法による診断の進め方
Diagnostic approach using ICG lymphography

4. 診　断

　前章でも述べられたように、リンパ浮腫の進行に合わせてICG所見は変化してゆく（**Fig. 5-5-2, 3**）。リンパ節郭清直後はほぼすべての症例で下腹部から大腿の浮腫を認める。腫脹部に一致したICGの貯留も認める。しかし、これは組織間隙に一時的に間質液が貯留しただけに過ぎず、リンパ管の機能破綻にはまだ至っていない。この状態は1〜2ヵ月程度で改善する（**Fig. 5-5-4**）。しかし、一部は術直後の浮腫が改善した後、もしくは改善しないまま「Dermal Backflow」が出現し、そのままリンパ浮腫へと移行してゆく（**Fig. 5-5-5**）。したがって、「Dermal Backflow」を認めた時点で、リンパ管機能は破綻しており、リンパ浮腫が発症していると考え、治療が必要となる。この時点では、リンパ管の変化はまだ可逆的な変化と考えられる。

5. 早期治療

　リンパ浮腫が早期に診断され、症状が軽度な場合は、弾性装具の着用と用手的ドレナージのみとなることが多い。しかし、その後リンパ浮腫は緩やかに進行してゆき、リンパ管は不可逆的変化を遂げる。そのため、発症を早期に確認した時点（リンパ管のダメージが軽度な状態）でリンパ管静脈吻合術を行い、外科的に側副路をつくることで、完治の可能性が高くなると考える（**Fig. 5-5-6**）。

6. まとめ

　ICG蛍光リンパ管造影法を用いた早期診断は、腫瘍摘出術後や、それ以外でもリンパ浮腫の診断に用いることができる。そして、リンパ浮腫の早期治療の助けとなりうる。

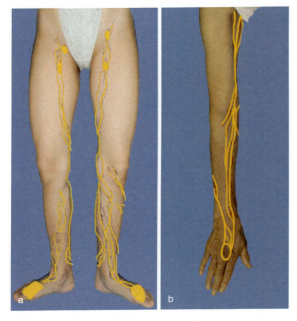

Fig. 5-5-2. 正常なリンパ流　Normal lymph flow
ICG 蛍光リンパ管造影法によって確認されたリンパ流を黄色線でマーキングした。
a：正常下肢
b：正常上肢
Lymph flow identified by ICG lymphography is drawn in yellow.
a：Normal lower extremity
b：Normal upper extremity

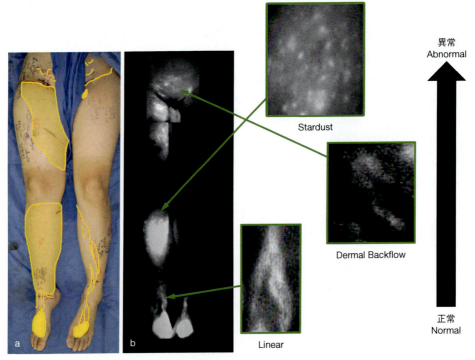

Fig. 5-5-3. リンパ浮腫の場合　ICG lymphography of lymphedema
ICG 蛍光リンパ管造影法により Dermal Backflow が確認される。
a：ICG 蛍光リンパ管造影法によって確認されたリンパ流を黄色線でマーキングした。
b：近赤外線カメラにて撮影した画像
Dermal Backflow is observed during ICG lymphography.
a：Lymph flow identified by ICG lymphography is drawn in yellow.
b：Image using an infrared camera system

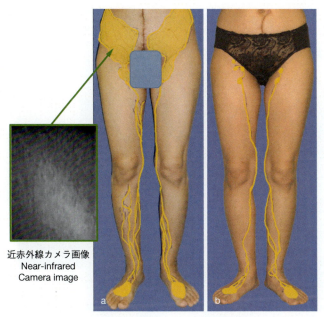

Fig. 5-5-4. リンパ節郭清後の経過：リンパ浮腫を発症しなかった症例
Progress after lymph node dissection : Case in which lymphedema did not develop

a：リンパ節郭清後1週間のリンパ流。下腹部から鼠径部にかけてICGの均一な貯留を認める。
b：リンパ節郭清後2ヵ月のリンパ流。正常化した。
a：Lymph flow seen one week postoperatively. Uniformly pooling of ICG was observed from the pubic region to the thighs.
b：Lymph flow seen at two months postoperatively. Lymph flow has normalized.

I. Early diagnosis of lymphography

Lymphedema was once considered to be an incurable condition without an effective treatment. Even with conservative treatment, lymphedema gradually progresses and patients may develop Stewart-Treves syndrome, a fatal angiosarcoma.

However, there are some patients that after lymphaticovenous anastamosis (LVA) go on to recover fully from their lymphedema without the need for further compression therapy. At this time, it is difficult to detect lymphedema at an early stage, because a diagnostic criterion of lymphedema has not yet been established. When the symptoms of lymphedema and increasing extremity circumferences are clinically apparent, the disease has progressed and unfortunately irreversible changes in lymphatic structures have occurred. In order to prevent this, it is necessary to establish a protocol for early diagnosis in order to identify patients with asymptomatic to mild forms of lymphedema such that treatment can be initiated prior to further progression of the disease. At our institution, we utilize indocyanine green (ICG) lymphography for early diagnosis.

1．**Staging classification**：There are several staging classifications of lymphedema. In our protocol, we use the International Society of Lymphology (ISL) (see **Table 4-3-1**). Early stage is considered stage 0-Ⅰ. It is important to detect and treat the patient in stage 0 who have no symptoms but are prone to develop refractory lymphedema in the future.

2．**Patients**：Patients were considered high-risk or developing lymphedema due to their prior surgical

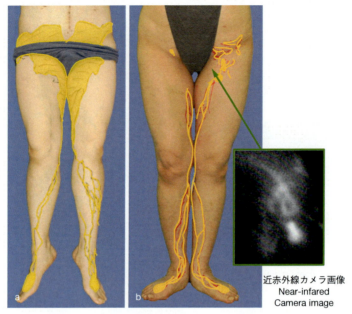

Fig. 5-5-5. リンパ節郭清後の経過：リンパ浮腫を発症した症例
Progress after lymph node dissection：Case in which lymphedema did develop
 a：リンパ節郭清後1週間のリンパ流。下腹部から鼠径部にかけてICGの均一な貯留を認める。
 b：リンパ節郭清後3ヵ月のリンパ流。Dermal Backflowが出現した。
 a：Lymph flow seen one week postoperatively. Uniformly pooling of ICG was observed from the pubic region to the thighs.
 b：Lymph flow seen at three months postoperatively. Dermal Backflow is present.

history(tumorectomy with lymphadenectomy in breast, gynecological or prostate cancer).

 3. Procedure：ICG is subcutaneously injected. After 4 hours, images are acquired using an infrared camera system (Photodynamic Eye, Hamamatsu Photonics, K. K., Hamamatsu, Japan). Lymph vessels observed through the camera are directly marked on the skin using a pen and photographed. These examinations are performed one week and one month after surgery, every month thereafter, every three months from postoperative month 6, and every six months from postoperative year 1. It is crucial to keep a close follow up, because lymphedema tend to develop within six months of the operation(**Fig. 5-5-1**).

 4. Diagnosis：As previous chapters have shown, observations of ICG lymphography change with progression of lymphedema. Immediately after the operation, most patients were swollen from the pubic region to the thighs(**Fig. 5-5-2, 3**). In the same area, ICG pooling is observed. However, this phase is transient and swelling improves in just a few months(**Fig. 5-5-4**). In some patients, "Dermal Backflow" appears even after swelling has improved(**Fig. 5-5-5**). This represents abnormal lymphatic circulation which with early treatment may be reversible.

 5. Early treatment：When lymphedema can be diagnosed early and the symptoms are mild, conservative treatments in the form of compression garments are utilized. However, given the pathophysiology of lymphedema, the disease progresses resulting in irreversible changes. If collateral pathways are surgically made by LVAs in early lymphedema, the likelihood of cure increases(**Fig. 5-5-6**).

 6. Summarization：Our method using ICG lymphography for diagnosis of early lymphedema can be used

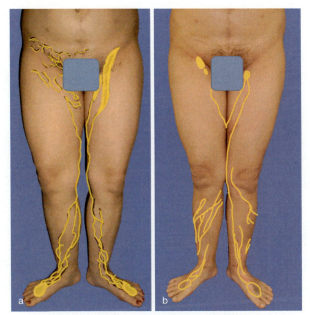

Fig. 5-5-6. 早期にLVAを施行し、完治した症例
Case in which LVA was performed early

a：リンパ節郭清後6ヵ月。Dermal Backflowが出現しリンパ浮腫と診断されたため、LVAを施行した。
b：リンパ節郭清後8ヵ月（LVA後2ヵ月）。Dermal Backflowは消失し、リンパ浮腫は完治した。
a：Lymph flow seen six months after lymph node dissection. Dermal Backflow is present. The patient developed lymphedema and LVA was subsequently performed.
b：Lymph flow seen two months after LVA. Dermal Backflow has disappeared and the patient recovered fully from lymphedema.

except for postoperative patients and become conductive to early treatment.

II 予測・予防

　続発性リンパ浮腫の危険因子をもつ患者には、十分な患者教育と自己ケアによってリンパ浮腫発症の予防を図らなくてはならない。最近では、リンパ節郭清を伴う乳癌や子宮癌の手術と同時に予防的リンパ管吻合術を行い、その良好な成績が報告されている。したがって、リンパ浮腫を高率で発症する手術を行う場合は、予防的リンパ管静脈吻合術を行うことを検討してもよいかも知れない。

　しかし、すべての患者に予防的に手術を行うことは困難である。続発性リンパ浮腫を発症するかどうかは生まれつきのリンパ側副路の発達によると考えられている。そのため、リンパ節郭清術を行う前の段階でスクリーニング検査を行い、リンパ浮腫を発症する可能性の高いものを見つけることが望ましい。このように、リンパ浮腫も他の多くの疾患と同様にスクリーニングに基づ

いて予防を行うことが理想的である。
　スクリーニングは、低侵襲で簡便であることが望ましい。リンパ流およびリンパ浮腫の評価方法には、リンパシンチグラフィやCTなどがあるが、ICG蛍光リンパ管造影法はこの条件を最も満たしている。ここでは、ICG蛍光リンパ管造影法を用いた、リンパ節郭清前におけるリンパ流が不良例のスクリーニング法を提示する。

1．方　法

リンパ節郭清前にICGリンパ管造影法を行う。ICG注射後4時間のリンパ流を評価する。

2．評　価

　リンパ流が正常なものはICGが鼠径部まで流れているのを確認できる。しかし、リンパ流が不良なものはICGが膝下までにとどまるというリンパ流の滞りを認める（**Fig. 5-5-7**）。このような症例は高率でリンパ浮腫を発症するため、予防的にリンパ管静脈吻合術を行うよい適応である。

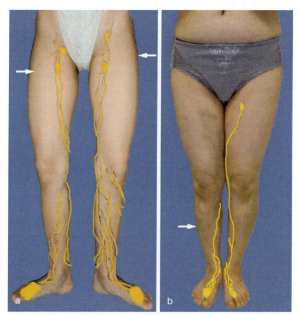

Fig. 5-5-7．ICG蛍光リンパ管造影法によるリンパ浮腫の予測
Prediction of development of lymphedema using ICG lymphography
術前にICG蛍光リンパ管造影法を施行した。
　a：リンパ流良好な症例。両鼠径部までのリンパ流を確認することができる。
　b：リンパ流不良な症例。リンパ流が膝下までにとどまる。
ICG lymphography was performed prior to lymph node dissection.
　a：In normal lymphatics, flow reaches the inguinal.
　b：In abnormal lymphatics, flow reaches only to below the knee.

3. まとめ

リンパ節郭清前にリンパ流が悪いと判断された症例では、リンパ節郭清と同時もしくは時間を空けず、予防的にリンパ管静脈吻合術を行うよい適応となりうる。

このスクリーニング法で陽性とならなかったものでも、リンパ浮腫となるものがある。これは、術後の放射線療法やリンパ節郭清手技などに左右されている可能性がある。そのため、たとえ術前のリンパ流が正常であってもリンパ節郭清後は定期的にICGリンパ管造影法を行い、リンパ浮腫を早期診断することが望ましい。

（大島　梓）

II. Prediction of development of lymphedema

High risk patients need to be educated about their disease and the importance of utilizing compression garments. Patients need to understand that despite conservative treatments, surgical intervention may be necessary to halt the progression of lymphedema. Recently in our institution, LVA is performed simultaneously in cases of tumorectomy with lymph node dissection, with the aim of lymphedema prevention. Although a small number of cases were performed, the long term results are excellent.

In terms of screening for lymphedema, ICG lymphography is a non-invasive and simple method and reveals more information regarding lymphatic flow than lymph scintigraphy and computed tomography (CT). Consequently our protocol utilizes ICG lymphography as a preoperative screening tool to predict the development of lymphedema after surgery.

1. Methods：ICG lymphography is performed before surgery. About 4 hours after injection of ICG, images of lymphatic flow are recorded and evaluated.

2. Evaluation：In normal lymphatic, flow reaches the inguinal region within 4 hours after injection of ICG. In abnormal lymphatics, flow reaches only below the knee at 4 hours after injection (**Fig. 5-5-7**). This signifies a higher possibility of developing of lymphedema postoperatively. As such we might consider performing LVA as a preventive measure.

3. Summarization：Poor lymph flow before lymph node dissection is another indication for LVA in conjunction with or shortly after dissection.

Some patients who were categorized as low risk subsequently developed lymphedema. This may be due to postoperative radiotherapy and the technique utilized for lymph node dissection. Therefore, even if normal lymph flow is identified before operation, it is preferable that ICG lymphography is regularly performed for early diagnosis of lymphedema after lymph node dissection.

(*Azusa Oshima*)

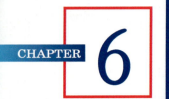

治療方針・適応
Treatment plan and indication
1. 二次性リンパ浮腫の治療方針
Management of secondary lymphedema

Ⅰ 二次性リンパ浮腫の病態

　二次性リンパ浮腫は手術・放射線・感染・外傷などによりリンパ流が閉塞することで発症する閉塞性リンパ浮腫である。リンパ流閉塞が原因となり、リンパ流うっ滞および内圧上昇が生じ、集合リンパ管が拡張する。リンパ管の拡張によりリンパ管内の弁不全をきたすようになり、逆行性リンパ流が生じる。逆行性リンパ流により前集合リンパ管・毛細リンパ管などの末梢リンパ管にも負荷がかかるようになり、リンパ管硬化・漏出をきたして間質にリンパ液が貯留しリンパ浮腫が顕在化する。貯留した蛋白に富んだリンパ液は間質に脂肪沈着をきたし不可逆的な形態変化を生じる。また、免疫細胞を含むリンパのうっ滞は局所免疫異常を生じ、蜂窩織炎などの炎症をきたし、患部の線維化を進行させる。末期には著しい形態変形と皮膚線維化を伴う象皮症となり、長期罹患により脈管肉腫をきたすこともある（Stewart-Treves 症候群）。

　最も重要な点は進行性であることである。圧迫療法により浮腫の進行が抑えられているようにみえてもリンパ循環の異常は徐々に増悪し、ある時期に急速に浮腫が増悪する、というリスクが常にある。リンパ管細静脈吻合術（LVA）や血管柄付きリンパ節移植術（LNT）などのリンパ循環を改善する治療を行った場合は、浮腫の進行が完全に制御され圧迫療法が不要となる"完治"の可能性があるが、基本的には生涯にわたり圧迫療法が必要となる。

I. Pathophysiology of secondary lymphedema

　Secondary lymphedema is obstructive lymphedema due to lymph flow obstruction caused by surgery, irradiation, infection, and trauma. Lymph flow obstruction leads to lymph congestion and lymphatic hypertension, which results in dilatation of collecting lymphatic vessels. Valves in dilated vessels become insufficient, and retrograde lymph flows take place. Lymphatic valvular insufficiency and retrograde flow cause dilatation of peripheral vessels, such as lymphatic precollectors and capillaries, and subsequent lymphosclerosis and lymph extravasation; at this time, edema becomes evident. Interstitial protein-rich lymph provokes fat deposition and results in irreversible morphological changes. Furthermore, congestion of lymph with immune cells leads to local immune abnormality, inflammation such as cellulitis, and tissue fibrosis. Finally, lymphedema causes elephantiasis with prominent morphology change and skin fibrosis, and some develop angiosarcoma (Stewart-Treves syndrome) with a very long history of lymphedema.

　Secondary lymphedema, the most importantly, is progressive in nature. Even if edema seems under control of compression therapy, lymph circulation does become worse gradually, and there is a risk of exacerbation of edema to occur suddenly at some point. Basically, life-long compression therapy is necessary. However, there would be a chance of "lymphedema cure" after physiological surgeries such as LVA and LNT, which represents complete control of lymphedema progression without maintenance compression.

Ⅱ 二次性リンパ浮腫の診断と重症度評価

リンパ節郭清や放射線照射などを伴うがん治療など、原因と考えられる機転が明らかであれば診断は比較的容易であるが、まずは静脈疾患など他の浮腫性疾患を除外することが必要である。他の浮腫性疾患が除外されリンパ流閉塞の原因となる機転が明らかであれば二次性リンパ浮腫と診断することも可能であるが、リンパ循環を精査しリンパ流閉塞に伴う所見があることを確認することが望ましく、また、最適な治療を提供するうえでもリンパ循環動態に基づいた重症度評価を行った方がよい。

リンパ循環の評価法としては、直接的リンパ管造影、リンパシンチグラフィ、SPECT/CT、MR および CT リンパ管造影、ICG リンパ管造影などがある。直接的リンパ管造影は、小切開からリンパ管にカニュレーションして造影剤を直接リンパ管内に注入して、X 線撮影することでリンパ管を造影する方法である。近年は単純 X 線ではなく CT を用いて撮影することで 3 次元的な評価も可能であるが、造影剤そのものにリンパ管を閉塞させる作用があるため基本的にはリンパ浮腫の評価としては用いられておらず、リンパ漏・乳び漏の診断・治療として使用されている。リンパシンチグラフィは最も標準的な評価法とされている検査法で、RI を皮下注射して骨シンチグラフィなどと同様の装置で撮像するものである。全身の深部リンパ流まで評価できるが、画像が粗く小さい組織（陰部・乳房・顔面など）の評価には不向きであり、読影者により評価が異なりやすいといった難点がある。SPECT/CT は同様に RI を皮下注射して撮像するが、CT のように 3 次元の評価が可能であり、最も詳細なリンパ流の評価ができる検査と考えられる。しかしながら、被曝線量も多くなるためルーチンのフォロー検査としては不適切である。MR リンパ管造影も 3 次元で詳細なリンパ流の評価が可能だが、造影剤の皮下注射による皮膚壊死のリスクがあること、および、1 回の撮像では限られた範囲しか撮像できないため広範囲の評価には長時間かかることが難点である。3 テスラの MR 装置であれば、造影剤なしでもリンパ管の描出が可能なこともあるが、0.3 mm 程度の細いリンパ管の描出は困難である。

ICG リンパ管造影は低侵襲に被曝なくリアルタイムに最も鮮明に浅リンパ流を可視化する検査法である。ICG を皮下注射してハンディタイプの近赤外線カメラで観察するのみであり、他の検査法と異なり手術中にも使用できるため手術のナビゲーションとしても重宝されている（**Fig. 6-1-1**）。ICG 注射によるアレルギーのリスクがあり、体表から 2 cm 以上深部のリンパ流を直接的には観察できないといったデメリットがあるが、陰部・顔面など小組織でも詳細にリンパ循環の評価が可能で（**Fig. 6-1-2**）、予後および治療効果の予測に有用な上肢・下肢・陰部・顔面の重症度分類が開発されており、臨床的には最も有用性が高い（**Table 6-1-1**）。ICG リンパ管造影所見は、リンパ流閉塞直後は Linear パターンであるが、逆行性リンパ流により末梢のリンパ管が拡張すると Splash パターンを呈し、リンパ管硬化やリンパ液の漏出が生じると Stardust パターン、高度のリンパ管硬化・リンパ液漏出・組織の線維化が生じると Diffuse パターンに変化していく（**Fig. 5-4-1**、135 頁参照）。ICG リンパ管造影所見をもとに病態生理的な重症度分類 DB stage が診断できる（Chap. 4-3、5-4 参照）。

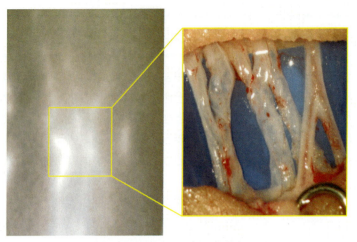

Fig. 6-1-1. ICGリンパ管造影による手術のナビゲーション
ICG lymphography-navigated surgery

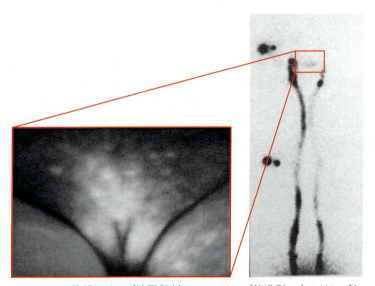

Fig. 6-1-2. 陰部のリンパ流評価（左：ICGリンパ管造影、右：リンパシンチグラフィ）
Evaluation of genital lymph flows using ICG lymphography (left), and lymphoscintigraphy (right)

II. Diagnosis and severity staging of secondary lymphedema

Edematous diseases other than lymphedema, especially venous edema such as deep venous thrombosis and varix, should be ruled out first. It is relatively easy to diagnose lymphedema when other edematous diseases are ruled out and there is a causative condition of lymph flow obstruction such as after lymph node dissection or therapeutic radiation against cancer. It is important and recommended to confirm abnormal lymph circulation with lymph flow imaging and to evaluate severity based on lymphodynamics.

There are several methods for evaluation of lymph circulation, including direct lymphangiography, lymphoscintigraphy, SPECT/CT, MR/CT lymphography, and ICG lymphography. In direct lymphangiogra-

Table 6-1-1. 各部位のリンパ浮腫評価に有用な病態生理的重症度評価
Pathophysiological severity evaluation systems for various parts of lymphedema

	ADB	LDB	FDB	GDB
Stage 0	DB（－）	DB（－）	DB（－）	DB（－）
Stage I	腋窩 Axilla Splash	鼠径部 Groin Splash	顎下部 Submandibular Splash	鼠径部 Groin Splash
Stage II	肘まで To elbows Stardust（＋）	膝まで To knees Stardust（＋）	顎下のみ Only submandibular Stardust（＋）	下腹部のみ Only lower abdomen Stardust（＋）
Stage III	肘より先も Beyond elbows Stardust（＋＋）	膝より先も Beyond knees Stardust（＋＋）	顔面も Face too Stardust（＋＋）	陰部も Genital area too Stardust（＋＋）
Stage IV	上肢全域 All upper extremities Stardust（＋＋＋）	下肢全域 All lower extremities Stardust（＋＋＋）	頭頸部全域 All head and neck Stardust（＋＋＋）	Diffuse
Stage V	Diffuse	Diffuse	Diffuse	－

phy, a lymphatic vessel is cannulated via a small skin incision and contrast medium is injected to visualize lymphatics with X-ray or CT；CT lymphangiography allows 3D evaluation. However, contrast medium itself causes lymphatic vessel's obstruction, and lymphangiography is only applied to diagnosis and treatment for lymphorrhea or chylorrhea. Lymphoscintigraphy is considered a gold standard for lymphedema evaluation, allowing systemic deep lymph flow evaluation. However, the images are obscure and not suitable for evaluation of small regions such as the genitalia, the breast, and the face, and interrater variability cannot be ignored. SPECT/CT allows the most precise evaluation of lymph circulation with 3D images, although not suitable for routine follow evaluation because of a large amount of radiation exposure. MR lymphography also allows 3D lymph flow evaluation, but contrast medium for MR lymphography can cause skin necrosis at the injection site. Another disadvantage is that it takes a long time when the region of interest is wide. When using a 3 Tesla MR device, lymphatic vessels can be visualized without contrast enhancement, but 0.3 mm or smaller lymphatic vessels are hardly visualized even with the 3 Tesla MR device.

ICG lymphography allows the clearest visualization of superficial lymph flows in real-time without radiation exposure. After subcutaneous injection of ICG, the image can be obtained using a handheld near-infrared camera. ICG lymphography is useful to navigate lymphatic surgery (**Fig. 6-1-1**). Although there is a risk of allergic reaction to ICG and lymphatic flow deeper than 2 cm from the body surface cannot be visualized, ICG lymphography enables precise evaluation of small regions such as the genitalia and the face (**Fig. 6-1-2**). Pathophysiological severity staging systems for arm, leg, genital, and facial lymphedema have been developed, that are useful to predict prognosis and results of therapeutic interventions (**Table 6-1-1**). ICG lymphography is considered the most useful clinical lymph imaging modality. Lymphography pattern changes from Linear pattern to Splash pattern when peripheral lymphatics are dilated, to Stardust pattern when lymphosclerosis and lymph extravasation take place, and finally to Diffuse pattern when lymphosclerosis, extravasation, and fibrosis are severe (see Chap. 4-5 & **Fig. 5-4-1**).

Ⅲ 二次性リンパ浮腫の治療戦略

二次性リンパ浮腫の治療の要は圧迫療法であり、リンパ浮腫の診断が確定したらまず行われる

治療である。しかしながら、圧迫療法では"リンパ流閉塞"という原因は解消されず、発症前の圧迫療法による予防効果はなく、対症療法であるため生涯にわたる治療を要する。また、進行性で圧迫療法抵抗例も少なくなく、さらなる外科治療が必要となることが多い。古典的な減量術やリンパ流再建術は侵襲が大きく効果も不安定であったため廃れていった。現在は、LVA、LNT、脂肪吸引(LS)が主に施行されている。

LVAは局所浸潤麻酔下で2cm程度の皮膚切開から施行可能な最も低侵襲な外科治療であり、まず最初に考慮される手術療法である。脂肪層(通常、浅筋膜下の深脂肪層)にある集合リンパ管を近傍の細い静脈に内皮同士が接合するように文字どおり吻合する。うっ滞したリンパを静脈系にバイパスする手術で、もともとリンパ系は静脈角で静脈系に流入しており生理的な再建術である。1990年代頃までに頻繁に行われていた古典的リンパ管静脈吻合術も生理的なリンパ流再建術ではあるが、LVAとは異なり内皮ではない組織が静脈内に露出するため血栓形成率が高く廃れてしまった。LVAでは細い静脈を用いるため、圧が低く静脈内に弁を有し逆流の可能性が低いこと、内皮同士が接合するように吻合されているため、仮に吻合部に静脈逆流をきたしても血栓形成を防げるといった利点がある(**Fig. 6-1-3**)。リンパ管は0.5mm前後であり、スーパーマイクロサージャリーの技術が不可欠である。浮腫容積減少、圧迫療法の軽減・解除、蜂窩織炎の予防といった効果があるが、重症例ではリンパ管硬化によりバイパス効果が低減するため早期での施行が望ましい。

LNTは健常部よりリンパ節を含む組織を血管柄付きで採取し、患部に血管吻合して移植する方法である。移植されたリンパ組織は患部の周囲組織との間にリンパ管新生を生じることで、患部のうっ滞したリンパを移植リンパ節内まで吸収し、リンパ節内のリンパ静脈シャントを介して栄養静脈に流れ、吻合静脈を通して静脈系にドレナージされる。LVAと同様にリンパ循環を改善するリンパ流再建術に分類され、浮腫容積減少、圧迫療法軽減・解除、蜂窩織炎予防といった効果がある。移植リンパ節に吸収されたリンパ液の半分程度は輸出リンパ管に流れるため、可能な限り輸出リンパ管も近傍の静脈などに吻合することが望ましい(**Fig. 6-1-4**)。LVAが効きづらいリンパ管硬化が著しい進行例でも効果が期待できるが、通常全身麻酔が必要であり、採取部のリンパ浮腫をきたすリスクがある。血管吻合のみの移植であればスーパーマイクロサージャリーは

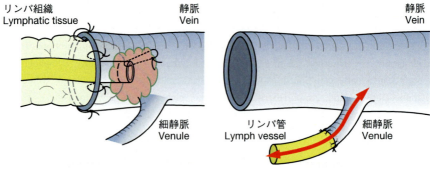

Fig. 6-1-3. 古典的リンパ管静脈吻合術(左)とスーパーマイクロサージャリーによるリンパ管細静脈吻合術(右)
Classical lymphaticovenous anastomosis (left) and supermicrosurgical lymphaticovenular anastomosis (right)

不要で技術的には LVA よりも容易であるが、輸出リンパ管を吻合する場合はリンパ節弁の挙上の時点で輸出リンパ管を剥離同定しておかなければならず LVA よりも技術的ハードルが高い。

LS は直接的に浮腫組織の脂肪を除去する方法で、即効性のある確実な容積減少効果を有するが、LVA・LNT と異なりリンパ循環は改善しない。むしろ、脂肪とともにリンパ組織も除去されるため、注意して施行しないと LS 術後にリンパ循環が悪化することとなる。主な適応はリンパのドレナージ能が廃絶した進行例となるが、LVA・LNT と組み合わせて施行することも可能である。LS 術後は強固な圧迫療法が不可欠であり、圧迫療法を怠ると 100％再増悪をきたす。圧迫療法を軽減・解除することは不可能で、蜂窩織炎予防効果も乏しい。通常、全身麻酔下に施行され、駆血下もしくはツメセント下に行われる。技術的には最も容易で再現性も高いが、出血・感染・皮膚壊死・静脈血栓・脂肪塞栓などのリスクがある。

各手術には欠点と利点があり、適応については各症例において十分に検討する必要がある（Table 6-1-2）。適応の判断には ICG リンパ管造影による重症度分類が有用である（Table 5-4-1、

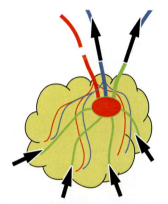

移植されたリンパ節はリンパ管新生により周囲のリンパを吸収
Transplanted LN drains lymph via lymphangiogenesis

吸収されたリンパはリンパ節の栄養静脈および輸出リンパ管より排出
Drained lymph flows into the nutrient vein and the efferent lymphatic vessel

Fig. 6-1-4. 血管柄付きリンパ節移植術によるリンパのドレナージ
Lymph drainage by vascularized lymph node transfer

Table 6-1-2. 各種外科治療の利点と欠点
Advantages and disadvantages of lymphatic surgeries

	LVA	LNT	LS
麻酔 Anesthesia	局所麻酔 Local infiltration	全身麻酔 General	全身麻酔 General
皮切 Incision	小さい 2 cm	長め 7 cm	最小 3 mm
入院期間 Hospitalization	0～7 日 Outpatient OK	3～14 日 About 1 week	1～7 日 About 3 days
リスク Risks	アレルギーのみ Allergy only	ドナーリンパ浮腫ほか Donor lymphedema, etc	血栓・脂肪塞栓ほか Embolism, etc
容積減少 Volume reduction	○ 可能 Possible	○ 可能 Possible	◎ 即効性 Immediate
リンパ循環改善 Circ. Improvement	○ 可能 Possible	◎ 良好 Good	× 不可能 Impossible
術後圧迫の減弱 Compression relief	○ 可能 Possible	○ 可能 Possible	× 不可能 Impossible

143 頁参照）。基本的には、手術による効果・リスクを勘案すると圧迫療法抵抗例では LVA が第一選択と考えられるが、ICG リンパ管造影で DB stage IV/V といった進行例では LVA が効果不十分となる確率も高くなってくるため、初回より LNT や LS を行うといった検討も必要であろう。

Ⅲ. Therapeutic strategy for secondary lymphedema

Compression therapy is a mainstay of secondary lymphedema treatment and should be commenced first after diagnosis of the disease. Since compression therapy is an anti-symptomatic treatment and does not address the cause of secondary lymphedema (lymph flow obstruction), prophylactic compression does not prevent lymphedema development, and compression therapy is required life-long. It is not rare that progressive lymphedema is refractory to compression therapy and requires further surgical treatment. Classical debulking and reconstructive surgeries are abandoned because of high invasiveness and unstable results. Lymphaticovenular anastomosis (LVA), vascularized lymph node transfer (LNT), and liposuction (LS) are currently applied into clinics in lymphedema surgery.

LVA is the least invasive lymphatic surgery, which can be performed via an approximately 2-cm-long skin incision under local anaesthesia, and is considered first for compression-refractory lymphedema. In LVA, a lymphatic vessel in the deep fat layer just under the superficial fascia is anastomosed to a nearby small vein or a venule in an intima-to-intima coaptation manner. LVA diverts congested lymph into venous circulation and is a physiological reconstructive surgery since lymph originally flows into venous circulation at the venous angles. Classical lymphovenous anastomosis is also a physiological surgery but is different from LVA ; in classical anastomosis, lymphatic tissues are inserted into a larger vein, and non-endothelial tissue is exposed into the venous lumen, which has a significantly higher risk of thrombosis formation. In LVA, a small vein or a venule with an intact valve and lower venous pressure is used and works for prevention of venous reflux, and anastomosis site thrombosis can be prevented even when venous reflux takes place thanks to intima-to-intima coaptation anastomosis (**Fig. 6-1-3**). Although the supermicrosurgical technique is necessary to anastomose 0.5 mm lymphatic vessels, LVA works to reduce lymphedematous volume, to reduce or even eliminate the necessity of maintenance compression, and to prevent cellulitis. Early LVA is preferable because LVA can hardly work for severe lymphedema cases, because less bypass effect can be expected with a sclerotic lymphatic vessel in progressed cases.

LNT is also a physiological lymph reconstruction, in which tissue containing lymph node (s) is harvested and transferred to a lymphedematous region with vascular anastomoses. Lymphangiogenesis takes place between a transferred lymph node flap and the surrounding tissue, and congested lymph is drained into the lymph node via the lymphangiogenesis and then into venous circulation through native lymphovenous shunts within the lymph node and via the anastomosed drainage vein of the lymph node. As LVA does, LNT works to reduce lymphedematous volume, to reduce compression, and to prevent cellulitis. Since approximately half of lymph drained into a lymph node flows into the efferent lymphatic vessel, the efferent lymphatic vessel of a lymph node should be anastomosed to a nearby recipient vessel (usually vein) as possible (**Fig. 6-1-4**). LNT is effective even for LVA-refractory cases with severe lymphosclerosis, but basically requires general anesthesia, and has a risk of donor site lymphedema. Without efferent lymphatic vessel anastomosis (ELVA), LNT is technically easier than LVA, but more difficult when ELVA is performed.

LS directly removes deposit fat, and its effect of volume reduction can be observed immediately after the operation. Unlike LVA and LNT, LS does not improve lymph circulation, and rather deteriorate ; lymphatic tissue is also removed with fat removal. LS is basically indicated for progressed cases with completely dysfunctional lymph drainage ability. LVA and LNT can be concomitantly performed with LS to achieve both volume reduction and improvement of lymph circulation. Strong compression is necessary after LS to maintain reduced volume, and lymphedema shall re-exacerbate once compression is released LS cannot reduce/release compression therapy, and hardly prevent cellulitis. LS is performed usually under general

6-1. 二次性リンパ浮腫の治療方針

anaesthesia with or without tourniquet or tumescent. LS is the easiest surgical treatment for lymphedema and reproducibility is high but has risks of bleeding, infection, skin necrosis, venous thrombosis, and fat embolism.

LVA, LNT, and LS have advantages and disadvantages (**Table 6-1-2**). ICG lymphography can be helpful to consider as an indication of each surgical treatment (see **Table 5-4-1**). Basically, LVA is considered a first-line surgical treatment for compression-refractory lymphedema based on its effectiveness and less invasiveness. However, LNT and/or LS can be an option for primary surgery for progressed lymphedema with DB stage Ⅳ/Ⅴ lymphedema, because LVA is likely to be less effective and not enough to improve the disease's conditions.

■ Ⅳ　不顕性リンパ浮腫の概念と予防的治療

　国際リンパ学会の分類（ISL stage）では、リンパ循環に異常があるものの浮腫が明らかでない状態を ISL stage 0 と定義している。ISL stage におけるリンパ循環評価はリンパシンチグラフィが基準となっており、リンパシンチグラフィで異常を認めない場合はリンパ浮腫でないため ISL stage では定義されていない。しかしながら、リンパシンチグラフィより異常リンパ流の検出感度の高い ICG リンパ管造影では、リンパシンチグラフィ正常例においても Splash パターンや Stardust パターンといった異常所見がみられることがある（**Fig. 4-3-13**、81 頁参照）。浮腫がない状態であっても、Splash パターンを伴う場合（DB stage Ⅰ）、浮腫が顕在化しリンパ浮腫が進行する確率は約 30％程度とされ、Stardust パターンを伴う場合（DB stage Ⅱ）は 90％以上が発症するとされるため、ICG リンパ管造影での異常所見は臨床上極めて重要である。DB stage Ⅰの約 30％は正常（DB stage 0）に改善することがあるが、DB stage Ⅱでは stage 0/Ⅰに改善することがない点も特記すべき特徴である（**Table 6-1-3**）。したがって、ISL stage 0 および ISL stage では定義がない超早期リンパ浮腫は ICG リンパ管造影による重症度分類では DB stage 0/Ⅰ/Ⅱの 3 つのステージに分類され、それぞれ予後が異なっている。

　DB stage 0 は正常所見でリンパ浮腫ではなく、リンパ浮腫発症リスクもほぼないため治療適応はない。DB stage Ⅱはほぼ全例が保存療法に抵抗して進行していくため、早期リンパ浮腫と

Table 6-1-3.　DB stage とリンパ浮腫の進行リスク
Risk of lymphedema progression according to DB stage

	ICG 所見 ICG findings	病態 Clinical condition	予後 Risk of progression
Stage 0	DB なし	リンパ浮腫なし No lymphedema	0〜%
Stage Ⅰ	Splash のみ	不顕性リンパ浮腫 Subclinical lymphedema	10〜40%
Stage Ⅱ	Stardust（＋）	早期リンパ浮腫 Early lymphedema	50〜95%
Stage Ⅲ	Stardust（＋＋）	進行リンパ浮腫 Progressed lymphedema	80〜100%
Stage Ⅳ	Stardust（＋＋＋）		
Stage Ⅴ	Diffuse（＋）		

163

呼ぶべき状態であり低侵襲外科治療であるLVAの適応となる。DB stage Iは一部は保存的に改善して正常になるため不顕性リンパ浮腫と定義され、早期介入による完治のメリットと過治療となるリスクを勘案しなければならない。保存療法による発症前の予防効果が立証されていないことを考慮すると、不顕性リンパ浮腫に対してはICGリンパ管造影による経過観察、もしくはLVAによる予防的介入が検討される。LVAを行う場合であっても、より低侵襲となるようICGリンパ管造影ナビゲーション下にmmレベルの皮膚切開からLVAを行う（最小侵襲リンパ超微小外科 Minimally Invasive Lymphatic Supermicrosurgery；MILS)、もしくは鼠径部1ヵ所の皮膚切開で輸出リンパ管を用いたLVA（輸出リンパ管静脈吻合 Efferent Lymphatic Vessel-to-venous Anastomosis；ELVA）を行うのが好ましい（**Fig. 6-1-5, 6**）。特に、ELVAは最もリンパ流閉塞部位に近い場所でバイパスし、リンパ節機能を温存する術式であり、経過観察に

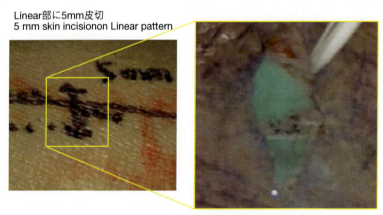

Fig. 6-1-5. 最小侵襲リンパ超微小外科（MILS）
Minimally invasive lymphatic supermicrosurgery（MILS）

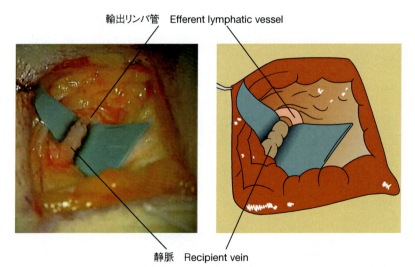

Fig. 6-1-6. 輸出リンパ管静脈吻合（ELVA）
Efferent lymphatic vessel-to-venous anastomosis（ELVA）

比較して完治率が有意に高いことが報告されており、不顕性リンパ浮腫に介入する際の第一選択と考えられる。

（山本　匠、山本奈奈、林　明辰、成島三長）

IV. The concept of subclinical lymphedema and prophylactic treatment

International Society of Lymphology defines a condition of no obvious edema with abnormal circulation on lymphoscintigraphy as ISL stage 0 ; there is no definition of ISL stage for cases where lymphoscintigraphy findings are normal. However, ICG lymphography, more sensitive than lymphoscintigraphy, can detect abnormal lymph circulation such as Splash pattern and Stardust pattern even in cases without abnormal findings on lymphoscintigraphy (see **Fig. 4-3-13**). Even without no findings of edema, patients with Splash pattern (DB stage Ⅰ) have 30% risk of developing progressive lymphedema and 30% possibility of spontaneous (non-surgical, even with compression) improvement to DB stage 0, and patients with Stardust pattern (DB stage Ⅱ) have more than 90% risk of progression and no possibility of spontaneous improvement (**Table 6-1-3**). Thus, differences in ICG lymphography findings are clinically very important to predict patients' prognosis. Very-early lymphedema (ISL stage 0 or earlier) can be subdivided into 3 stages in ICG lymphography-based DB stage, DB stage 0/ Ⅰ / Ⅱ.

In DB stage 0 (normal lymph flow), there is almost no risk of developing lymphedema, and no treatment is indicated. In DB stage Ⅱ, almost all cases will eventually develop progressive lymphedema even with conservative treatments, and thus least invasive surgery (LVA) is indicated for this early lymphedema. In DB stage Ⅰ, some may improve spontaneously, and others may develop progressive lymphedema ; DB stage Ⅰ lymphedema is defined as subclinical lymphedema. For subclinical lymphedema, watchful waiting followed with ICG lymphography, or prophylactic LVA is considered. When LVA is performed, a surgeon should pay attention to minimize morbidity ; ICG lymphography-navigated millimeter-incision LVA (minimally invasive lymphatic supermicrosurgery ; MILS), or efferent lymphatic vessel-to-venous anastomosis (ELVA) is recommended (**Fig. 6-1-5, 6**). Unlike conventional LVA, ELVA can preserve lymph node function, since LVA is performed at the most proximal region to the lymph flow obstruction site and distal to lymph nodes. ELVA has been reported to have higher cure rate compared with watchful waiting and can be considered a first-line surgical treatment for subclinical lymphedema.

(Takumi Yamamoto, Nana Yamamoto, Akitatsu Hayashi, Mitsunaga Narushima)

1) International Society of Lymphology : The diagnosis and treatment of peripheral lymphedema ; 2013 Consensus Document of the International Society of Lymphology. Lymphology 46 (1) : 1-11, 2013.
2) Lee BB, Antignani PL, Baroncelli TA, et al : IUA-ISVI consensus for diagnosis guideline of chronic lymphedema of the limbs. Int Angiol 34 (4) : 311-332, 2015.
3) Yamamoto T, Narushima M, Doi K, et al : Characteristic indocyanine green lymphography findings in lower extremity lymphedema : the generation of a novel lymphedema severity staging system using dermal backflow patterns. Plast Reconstr Surg 127 (5) : 1979-1986, 2011.
4) Yamamoto T, Koshima I : Subclinical lymphedema ; understanding is the clue to decision making. Plast Reconstr Surg 132 (3) : 472e-473e, 2013.
5) Yamamoto T, Yamamoto N, Doi K, et al : Indocyanine green (ICG)-enhanced lymphography for upper extremity lymphedema ; a novel severity staging system using dermal backflow (DB) patterns. Plast Reconstr Surg 128 (4) : 941-947, 2011.
6) Yamamoto T, Matsuda N, Doi K, et al : The earliest finding of indocyanine green (ICG) lymphography in asymptomatic limbs of lower extremity lymphedema patients secondary to cancer treatment : the modified dermal backflow (DB) stage and concept of subclinical lymphedema. Plast Reconstr Surg 128 (4) : 314e-321e, 2011.

7) Yamamoto T, Yamamoto N, Yoshimatsu H, et al：Indocyanine green lymphography for evaluation of genital lymphedema in secondary lower extremity lymphedema patients. J Vasc Surg：Venous and Lym Dis 1(4)：400-405, 2013.

8) Yamamoto T, Narushima M, Yoshimatsu H, et al：Indocyanine green velocity；Lymph transportation capacity deterioration with progression of lymphedema. Ann Plast Surg 71(5)：591-594, 2013.

9) Yamamoto T, Narushima M, Yoshimatsu H, et al：Dynamic indocyanine green(ICG) lymphography for breast cancer-related arm lymphedema. Ann Plast Surg 73(6)：706-709, 2014.

10) 山本　匠, 山本奈奈, 成島三長, 光嶋　勲：ICG リンパ管造影ガイド下リンパ管細静脈吻合術. 脈管学 52：327-331, 2012

11) 山本　匠, 成島三長, 光嶋　勲：ICG リンパ管造影を用いた下腹部・陰部リンパ浮腫評価. 静脈学 25：43-47, 2014.

12) Szuba A, Cooke JP, Yousuf S, et al：Decongestive lymphatic therapy for patients with cancer-related or primary lymphedema. Am J Med 109：296-300, 2000.

13) Yamamoto T, Narushima M, Kikuchi K, et al：Lambda-shaped anastomosis with intravascular stenting method for safe and effective lymphaticovenular anastomosis. Plast Reconstr Surg 127(5)：1987-1992, 2011.

14) Yamamoto T, Yoshimatsu H, Narushima M, et al：A modified side-to-end lymphaticovenular anastomosis. Microsurgery 33(2)：130-133, 2013.

15) Yamamoto T, Narushima M, Yoshimatsu H, et al：Minimally invasive lymphatic supermicrosurgery (MILS)；indocyanine green lymphography-guided simultaneous multi-site lymphaticovenular anastomoses via millimeter skin incisions. Ann Plast Surg 72(1)：67-70, 2014.

16) Becker C, Assouad J, Riquet M, et al：Postmastectomy lymphedema；long-term results following microsurgical lymph node transplantation. Ann Surg 243(3)：313-315, 2006.

17) Vignes S, Blanchard M, Yannoutsos A, et al：Complications of autologous lymph-node transplantation for limb lymphedema. Eur J Vasc Endovasc Surg 45(5)：516-520, 2013.

18) Yamamoto T, Yoshimatsu H, Narushima M, et al：Sequential anastomosis for lymphatic supermicrosurgery；multiple lymphaticovenular anastomoses on one venule. Ann Plast Surg 73(1)：46-49, 2014.

19) Yamamoto T, Yamamoto N, Azuma S, et al：Near-infrared illumination system-integrated microscope for supermicrosurgical lymphaticovenular anastomosis. Microsurgery 34(1)：23-27, 2014.

20) Brorson H, Svensson H：Liposuction combined with controlled compression therapy reduces arm lymphedema more effectively than controlled compression therapy alone. Plast Reconstr Surg 102：1058-1067, 1998.

21) Yamamoto T, Yamamoto N, Yoshimatsu H, et al：Indocyanine green lymphography for evaluation of genital lymphedema in secondary lower extremity lymphedema patients. J Vasc Surg：Venous and Lym Dis 1(4)：400-405, 2013.

22) Yamamoto T, Iida T, Matsuda N, et al：Indocyanine green (ICG)-enhanced lymphography for evaluation of facial lymphoedema. J Plast Reconstr Aesthet Surg 64(11)：1541-1544, 2011.

23) Yamamoto T, Yoshimatsu H, Narushima M, et al：Split intravascular stents for side-to-end lymphaticovenular anastomosis. Ann Plast Surg 71(5)：538-540, 2013.

24) Yamamoto T, Yamamoto N, Yamashita M, et al：Efferent lymphatic vessel anastomosis(ELVA)；supermicrosurgical efferent lymphatic vessel-to-venous anastomosis for the prophylactic treatment of subclinical lymphedema. Ann Plast Surg 76(4)：424-427, 2016.

CHAPTER 6

治療方針・適応
Treatment plan and indication

2. 原発性リンパ浮腫の治療方針
Management of primary lymphedema

I 原発性リンパ浮腫の病態

　原発性リンパ浮腫はさまざまな病態を含む疾患群で、二次性リンパ浮腫や他の浮腫性疾患の除外診断で診断される。Milroy病における *VEGFR3* などさまざまな原因遺伝子が報告されているが、原因が解明されているのは原発性リンパ浮腫の一部のみで、大部分は孤発性かつ多因子による疾患で病態が明らかになっていない。毛細リンパ管・前集合リンパ管・集合リンパ管・リンパ管内の弁やリンパ節・乳び槽・胸管などさまざまなレベル・部位における無形成・低形成・過形成などの多様な奇形成因と考えられている。奇形の種類・程度・範囲により臨床象は多彩であり、浮腫を伴わないリンパ管奇形(リンパ嚢胞)、血管奇形・リンパ管奇形に合併したリンパ浮腫、明らかな他の奇形を伴わない原因不明のリンパ浮腫など、さまざまなリンパ系の奇形のうち他の浮腫性疾患が除外されリンパ循環異常を伴った浮腫を呈する病態が原発性リンパ浮腫と呼ばれる。

　分類法としては発症年齢による分類が一般的だが、病態には基づいておらず治療方針の参考にならないことも少なくない。各種画像検査を駆使してリンパ系の構造および循環動態を把握することが重要である。基本的には、奇形などによりある部位で(もしくは全身的に)リンパ流が異常となり、その部位およびその末梢領域にリンパうっ滞を生じることでリンパ浮腫を発症するものと考えられる。成因は異なるが、リンパ流閉塞が原因である場合は病態・治療方針共に二次性リンパ浮腫に準じたものとなる。

I. Pathophysiology of primary lymphedema

　Primary lymphedema is a category of diseases including a variety of etiologies, and is diagnosed by excluding other edematous diseases. Although genetic mutations are reported to be causes of some primary lymphedema such as *VEGFR3* gene for Milroy disease, majority of primary lymphedemas are sporadic and multifactorial, and their pathogeneses are yet to be clarified. Various malformations are considered causes of primary lymphedema, and there are a wide variety of clinical manifestations according to severity, type, and distribution of malformation. Edematous diseases with lymph malformation and lymph flow abnormality in which other edematous diseases are excluded are called primary lymphedema. Classification according to onset age (congenital lymphedema, lymphedema precox, and lymphedema tarda) is the most common, but does not address pathophysiology of the disease. It is important to elucidate pathophysiology using various imaging tests. Symptom of primary lymphedema manifests by lymph congestion in and distal to malformation site (s). Although pathology is different, primary lymphedema due to lymph flow obstruction is similarly evaluated and treated to secondary lymphedema.

Ⅱ 原発性リンパ浮腫の診断と ICG リンパ管造影分類

　原発性リンパ浮腫の診断は、まず浮腫をきたしうる疾患・病態を除外していくことから始まる。問診により外傷・感染・薬剤・月経・遺伝疾患による浮腫を、身体所見・胸部 X 線写真・血液検査により心不全・肝硬変・ネフローゼ・腎不全・低蛋白血症・内分泌疾患を、超音波検査により深部静脈血栓・静脈瘤を、CT・MRI などにより悪性疾患による二次性リンパ浮腫を除外する。これらの精査によっても原因が不明な浮腫が原発性リンパ浮腫と呼ばれるが、リンパ浮腫と確定診断するためにはリンパ循環の評価が不可欠であり、リンパシンチグラフィや ICG リンパ管造影により評価される。リンパシンチグラフィではリンパ逆流やトレーサーの取り込み・移動速度の低下などさまざまな異常所見が報告されている。深部のリンパ流も評価できる最も基本的なリンパ流評価法であるが、臨床上有用な分類方法は報告されていない。後述のとおり、ICG リンパ管造影では特徴的な所見に基づいた分類法が報告されており、治療適応の判断材料となりうる。MR リンパ管造影や SPECT/CT など新しい検査方法の臨床使用例も報告されており、これらは深部リンパ流や構造を 3 次元的に評価できるため、病態の把握に極めて有用と考えられる。原発性リンパ浮腫の分類法は報告されていないため、今後の研究が待たれる。

　原発性リンパ浮腫における ICG リンパ管造影の感度・特異度は極めて高く、症候性である下肢リンパ浮腫に対してはいずれも 100%である。また、原発性リンパ浮腫の特徴的な ICG リンパ管造影所見が明らかにされており、原発性リンパ浮腫は ICG リンパ管造影所見から、proximal DB（PDB）パターン、distal DB（DDB）パターン、less enhancement（LE）パターン、no enhancement（NE）パターンの 4 群に分類される（**Fig. 6-2-1**）。PDB パターンは近位から DB パターンが遠位に拡大していくもので、中枢でのリンパ流閉塞をきたすリンパ管・リンパ節の低・無形成などが原因と考えられる。DDB パターンでは、下腿など末梢のみに DB パターンを認めるもので、末梢でのリンパ流閉塞が原因と考えられ蜂窩織炎を頻発する例が多い。LE パターンでは末梢のみに Linear パターンを認め、中枢のリンパ節が造影されず DB パターンも認めない。NE パターンでは Linear パターンも DB パターンもみられないまったく造影されない所見で、重度の低形成・無形成・吸収障害が原因と考えられる（Chap. 4-3 参照）。

II. Diagnosis and classification of primary lymphedema

　Diagnosis of primary lymphedema starts from ruling out other edematous diseases. History taking, physical examinations, chest-X-ray, blood tests, ultrasound, CT, and/or MRI are used to rule out drug-induced edema, menstrual edema, heart failure, liver cirrhosis, nephrosis, renal failure, endocrine disorders, hypoproteinemia, deep vein thrombosis, varix, and malignant diseases involving lymphatic systems. Then, lymph circulation is evaluated with lymph imaging tests such as lymphoscintigraphy and ICG lymphography to confirm the diagnosis of primary lymphedema. Lymphoscintigraphy may show various abnormalities such as dermal backflow and impaired uptake and/or movement of the tracer. Although the most basic evaluation methods to visualize superficial and deep lymph flows, lymphoscintigraphy lacks clinically useful classification for primary lymphedema. As described later, ICG lymphography is useful to classify primary lymphedema, which can be applied in decision making for primary lymphedema management. New methods such as MR lymphography and SPECT/CT have been developed to evaluate lymphedema, which allows three-dimensional evaluations of deep lymph flows and structures. Although considered the most precise

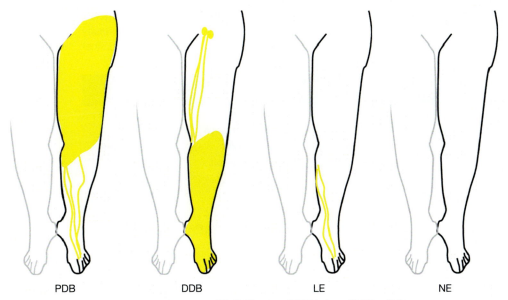

Fig. 6-2-1. ICG リンパ管造影による原発性リンパ浮腫の分類
ICG lymphography classification for primary lymphedema

methods to evaluate lymph flows and structures, MR lymphography and SPECT/CT lacks classification of primary lymphedema, and further studies are warranted.

ICG lymphography has an extremity high sensitivity/specificity for diagnosis of primary lymphedema, especially regarding symptomatic leg lymphedema ; both are 100%. Characteristic findings of primary lymphedema on ICG lymphography have been clarified. Primary lymphedema is classified into 4 patterns ; proximal DB (PDB) pattern, distal DB (DDB) pattern, less enhancement (LE) pattern, and no enhancement (NE) pattern (**Fig. 6-2-1**). In PDB pattern, DB pattern extends distally from a proximal obstruction site due to lymphatic hypoplasia/aplasia. In DDB pattern, DB pattern is seen only in the distal region and not in the proximal region. Cellulitis is usually associated, and would affect its pathophysiology. In LE pattern, Linear pattern is seen only in the distal region, and there is no DB pattern or enhanced lymph nodes in the proximal region. In NE pattern, there is no enhanced image such as Linear pattern nor DB pattern, resulting from severe hypoplasia/aplasia or malabsorption (see Chap. 4-3).

III 原発性リンパ浮腫の治療戦略

まずは確実な診断が治療開始には不可欠であり、静脈性浮腫や隠れた悪性腫瘍による二次性リンパ浮腫を見逃してはならない。原発性リンパ浮腫の診断が確定した場合は、二次性リンパ浮腫と同様にまず圧迫療法を開始する。圧迫療法に抵抗する場合は外科治療を検討するが、手術方法の選択においては現在のところ ICG 分類が最も有用と考えられる (**Table 6-2-1**)。PDB パターン・DDB パターンでは二次性リンパ浮腫と同様に閉塞性リンパ浮腫であるため、うっ滞したリンパを減圧するリンパ管細静脈吻合術 (LVA) が効果的と考えられる。リンパ管硬化が著しくバイパス効果が見込めない、もしくは LVA で効果が不十分な場合はリンパ節移植が検討される。一

Table 6-2-1. ICGリンパ管造影分類と原発性リンパ浮腫の病態と治療
Pathophysiology and suggested treatments of primary lymphedema according to ICG lymphography classification

ICG分類 ICG classification	病態 Pathophysiology	治療 Treatment
PDBパターン	近位での閉塞 Proximal obstruction	リンパ静脈吻合 LVA
DDBパターン	遠位での閉塞 Distal obstruction	リンパ静脈吻合 LVA
LEパターン	ポンプ不全など Pump failure, etc	厳格な圧迫 Strict compression
NEパターン	無形成・吸収不全など Aplasia, malabsorption, etc	リンパ節移植 LNT

方、LEパターンでは閉塞機序が明らかではなく、通常は浮腫も軽度であるため、厳格な圧迫療法のみでコントロールしていくのが望ましい。しかし、LVAによる治療効果を認める例もあるため、強固な圧迫療法でも効果が乏しい際はLVAを検討してもよい。NEパターンでは無形成の可能性もあり、患部ではリンパ管を認めないことがある。低侵襲なLVAを試験的に行ってもよいが、多くは治療効果が乏しいため、別部位に健常なリンパ節があることを画像検査で確認したうえでリンパ節移植を行う方が効果が見込める。多くは先天性であり、脂肪沈着がメインである場合は、術後の強固な圧迫療法が不可欠であるが脂肪吸引による治療も検討すべきである。

(山本　匠、山本奈奈、林　明辰、成島三長)

III. Therapeutic strategy for primary lymphedema

Definitive diagnosis should be confirmed before the commencement of treatment for primary lymphedema, and venous edema and lymphedema secondary to occult cancer should not be overlooked. After confirmation of diagnosis, compression therapy is performed first for the treatment of primary lymphedema as for secondary lymphedema treatment. Surgical treatments are considered for compression-refractory cases. ICG classification is considered the most useful one to consider optimal surgery for progressive primary lymphedema (**Table 6-2-1**). In PDB pattern and DDB pattern, obstructive mechanism plays an important role in pathophysiology, and LVA is considered effective to decongest stagnated lymph. When lymphosclerosis is severe or LVA is not enough to improve lymphedema in patients with PDB or DDB pattern, LNT can be applied as a further treatment. Since obstructive mechanism is not apparent in LE pattern, rigorous compression therapy is usually effective. In NE pattern, lymphatic vessels suitable for LVA are rarely found because of severe hypoplasia or aplasia, and LNT may be better when there are intact lymph nodes in other regions. Most NE pattern cases are congenital, and liposuction can be applied for cases where the main pathology is fat deposition, although liposuction necessitates postoperative strong compression therapy for a life-long time.

(*Takumi Yamamoto, Nana Yamamoto, Akitatsu Hayashi, Mitsunaga Narushima*)

1) Connell FC, Gordon K, et al : The classification and diagnostic algorithm for primary lymphatic dysplasia ; an update from 2010 to include molecular findings. Clin Genet 84(4) : 303-314, 2013.

6-2. 原発性リンパ浮腫の治療方針

2) Yamamoto T, Narushima M, et al：Characteristic indocyanine green lymphography findings in lower extremity lymphedema；the generation of a novel lymphedema severity staging system using dermal backflow patterns. Plast Reconstr Surg 127(5)：1979-1986, 2011.

3) Yamamoto T, Matsuda N, et al：The earliest finding of indocyanine green (ICG) lymphography in asymptomatic limbs of lower extremity lymphedema patients secondary to cancer treatment；the modified dermal backflow (DB) stage and concept of subclinical lymphedema. Plast Reconstr Surg 128(4)：314e-321e, 2011.

4) Lee BB, Villavicencio JL：Primary lymphoedema and lymphatic malformation；are they the two sides of the same coin? Eur J Vasc Endovasc Surg 39(5)：646-653, 2010.

5) Yamamoto T, Yoshimatsu H, et al：Indocyanine green lymphography findings in primary leg lymphedema. Eur J Vasc Endovasc Surg 49：95-102, 2015.

6) Zhibin Y, Quanyong L, Libo C, et al：The role of radionuclide lymphoscintigraphy in extremity lymphedema. Ann Nucl Med 20：341-344, 2006.

7) Gamba JL, Silverman PM, Ling D, et al：Primary lower extremity lymphedema；CT diagnosis. Radiology 149：218, 1983.

8) Case TC, Witte CL, Witte MH, et al：Magnetic resonance imaging in human lymphedema；comparison with lymphangioscintigraphy. Magn Reson Imaging 10：549-558, 1992.

9) Yamamoto T, Narushima M, et al：Characteristic indocyanine green lymphography findings in lower extremity lymphedema；the generation of a novel lymphedema severity staging system using dermal backflow patterns. Plast Reconstr Surg 127(5)：1979-1986, 2011.

10) Yamamoto T, Yamamoto N, Azuma S, et al：Near-infrared illumination system-integrated microscope for supermicrosurgical lymphaticovenular anastomosis. Microsurgery 34(1)：23-27, 2014.

11) Yamamoto T, Koshima I, Yoshimatsu H, et al：Simultaneous multi-site lymphaticovenular anastomoses for primary lower extremity and genital lymphoedema complicated with severe lymphorrhea. J Plast Reconstr Aesthet Surg 64(6)：812-815, 2011.

12) Yamamoto T, Yamamoto N, Doi K, et al：Indocyanine green (ICG)-enhanced lymphography for upper extremity lymphedema；a novel severity staging system using dermal backflow (DB) patterns. Plast Reconstr Surg 128(4)：941-947, 2011.

13) Yamamoto T, Narushima M, Yoshimatsu H, et al：Minimally invasive lymphatic supermicrosurgery (MILS)；indocyanine green lymphography-guided simultaneous multi-site lymphaticovenular anastomoses via millimeter skin incisions. Ann Plast Surg 72(1)：67-70, 2014.

14) Yamamoto T, Yamamoto N, Numahata T, et al：Navigation lymphatic supermicrosurgery for the treatment of cancer-related peripheral lymphedema. Vasc Endovasc Surg 48(2)：139-143, 2014.

171

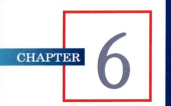

治療方針・適応
Treatment plan and indication

3. 骨盤リンパ嚢胞の治療
Treatment of pelvic lymphocele

I 骨盤リンパ嚢胞とは

1. 定義および病態

　骨盤リンパ嚢胞とは、上皮に覆われていないリンパ液の貯留した嚢胞が、骨盤内に存在したものと定義される。多くは、前立腺癌や婦人科癌などの骨盤部リンパ節郭清を伴うものや、腎移植といった腹腔内手術の術後合併症として発生する。

2. 発生機序

発生機序は、以下のような連鎖により説明される。
①前述の手術で下肢から骨盤内に流入する主たるリンパ経路である深鼠径・外腸骨・閉鎖リンパ節を含むリンパ系が手術的に郭清されることで、下肢からの上行リンパ路が遮断される。
②下肢リンパ系へのリンパ液流入量（生理学的には 2〜4 L/日といわれる）はほぼ変わらないため、代償経路である側副リンパ路に流路が求められるが、側副リンパ路の処理能力が下肢から上行するリンパ流を賄い切れない状態となり、下肢リンパ流のうっ滞が生じる（術後から持続的に賄えない場合もあれば、術後一定期間賄えていたものの感染や加齢によって賄えられなくなる場合もある）。
③うっ滞により、リンパ路内圧の上昇と、リンパ路に流入できなかったリンパ液の間質への貯留が生じる（この貯留状態がリンパ浮腫である）。
④リンパ路内圧の上昇により、手術後閉鎖状態だったリンパ管断端が開放され、腹腔内に流入し、リンパ嚢胞を形成する。

3. 発生頻度

　骨盤リンパ嚢胞の発生頻度としては、1〜49％と、報告によりかなりのばらつきがある。術後の短期間においては、ほぼ必発であるとの報告さえある。これは、術後急激に処理能の増大を求められた側副リンパ路の慣らし期間中に、オーバーフローになってしまったリンパ液が一過性に嚢胞を形成したものと理解される。

I. What is a pelvic lymphocele?

1. The definition and condition：A pelvic lymphocele (PLC) is defined as an abnormal collection of lymph fluid in the pelvic cavity that lacks an epithelial lining. A PLC mainly occurs as a complication of a surgical procedure such as a pelvic lymphadenectomy for gynecologic or prostatic malignancies or a renal transplantation.

2. The mechanism of occurrence：The mechanism of occurrence is explained by the following chain reaction of events：

①Following an operation, as described above, the damage to the deep inguinal, external iliac, and obturator lymph nodes causes the main lymphatic flow pathways from the lower limbs to the pelvic site to be obstructed.

②Because the lymphatic inflow from the lower limbs (estimated to be 2-4 L/day physiologically) is almost constant, the collateral lymphatic flow must compensate for the entire lymphatic inflow. However, the collateral flow is insufficient, as its capability can increase only gradually, thus the lymphatic flow becomes congested.

③This congestion leads to rising lymphatic internal pressure and interstitial accumulation of lymph fluid, which cannot flow into lymph vessels (This condition is known as lymphedema).

④The increasing pressure leads to the re-opening of the lymph vessels' end, which was closed during the operation. From the open end, lymphatic flow drains into the pelvic cavity and forms a PLC.

3. The incidence：The reported incidence of PLC varies widely, from 1-49%. Especially in the acute postoperative phase, some reports have found that a PLC must always occur. This is due to the adaptation period during which the capacity of the collateral pathways slowly increases to accommodate the entire lymphatic flow. During this period immediately post-operation, some of the lymphatic flow cannot be drained, and a temporary PLC forms.

Ⅱ　随伴症状

リンパ嚢胞が小さい場合、特に自覚症状はない。貯留が多くなり、他の臓器を圧迫するようになると諸症状が出現する。具体的には、膀胱圧迫による頻尿・残尿感、下大静脈の圧迫による静脈うっ滞や深部静脈血栓、尿管圧迫による水腎症や尿路感染症といったものである。また、嚢胞感染は、リンパ嚢胞が大きい場合はもちろん、小さくても生じることがある。嚢胞では抗生剤の効果が発現しづらいため、嚢胞感染を繰り返すこともあり、重症化をきたし敗血症に至ることもある。

嚢胞自体が消失したとしても、それは嚢胞へのリンパ液の流入がなくなっただけであり、下肢リンパ流がうっ滞なく排出されるようになったわけではない。実際、骨盤リンパ嚢胞消失後に下肢リンパ浮腫を発症する患者は多く、嚢胞形成経験者の5割程度と報告される。これは、一般的なリンパ浮腫発症率よりも高率である。

Ⅱ. Accompanying symptoms

When PLCs are small enough, there are no symptoms. However, when the PLC is large enough to compress other organs, some symptoms appear, such as urinary frequency and a feeling of residual urine from the compressed bladder, venous congestion and deep venous thrombosis from the compressed vein, and hydronephrosis from the compressed urinary duct. Moreover, an infection can occur in a PLC of any size.

Because antibiotics are less effective for PLCs, such infections can occur repeatedly, and sometimes become severe even to the point of sepsis.

The disappearance of a PLC only means that there is no more inflow into the PLC. PLC disappearance is independent of whether or not the lymphatic pathways from the lower limbs flow smoothly to the pelvic site. Indeed, approximately 50% of PLC patients often develop lymphedema after the PLC disappears. This is higher than the common lymphedema incidence rate.

Ⅲ　既存の治療法について

　無症状の場合は経過観察が第一選択となる。一方、有症状の場合や嚢胞感染が疑われる場合には加療の対象となる。既存の治療法としては、経皮的カテーテル留置が行われることが多い。これは貯留液をドレナージすることでスペースの減少を狙うとともにその間に側副路への流量増加を待つものと理解される。この治療法で80%程度はいったん治癒するが、再発率も80%程度と高く、また穿刺経路からの感染を惹起しうる点で、最善の治療とは言い難い。その他には、硬化剤の注入や流入リンパ管結紮術といった嚢胞への流入を途絶することを目的とした治療法も行われる。これらの治療はすべて、嚢胞に流入していたリンパ液全量を側副リンパ路で代償することが治癒の前提となっている。

　上記とは別機序の治療法としては、開窓術がある。これは、後腹膜に存在する嚢胞を腹腔と交通させることで、腹膜からリンパ液を吸収させるものである。下肢リンパ流の上行経路に腹膜の経路が追加されるため、側副リンパ路の代償能が小さい場合でも有用と考えられるが、次第に開窓部分が腹膜で被覆されて閉鎖されてしまうため、長期的には効果が期待できない、との報告もある。

Ⅲ.　Existing treatment of PLC

When no symptoms are present, a period of observation is the first choice. When one or more symptoms are present or PLC infection is suspected, some treatments are considered. Needle aspiration and percutaneous catheter drainage are commonly used for the initial management. These treatments have high initial cure rates of approximately 80%, but the PLC often recurs and infection can be introduced because a pathway is created from outside the body to the inside of the PLC. Sclerotherapy is also reported as a treatment with a high cure rate. However, its success rate is inversely related to the size of the PLC. Thus, a PLC that is large enough to be symptomatic and require treatment is less likely to be cured with sclerotherapy. Furthermore, both therapies only stop lymphatic inflow into the PLC. Therefore, a successful cure is dependent on the ability of the collateral lymphatic flow.

Laparoscopic or surgical fenestration is effective even for PLCs resistant to other therapies, but this is the most invasive form of treatment.

Ⅳ LVA の適応について

　LVA（lymphaticovenular anastomosis）は、主に四肢のリンパ浮腫に対して行われる手術で、解剖的には左鎖骨下の静脈角で静脈に流入する下肢リンパ流を、下肢の手術部位で静脈に流入させる治療法である。下肢においてリンパ管と静脈を吻合することで、リンパ管にうっ滞したリンパ液を直接静脈に流入させているため、側副リンパ路の代償能とは独立してリンパ液を循環系に乗せることができる。

　LVA 施行時、一番問題となる点は、①リンパ管が同定できるか、と②同定したリンパ管に十分なリンパ流量があるか、である。下肢リンパ浮腫患者に LVA を施行する際には、多くの場合鼠径部までは ICG 蛍光造影法でリンパ管の走行を視認できず（つまり Linear pattern を呈していない）、またリンパ浮腫の進行度合いによってリンパ管がダメージを負って変性していたり、流量が乏しいことも多い。これに対し、リンパ嚢胞の場合には、嚢胞への流入路が存在していることは確実であり（でないと嚢胞を形成し得ない）、実際 ICG 蛍光造影法でも鼠径部まできれいに Linear pattern が描出されることと、嚢胞に穿刺したカテーテルにも蛍光されることからも確認される（詳細後述）。主経路が Linear に描出されるため、同部位に対して LVA を行うことで、上述の 2 つの問題点をクリアすることが可能であり、効果的かつ効率的に LVA を施行できる。

Ⅳ. Lymphatico-venular anastomosis(LVA) as a current treatment for PLC

　LVA is an operation primarily performed for lymphedema of the extremities. The main procedure involves draining the peripheral lymphatic flow into the venous flow directly at the operating site, instead of its anatomical site at the venous angle. Therefore, the lymphatic fluid does not need to pass through the lymphadenectomy lesion, and it can enter the venous flow independent of the ability of the collateral lymphatic flow.

　When performing LVA, the most important factors are ①locating the lymph vessel and ②ensuring that the vessel provides adequate flow. When performing this operation for lymphedema, typically the lymph vessels cannot be detected with lymphatic indocyanine green(ICG) fluorescence imaging of the upper to lower leg because of the back-flow to the peripheral areas and the damage to the lymph vessels(see the ICG stages section). However, when using this technique for PLC, it is easy to detect the lymph vessel using ICG imaging, because the lymphatic flow drains almost directly into the PLC. The detected lymph vessel is a primary route of lymphatic flow ; therefore, this is an effective vessel to use for LVA, which satisfies the two important criteria. In addition, the inner fluid drained by the catheter fluorescing within 5 minutes after ICG injection indicates less damage in the lymph vessel.

Ⅴ 治療プロトコール

　リンパ嚢胞の治療としては、流入を遮断することと、嚢胞の内容液を除去することが必要となる。流入を遮断する手段が LVA であるが、LVA では手術部位よりも下流に存在する嚢胞内容液を効率的に除去できるとは限らない（LVA での内容液除去には、嚢胞から下肢に向けてのリンパ流の逆流が前提となる）。そのため、われわれは経皮的カテーテルを併用することで内容液の除去

を促している。またカテーテル留置には、排液量＝囊胞流入量を計測できるメリットもある。具体的には、以下のようなことである。

①リンパ囊胞が疑われた後、確定診断のための検査を施行する。検査としては、容量や位置を評価しやすく、また経時変化を捉えやすい点でも CT が望ましい。

②内容液除去による症状軽減のため、カテーテルを留置する。排液量は毎日計測する。

③LVA 手術前日に、ICG を第 1 趾間に注射する。PDE で流路を確認してマーキングした後、カテーテルをいったんクランプする。これは、リンパ管内にリンパ液をうっ滞させることでリンパ管の拡張を図り、手術を施行しやすくするためである。

④LVA を施行し、クランプを解除する。LVA の術後管理は通常どおりとし、またカテーテルの排液量は毎日計測する。

⑤数日後、画像検査でリンパ囊胞の大きさを再評価する。囊胞の縮小および排液量の減少（20 mL/日以下）を認めた場合に、ドレーンを抜去する（**Fig. 6-3-1**）。

なおリンパ囊胞に対する LVA は、手術部位・手技その他すべてにおいて、リンパ浮腫に対する LVA となんら変わりがない。詳細は別章（Chap. 7-1「リンパ管細静脈吻合術」）を参照されたい。

V. The detailed protocol

For the treatment of a PLC, stopping the inflow and removing the fluid contents is necessary. LVA is used to stop the inflow, and the percutaneous catheter is used to remove the fluid. Therefore, the procedure is performed as follows：

①When a PLC is suspected due to the patient's symptoms, it is detected using a clinical examination, such as ultrasonography or computed tomography（CT）. Computed tomography（CT）is useful for calculating the volume and enabling an objective follow-up.

②To diminish the symptoms by removing the fluid contents, a percutaneous catheter is inserted. The drainage volume must be measured every day.

③The day before LVA, ICG is injected in the first web. After the fluorescent lines are marked with the imaging device, the catheter is cramped. This procedure is performed to expand the lymph vessels by increasing congestion, thus facilitating the LVA operation.

④LVA is performed in the same manner as it is for lymphedema. After the operation, the cramp is released and the volume measurement is restarted.

⑤A few days after LVA, a follow-up examination is performed that involves a physical examination, CT, or ultrasonography. When the output volume is less than 20 mL/day and the size of the PLC is reduced, the catheter is removed（**Fig. 6-3-1**）.

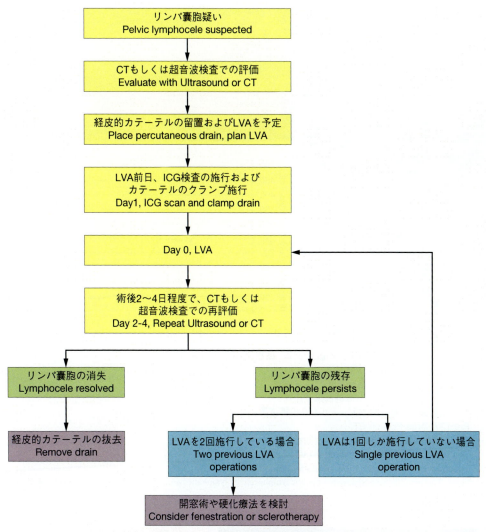

Fig. 6-3-1. リンパ嚢胞の治療方法アルゴリズム　Algorithm for the namagement of pelvic lymphocele
(Todokoro T, et al：Effective treatment of pelvic lymphocele by lymphaticovenular anastomosis. Gynecol Oncol 128（2）：209-214, 2013による)

VI 症例・結果

　53歳、女性。子宮体癌に対して準広汎子宮全摘＋両側卵巣摘出＋骨盤リンパ節郭清術を行った。POD 2よりリンパ嚢胞を認めたため、婦人科にて経皮的カテーテル留置が施行された。しかしながら、嚢胞の縮小や症状の改善を認めなかったため、POD 29に形成外科にコンサルトされた。同日施行のCTでは15×12×11 cm大のリンパ嚢胞を認めた(**Fig. 6-3-2-a**)。POD 38のICG検査では、注射後5分の検査で、カテーテル内リンパ液の蛍光を認め、下肢リンパ管機能が良好であることおよび下肢リンパ流が嚢胞に流入していることが確認できた(**Fig. 6-3-3-a, b**)。POD 39にLVAを施行した(**Fig. 6-3-2-b**)。術後のドレーン排液量は、翌日より著減した(**Fig. 6-3-2-d**)。

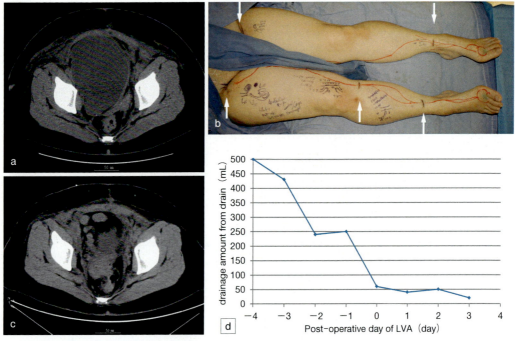

Fig. 6-3-2. 症例提示　A case report
a：術前。巨大囊胞を CT で認めた。
b：術直後。白矢印が LVA 施行部位。
c：術後 3 日での CT 検査。a と同部位で比較。
d：LVA 術前後での経皮的カテーテルからの排液量。
a：Pre-LVA large PLC on CT.
b：Post-operative view. White arrows are operation sites.
c：The same height as a 3 days after LVA.
d：The drainage chart from the percutaneous catheter.
（Todokoro T, et al：Effective treatment of pelvic lymphocele by lymphaticovenular anastomosis. Gynecol Oncol 128(2)：209-214, 2013 による）

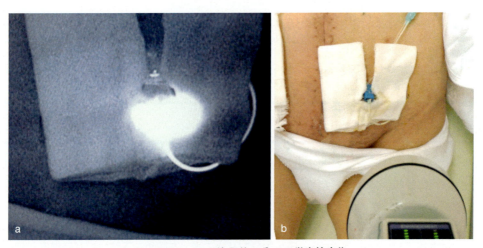

Fig. 6-3-3. ICG 注入後 5 分での蛍光検査像
The fluorescent image of the percutaneous catheter, 5 minutes after ICG injection
（Todokoro T, et al：Effective treatment of pelvic lymphocele by lymphaticovenular anastomosis. Gynecol Oncol 128(2)：209-214, 2013 による）

POD 42 に術後 CT を撮影した際には、リンパ嚢胞の消失を認めたため(**Fig. 6-3-2-c**)、ドレーン排液量と合わせて、抜去可能と判断し、カテーテルを抜去した。経過は良好であり、以降リンパ嚢胞の再発は認めていない。

(戸所　健)

VI. Case example and result

A 53-year-old female patient underwent a total abdominal hysterectomy, bilateral salpingo-oophorectomy, and pelvic lymphadenectomy for the treatment of endometrial cancer. On the second postoperative day (2 POD), a gynecologist detected a PLC and inserted a percutaneous catheter. However, the PLC was not reduced, and the gynecologist consulted us on 29 POD. We detected a PLC measuring $15 \times 12 \times 11$ cm on CT (**Fig. 6-3-2-a**). On 38 POD, ICG was injected and the fluorescent flow was found in the catheter after 5 minutes (**Fig. 6-3-3-a, b**). On 39 POD, LVA was performed (**Fig. 6-3-2-b**). The amount of drainage was dramatically reduced (**Fig. 6-3-2-d**). On 42 POD, the PLC was not visible on CT (**Fig. 6-3-2-c**) and the catheter was removed. During the follow-up period, there was no recurrence of PLCs.

(*Takeshi Todokoro*)

＊*We would like to thank Editage (www.editage.jp) for English language editing.*

1) Todokoro T, et al : Effective treatment of pelvic lymphocele by lymphaticovenular anastomosis. Gynecol Oncol 128(2) : 209-214, 2013.

CHAPTER 7 外科治療 Surgical treatment

1. リンパ管細静脈吻合術（LVA）
Lymphaticovenular anastomosis（LVA）

■ はじめに

　四肢のリンパ管は、一般的に左右の鎖骨下静脈角において静脈に流入するまでは独立した経路を通る。二次性リンパ浮腫の場合、この経路のどこかにおいてリンパが遮断されると浮腫を生じることとなる。リンパ管静脈吻合術は、この遮断された部位より遠位において、リンパ管を静脈にバイパスしリンパ液を静脈に流すことによってリンパ液のうっ滞を解除するリンパ管の機能的再建法である（Fig. 7-1-1）。

　リンパ管静脈吻合の歴史を遡ると、リンパ管静脈吻合法が 1969 年に山田らにより世界で初めて報告され、その後 O'Brien らにより発展していった。しかしリンパ管静脈吻合術は、リンパ組織を静脈内に挿入する術式であり、手技としては容易ではある一方で吻合部の血栓形成リスクが高く効果も不安定であった。

　リンパ管径は四肢において 0.2～1.0 mm と非常に細いことがこの手術の技術的課題であったが、近年の手術器具や技術の向上に伴い、0.5 mm 未満の確実な管腔吻合を可能とする super-microsurgery の発達により、リンパ管と細静脈の内皮同士が接合するように吻合するリンパ管細静脈吻合術（lymphaticovenular anastomosis；LVA）が本邦で開発された（Fig. 7-1-2）。LVA は、吻合部の閉塞リスクや血栓形成を低減させ、その低侵襲性と有効性から現在は世界中に広まっている。

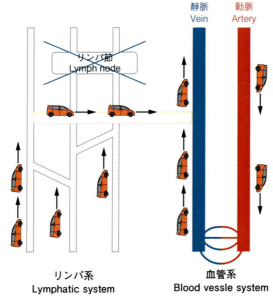

Fig. 7-1-1. リンパ管静脈吻合の概念　Concept of LVA

7-1. リンパ管細静脈吻合術(LVA)

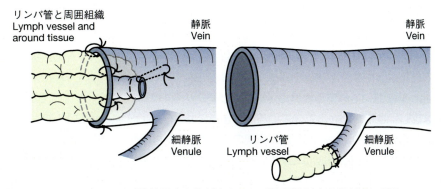

Fig. 7-1-2. リンパ管静脈吻合術(左)とリンパ管細静脈吻合術(右)の対比
Comparison between Lymphatic-Vein anastomosis(left) and Lymphatic-Venule anastomosis(right)

■Introduction

The lymphatic vessel system of four extremities goes along the independent course until it generally flows into the vein in the right and left infraclavicular angulus venosus. When lymph is intercepted in somewhere in this course, in the case of secondary lymphedema, edema of limbs will be noted. The lymphatic vessel phlebophlebostomy is the functional reconstruction which decreases congestion of the lymph fluid by the anastomosis between a vein and a lymphatic vessel. The lymph fluid will spread into the venous system theoretically (**Fig. 7-1-1**).

The lymphatic vessel venovenostomy was reported first time in the world by Yamada et al. in 1969 and developed by O'Brien et al. subsequently. The lymphatic vessel phlebophlebostomy is the technique of inserting lymphoid tissues into venous, lumen and risk of anastomotic thrombosis is high. Although it is an easy a maneuver, the effect was unstable.

Lymphaticovenular anastomosis (LVA) is the anastomosis between lymphatic vessels and small venous vessels. The diameter of the lumens is between 0.2 to 1.0 mm, so it is technique dependent of this surgery. By the development of supermicrosurgery and improvement of modern surgical instrument and technique, it can make the lumen still patency even the diameter is less than 0.5 mm (**Fig. 7-1-2**). We extend this technology to the whole world with low invensiveness and high effectiveness. We also reduce the risk of occlusion and thrombogenesis.

I 術前評価・適応

手術の適応決定にあたっては、これまで国際リンパ学会が定める ISL stage 分類や Campisi らの病期分類を参考にすることが多かった。しかし、リンパ浮腫となる症例のリンパ系の還流障害はかなり早期(ISL stage 0)から進行しているケースも多く、より正確なリンパ管還流機能の評価のために、新たにインドシアニングリーン(ICG)と赤外線照射を用いた ICG リンパ管造影によるリンパ管還流能の評価法が本邦において開発され、その有用性が確認されている。ICG リンパ管造影は被曝なくリアルタイムでリンパ流を可視化し、リンパ浮腫の重症度を病態生理的に評価できると同時に、リンパ管変性を予測する LVA 術前検査としても極めて有用である。

リンパ浮腫の進行に伴い、ICGリンパ管造影所見は、Linear、Splash、Stardust、Diffuse と変化していく。現在では、その所見をもとに、上肢と下肢それぞれにおいて、Dermal Back-flow stageを診断する（上肢：ADB stage、下肢：LDB stage）ことで、LVAの治療効果をある程度予測できるようになった（**Fig. 7-1-3, 4**）。DB stage Ⅰ〜Ⅲにおいては LVA による高い治療効果、stage Ⅳにおいてはある程度の治療効果が見込めるものの、stage Ⅴでは LVA 単独での治療効果は乏しいことがわかってきている。つまり、すべての DB stage において LVA の治療適応があるものの、DB stage Ⅰ〜Ⅲの早期の段階で LVA を行うことが望ましい。それに対し、stage Ⅳ〜Ⅴにおいては、初回は LVA のみで経過を見ることも可能であるが、効果が不十分であることも多く、近年は血管柄付きリンパ組織（リンパ節やリンパ管などを含む組織）移植や脂肪吸引を初回から LVA と同時に行う combined therapy の症例が増えている。

これまでの考え方では、外科的治療の適応の基準として、圧迫療法をある期間試みて改善がみられない場合に手術的療法を行うというのが一般的であった。しかし現在では、圧迫療法と同時に ICG リンパ管造影の検査を定期的に行うことで LVA の適応時期を逃さず、浮腫の進行・増悪を阻止することが可能であるため、形成外科・婦人科・乳腺外科をはじめとする外科医や保存療法を行う医師・コメディカルスタッフがリンパ浮腫の早期発見を行う検査や LVA などの早期外科治療を患者に提案できることが求められている。それと同時に、ある程度進行が進んだリンパ浮腫に対しては、LVA のみでは改善がみられない可能性があることを術前からあらかじめ患者に説明することも重要である。

I. Evaluation of preoperative condition

We are often according to International Society of Lymphology (ISL) stage and the staging of Campisi et al. to decide the adaptive surgery. For evaluating of a more correct lymphatic vessel function, indocyanine green (ICG) lymphangiogram was developed and used under infrared radiation. It is useful in confirming the early stage (ISL stage 0) of lymphedema. It is also useful in pre-operative examination to predict lymphatic vessel denaturation. Besides, ICG lymphangiogram can be used to evaluate the disease severity of lymphedema. If the progression of lymphedema, the ICG lymphangiogram showed gradual change with Linear, Splash, Stardust and Diffuse.

From this point of view, we are able to predict the effect of treatment of LVA in the arms and lower limbs (**Fig. 7-1-3, 4**) by Dermal Backflow stage (arms : ADB stage, lower limbs : LDB stage). The LVA is highly effective in ISL stage Ⅳ with DB stage Ⅰ-Ⅲ. However, the effect of treatment with LVA is poor in ISL stage Ⅴ. In other words, it is reasonable to perform LVA in ISL early stage with DB stage Ⅰ-Ⅲ. Though there is adaptation of LVA treatment in all DB stage.

In contrast, we can observe the insufficient effect in LVA treatment in ISL stage Ⅳ-Ⅴ initially. These patients can accept combine therapy with lymphoid tissues (tissue including lymph node or lymphatic vessel) transplant and liposuction in late years. In the past, we would arrange pressure therapy after surgical treatment for a period of time, but it was common no improvement. Now, we can suggest the patients in early stage lymphedema to receive surgical treatment such as LVA and conservative therapy. We can inhibit the progression of lymphedema, if lymphedema is detected early. So, plastic surgeon, breast surgeon and gynecologist are the stuffs of detecting the early lymphedema. If lymphedema is conducted the examination of ICG lymphangiogram and treated with LVA without missing the adaptive time, pressure therapy can be performed regularly. Besides, it is important to explain that improvement of lymphedema may not be found to the patients with the lymphedema is worse to some extent. The effect of LVA cannot be beforehand preoperatively.

7-1. リンパ管細静脈吻合術(LVA)

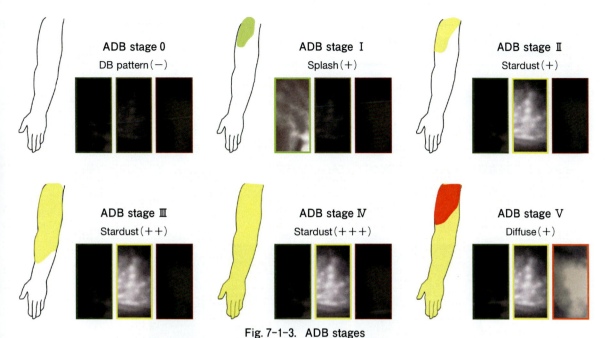

Fig. 7-1-3. ADB stages
(Chap. 4-3「ICG リンパ管造影による病態生理的重症度評価」Fig. 4-3-10 による　By Chap. 4-3 "Pathophysiological severity staging using dynamic ICG lymphography" Fig. 4-3-10)

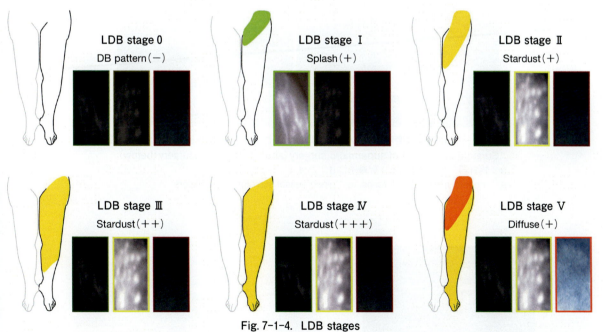

Fig. 7-1-4. LDB stages
(Chap. 4-3「ICG リンパ管造影による病態生理的重症度評価」Fig. 4-3-11 による　By Chap. 4-3 "Pathophysiological severity staging using dynamic ICG lymphography" Fig. 4-3-11)

II 必要な器具・技術

1. 必要な器具

　形成外科基本セット、マイクロサージャリー手術セット、マイクロ吻合針糸（10-0、11-0、12-0：30〜80μ）、移動式顕微鏡、電気メス、バイポーラは必須である。その他に、超微細血管吻合手術セット、超微細血管剥離子、血管クリップ、リンパ管クリップ、エコー、ルーペなどが揃っていると万全である（**Fig. 7-1-5, 6**）。

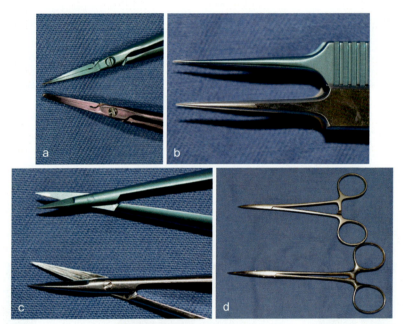

Fig. 7-1-5. 超微細血管吻合吻合手術器具（上）と微細血管吻合手術器具（下）の比較
Surgical instrument of supermicro surgery (above) and microsurgery (below)
a：持針器、b：攝子、c：剥離子、d：ハサミ
a：needle-holder, b：forceps, c：blood vessel elevator, d：scissors

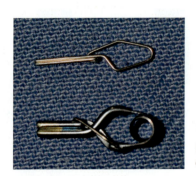

Fig. 7-1-6. リンパ管クリップ（上）と血管クリップ（下）
Clip for lymphatic vessel (above) and venule (below)

2. 必要な技術

　LVA においては、平均 0.5 mm 前後のリンパ管・細静脈を吻合することが一般的であり、さらには中等症から重症なリンパ浮腫においては、0.3 mm を切るリンパ管しか残っていないケースも多く、手術に先立ち 0.5 mm 前後の超微小血管吻合（スーパーマイクロサージャリー）の技術に精通している必要がある。臨床例では、subzone Ⅱ 以遠の指尖部再接着に成功するレベルの吻合技術をもつことが望ましい。また、トレーニング例ではラットの浅下腹壁動静脈吻合を用いた遊離鼠径皮弁移植に成功する程度の吻合技術をもっているのが理想である（**Fig. 7-1-7**）。またその準備段階としては、鶏手羽の tip section（手羽先）における 0.3 mm 前後の血管を用いた日常のトレーニングが有用である（**Fig. 7-1-8**）。

Ⅱ．Instruments & techniques

　1．**Instruments**：Plastic surgery unit set, microsurgery surgery set, microanastomosis needle thread（10-0, 11-0, 12-0：30-80 μ）, travelling microscope, electric scalpel, bipolar, super-mini anastomosis vasorum surgery set, super-mini blood vessel elevator, blood vessel clip, lymphatic vessel clip, echo, loupe（**Fig. 7-1-5, 6**）.

　2．**Techniques**：The diameter of anastomosis between lymphatic vessel and venule is about 0.5 mm. In severe lymphedema, the cutting end of lymphatic vessel is only about 0.3 mm. In LVA, it is necessary to be familiar with the super microvascular anastomosis（super microsurgery）prior to surgery. It is necessary to have good anastomosis technology when finger amputation in the zone Ⅱ of hand. We have a training program by using free groin dermal flap transfer of rat to anastomose the superior inferior epigastric artery（SIEA）（**Fig. 7-1-7**）. Besides, we also practice the blood vessel of chicken wings and it is about 0.3 mm in the tip section of chicken wing（**Fig. 7-1-8**）.

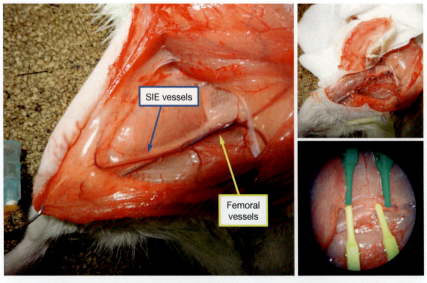

Fig. 7-1-7．ラットの浅下腹壁動静脈吻合を用いた遊離鼠径皮弁移植
Free groin flap transplantation of rat using the technique of anastomosis of superior inferior epigastric artery and vein

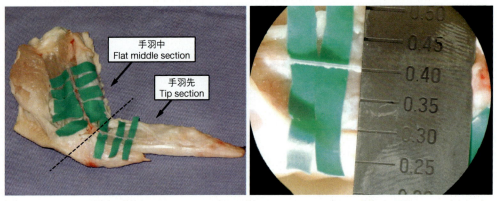

Fig. 7-1-8. 鶏手羽の tip section（手羽先）における 0.3 mm 前後の血管
The vessel (around 0.3 mm) in the tip section of chicken wings

III　手術手技

1.　麻　酔

　LVA の手術においては、局所麻酔・腰椎麻酔・全身麻酔が麻酔法の選択肢となるが、それぞれの賛否に関しては意見が分かれるところである。個々のケースに準じて麻酔法を選択すればよいと考えるが、基礎的疾患がないケースであれば、4 時間以内に手術を終わらせることができれば局所麻酔のみで十分可能である。また局所麻酔下では、患者に顕微鏡の付属モニターを通して、手術をリアルタイムで供覧してもらうことが可能となるため、患者の満足度向上につながる。
　皮切部位の局所浸潤麻酔について説明する。選択した皮切部位にエピネフリン添加 1%リドカインを、膨疹をつくるように皮内注射する。この際の注意点としては、真皮直下の細静脈を吻合に使用することもあるため、損傷しないよう必ず皮内に注射することが挙げられる。通常皮切は

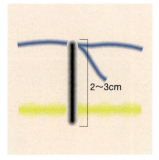

Fig. 7-1-9. 皮切デザイン
Design of skin incision

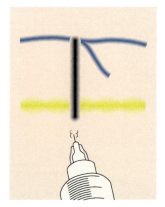

Fig. 7-1-10. 皮切部の局所麻酔
Local anesthesia in skin incision part

2～3 cm 以内でデザインするが、デザインよりも 1～2 cm 程度広く麻酔をしておくことがポイントである(**Fig. 7-1-9, 10**)。それは、デザインした皮切長で脈管が確保できなかった場合に、すぐに皮切を延長できるようにするためである。1 皮切につき 4～5 mL のエピネフリン添加 1%リドカインを要するが、剥離範囲が深筋膜周囲など深くなる場合は適宜 1～2 mL ずつ該当範囲に追加していくことをお勧めする。

2. リンパ管と静脈の剥離

まず、透明なリンパ管は血液で染まると判別しにくくなるため、皮切後は低出力の電気メスやバイポーラなどを用い出血を極力避けるように細心の注意を払わなければならない。また、リンパ管や血管、神経は脂肪隔壁間に存在することが多く、脂肪隔壁の間を分け入るように剥離していくと、リンパ管や細静脈を発見・確保しやすい。

次に、リンパ管の剥離であるが、通常吻合に適したリンパ集合管は浅筋膜直下に存在することが多いため、まず真皮直下の細静脈を確保しながら浅筋膜上の層を十分に剥離しておく必要がある。原発性リンパ浮腫を除き二次性リンパ浮腫では、浅筋膜上に吻合に適するリンパ集合管を認めることはほとんどないため、浅筋膜上では主に細静脈の確保にのみ注意すればよく、リンパ管の検索に必要以上に時間を費やすことは避けるべきである(原発性リンパ浮腫では、リンパ管の走行が正常とまったく異なるケースが多く、真皮直下にリンパ管を認めることもあり、皮切直後からリンパ管に注意しながら剥離する必要がある)。浅筋膜が広く剥離されたら、浅筋膜を切開し浅筋膜下の脂肪間を剥離しリンパ管を検索する。浅筋膜直下にリンパ管が見つからない場合は、その部分にリンパ管はないため、SPECT などの術前検査を用い深部リンパ管の優位性がわかっていない限りは、無駄に深筋膜下などの深部を剥離することなく、すぐに皮切を延長するか他部位に変更するのが妥当である。リンパ管を剥離したら、リンパ管は容易に見失いやすいためすぐに血管テープまたはナイロン糸を用い確保することをお勧めする。

最後に静脈の剥離であるが、LVA では弁があり逆流しない静脈を用いることが重要である。真皮直下の細静脈は剥離が容易でありリンパ管のサイズにマッチするものが多い一方、弁がなく逆流するものが多いのが事実である。それに対し、伏在静脈などの太いメインの静脈などから直接分岐する静脈は、弁を有するものが多く逆流する確率は低い。集合リンパ管と吻合可能なサイズであれば、吻合にやや困難が伴う場合でもこちらの静脈を使用する方が、吻合後の開存率は高いと考えられる。

吻合前のリンパ管・細静脈の選択・剥離は、手術の成否に直結するため、LVA において最も重要な過程である(**Fig. 7-1-11**)。

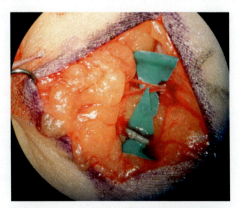

Fig. 7-1-11. リンパ管と静脈の剥離
Disection of lymphatic vessels and venules

3. 吻合

剝離し確保したリンパ管と静脈の本数や性状、位置関係などから、4つの吻合方法(端々・端側・側端・側々)(**Fig. 7-1-12**)を組み合わせて、最も効率的なバイパスとなるようにデザインする。リンパ管径は 0.5 mm 前後であることが多く、吻合には基本的に 11-0 を用いるが、拡張し 0.8 mm 以上になっている場合には 10-0、ダメージが強く 0.3 mm 未満の場合には 12-0 と適宜使用する針糸を変更するとよい。

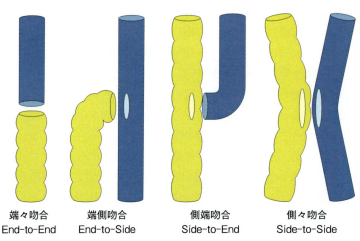

Fig. 7-1-12. 4つの基本吻合型(黄：リンパ管、青：静脈)
Four basic type of LVA (yellow：lymphatic vessel, blue：venule)

4. 閉創

通常、真皮縫合・表皮縫合により閉創するが、真皮縫合の結紮部が吻合部に干渉しないように注意する必要がある。足背や足首など吻合部が比較的浅層になりやすい部位では、顕微鏡下に真皮縫合を行うのが望ましい。また、リンパ管静脈吻合を行ったものと同一術者がその部位の閉創を行う方が安全であることは言うまでもない。

III. Operative techniques

1. **Anesthesia**：In the LVA, local anesthesia, lumber anesthesia, and general anesthesia are the options during peri operation. We are according to individual to choice the anesthetic method. If the patient is without underlying disease, it is possible to finish the operation under local anesthesia. The operation time must be less than 4 hours. The patients are satisfied with the detector proving the operation is successful in real time.

We perform the local anesthesia in the surgical site. We inject lidocaine intradermally with 1% epinephrine. We must remind that subcutaneous injection of local anesthetics may damage the small vessels that we want to anastomoses.

The skin incision is generally between 2-3 cm and local anesthesia injection must be extended 1-2 cm in length (**Fig. 7-1-9, 10**). When we cannot find the small vessels in the wound, we can immediately incise the wound longer. We need 4-5 mL lidocaine with 1% epinephrine in a incisional wound. We will add 1-2 mL lidocaine appropriately if we have to cut to deeper fascia or surrounding tissue.

7-1. リンパ管細静脈吻合術(LVA)

2. Dissection of lymphatic vessels and venules : First of all, we must note how to distinguish lymphatic vessels from venules, especially when the lymphatic vessels are stained with blood. Hemostasis is made by electric scalpel or bipolar after skin incision. Nerves are usually found when fat is separated then lymphatic vessels and venules are easy found.

The venules are under the dermis. The lymph collecting tubules are suitable for anastomoses usually under superficial fascia. It is rare in secondary lymphedema that lymph collecting tubules are suitable for anastomoses on superficial fascia. But, primary lymphedema may show lymphatic vessels just under dermis and it is necessary to exfoliate the lymphatic vessel from the skin dermis. We extend the skin incision immediately or change in other parts when the lymphatic vessel is not found under superficial fascia. We seldom approach to deep fascia, because the part does not have the lymphatic vessel. Unless the deep part lymphatic vessel is found by using pre-operative examination such as SPECT, we may approach to deep fascia. We recommend to use the blood vessel loop or a nylon suture when we finding out a lymphatic vessel. Because it is easy to lose sight the lymphatic vessel when we exfoliating it from fascia or dermis. Finally it is venous detachment. We should know that the vein with the valve inside the lumen to prevent blood flow backward. The venule is just under the dermis and it is easy to separate the venule and match the diameter of lymphatic vessel we have found.

In contrast, if we are engaged in the LVA and the venule is confluent to the large vein such as saphenous vein, it can be expected to higher patency rate. Because of the counter-flow of venule is smaller.

Selecting the appropriate lymphatic vessels and venules will directly affect the success or failure of LVA surgery (**Fig. 7-1-11**).

3. Anastomosis : We use the four methods (end-to-end, end-to-side, side-to-end, side-to-side) for the relative bond relationship between lymphatic vessel and venule (**Fig. 7-1-12**). The diameter of lymphatic vessel is often around 0.5 mm and 11-0 Nylon was used for LVA anastomosis basically. We expand the technique to anastomosis as small as 0.3 mm in diameter by 12-0 Nylon. If the diameter is 0.8 mm or larger, we use 10-0 Nylon for anastomosis.

4. Closure : We make wound closure by intradermal suture. The intradermal suture should not interfere with the anastomotic region, espeially dorsal foot and ankle. So, we should perform the intradermal suture under a microscope. Also, it does not need to say that it performed lymphatic vessel venovenostomy that the one where the same practiced hand performs the shut wound of the part in is safe.

Ⅳ　吻合方法

　閉塞したリンパ管やリンパ管内のリンパ圧が高い例では、リンパ管の弁不全が起こっているケースが多く、中枢側からの逆流を認めることがある。LVAの際には、この逆流も取り込むように、4つの吻合方法(端々・端側・側端・側々)を組み合わせてリンパ管の末梢側のみではなくできるだけ中枢側も吻合するようにすることが重要である。

　より実践的な吻合方法としては、下記が挙げられる。術野の状況と脈管の状態、術者の技量に応じて、それぞれを使い分けることが求められる(**Fig. 7-1-13～16**)。

Ⅳ. Anastomosis method

It is often happened of the valvular incompetence of the lymphatic vessel. The lymphatic vessel occlusion rate may also be increased due to the backflow of lymph fluid from the central side. In the case of LVA, we use the four methods (end-to-end, end-to-side, side-to-end, side-to-side) as possible for peripheral lymph fluid drainage. This may also let the backflow of lymph fluid from the central side import to venule.

189

According to the situation of the surgical field to choose more methods to anastomose lymphatic vessels and venules, this is our current policy of treatment of lymphedema (**Fig. 7-1-13 to 16**).

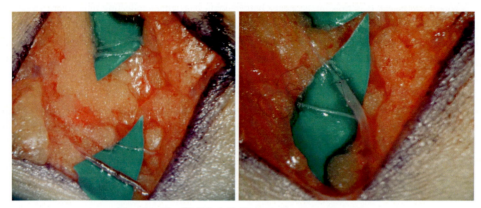

Fig. 7-1-13. 基本となる End-to-End anastomosis

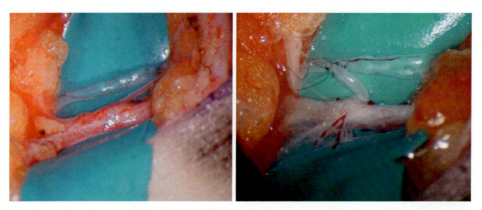

Fig. 7-1-14. Side-to-End anastomosis

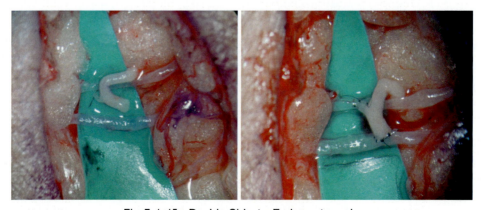

Fig. 7-1-15. Double Side-to-End anastomosis

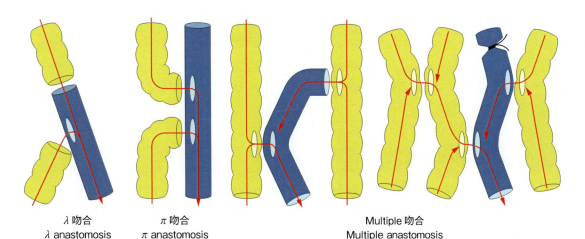

Fig. 7-1-16. 吻合型（黄：リンパ管、青：静脈）
Applied type of LVA (yellow：lymphatic vessel, blue：venule)

1. Double End-to-End

リンパ管の近位側と遠位側それぞれを細静脈に End-to-End で吻合する方法である。この方法は、リンパ管・静脈が共に細い場合に有効である。

2. Flow-through

術野において Y 字に分岐している静脈の枝を見つけた場合に、リンパ管の近位側と遠位側それぞれを End-to-End で吻合する方法である。

3. Side-to-End

リンパ管がある程度拡張している場合に有効で、リンパ管の側壁に静脈の断端を吻合する方法である。静脈側との吻合部において万が一血栓を生じ吻合部が閉塞しても、オリジナルのリンパ流を障害しないことがこの方法の利点である。リンパ管があまり拡張していないあるいはリンパ管の内腔が狭窄している症例においては、吻合が極端に難しくなることが多いため IVaS を用いることを勧めるが、吻合に時間がかかることが予想される場合は無理をせず、すぐに End-to-End に切り替える判断も重要である。

4. π 吻合 (End-to-Side×2)

術野においてリンパ管の 2 倍以上の径である太い静脈のみしか見つからない場合、その静脈の側壁にリンパ管の近位側と遠位側の両端を吻合する方法である。静脈からリンパ管への逆流が強過ぎる場合は、静脈の遠位側を 6-0 ナイロンなどで結紮する必要がある。

5. λ吻合（End-to-End＋End-to-Side）

End-to-End と End-to-Side を組み合わせたこの吻合方法は、手頃なサイズの静脈が術野に1本しか見つからない場合でも、IVaS法を併用すれば初心者でも確実に両方向のリンパ流をバイパスできる有用な方法である。

6. Multiple 吻合

原発性リンパ浮腫の原因の1つであるリンパ管奇形を有する症例においては、1ヵ所の術野に拡張したたくさんのリンパ管が剖出されることがある。静脈の数に対してリンパ管の数が明らかに多い場合は、Side-to-Side を含め上記の吻合方法すべてを駆使し、できる限り有効なバイパスを多くつくるのが本方法である。

1. **Double End-to-End**：It is a way to anastomose each distal side of lymphatic vessel to proximal side of venule with end-to end method. This method is effective when venule is thin.

2. **Flow-through**：It is a way to anastomose distal side of lymphatic vessel to the branch of vein in Y shape with end-to end method.

3. **Side-to-End**：It is a way to anastomose a venous stump to side wall of the lymphatic vessel. This method is effective when the lymphatics expand to a certain extent. The advantage of this method is that even if the embolization in the anastomotic site, it does not affect the original lymphatic flow. In the case of lymphatic vessel that is not too expended or the lymphatic vessel has constricted, and we recommend IVaS is used. Because of in this situation, the anastomosis will be extremely difficult, or even make the conversion to end-to end method immediately without wasting too much time.

4. **π anastomosis（End-to-Side×2）**：When the diameter of the venule is greater than two times the diameter of lymphatic vessel, it is a way to anastomose the proximal and distal stumps of lymphatic vessel to venule side wall. If the backflow of venule is too strong, it is necessary to ligate the distal side of venule with 6-0 nylon.

5. **λ anastomosis（End-to-End＋End-to-Side）**：This method is available when only one of the venule and the lymphatic vessel is found. The distal stump of lymphatic vessel is anastomosed to the proximal stump of venule with end-to end method and the proximal stump of lymphatic vessel is anastomosed to to side wall of venule with end-to-sidemethod, so that two-way lymph fluid can be resolved. The beginner can combine the IVaS method to complete the operation.

6. **Multiple anastomosis**：In the patients of primary lymphedema with lymphatic vessel deformity, it is a way to anastomose of several lymphatic vessels and only one venule can be found in the surgical field. We can use all of the previously mentioned ways including side-to-side to make the lymphatic reflow more efficient.

Ⅴ 周術期管理

吻合部の血栓形成、吻合部狭窄をできる限り予防するために、術直後より1週間ほどプロスタグランディン E_1（PGE_1）やヘパリンを使用する。その後1週間ほどは経口で PGE_1 を服用する。

局所麻酔下での LVA 後において、上肢は術直後から日常動作が可能であり、下肢においては歩行可能であるが、術後1週間はトイレ動作など以外はできる限りベッド上での安静が勧められ

る。患肢は挙上位とする。術後1週後の退院時からストッキング装着を再開し、術後1ヵ月はある程度患者の可能な範囲内で日常生活において下肢を横にする時間をつくってもらうようにしている。

　術後の圧迫療法やリンパマッサージ再開時期については、依然としてきちんとしたエビデンスは出ていない。術直後から弾性包帯による圧迫を再開するべきとする意見と、術後1週後より使い古した弾性ストッキングなどを使用した軽度の圧迫から徐々に再開するべきとする意見に大きく分かれる。リンパマッサージに関しても同様であり、術後数日から再開する施設もあれば、術後1ヵ月後から再開する施設もある。術者の吻合技術や弾性包帯の圧迫技術、リンパ浮腫の治療に対する知識はそれぞれにおいて違うため、一概にどのプロトコールがよいか決定できないのが現状であり、術後のより正しい保存療法の再開方法に関しては今後さらなる研究が必要とされている。

V. Perioperative care

　We prescribe intravenous form prostaglandin E_1 (PGE_1) and heparin after operating immediately. The duration is 1 week to prevent anastomotic throbogenesis and anastomotic stricture as possible. Then we prescribe oral form PGE_1 for the following 1 week. The LVA is performed under local anesthesia. Lower extremity activities can begin as soon as possible after surgery. Upper limb activity is recommended with bed rest for a week after surgery, then start normal activities. The limb is still necessary to elevation after surgery. The stocking can be worn after surgery one week. The lower limbs can be raised as possible within one month after surgery except daily life.

　About the pressure therapy and lymph massage after surgery, there is still no appropriate evidence to support. There are two factions. One option is wearing compression garment after surgery one week and the other option is that elastic bandage can be wrapped around immediately after surgery. A few days to a month after surgery can begin lymph massage. It is still not possible to determine which one is the best protocol. Surgical techniques, compression technique of elastic bandages and knowledge of treating lymphedema affect the prognosis of lymphedema. In the future, there is still a need for further research of conservative treatment after surgery.

Ⅵ　術後評価

　LVA はバイパス手術であるため、術後に著明な改善が得られたとしても、基本的には保存療法の継続を要する。そのため、最終的なリンパ浮腫の治癒を目的とするには、患者自身の治療継続に対するモチベーションの持続が重要となる。患者にとって、手術による直接的効果（つまり客観的評価）を知ることは、保存療法の継続や LVA の追加希望などの今後の治療にとって非常に重要である。さらに、術者にとっても、客観的な評価によって術後のリンパ管機能の改善を知ることができれば、保存療法の継続または軽減、リンパ移植や脂肪吸引の追加など次の治療方針の決定において重要な情報となり、正確な治療方針の計画が可能となる。ここでは、有用な客観的評価の方法とその注意点について述べる。

1. 写真撮影

　患者に手術の効果を知ってもらううえで最も簡便で有用な評価方法である。それだけに、撮影条件や撮影時間、撮影時期をしっかり考慮して撮影しなければならない。

　まず、撮影条件であるが、立位か仰臥位どちらにするか体位を一致させなければならない。基本的にはどちらもしっかりと評価できるが、仰臥位の場合、LVA の効果で軟らかくなった分ベッドへの接触面積が増え、周径が小さくなっているのに写真上は横に広がって悪く見える場合も少なからずあるので注意が必要である。また、膝や足関節の角度によっても異なった写真になりやすいので同条件になるようにするべきである。立位の長時間の写真撮影は、患者によっては精神的負担が大きい場合もあり医療不信につながる恐れがあるので、こちらも注意されたい。

　次に、撮影時間であるが、外来で測定する場合、いつも同じ時間に測定することはもちろん困難であり、また受診して長時間診察を待っていたりそれ以前の病院までの歩行距離などにより大きく条件は異なる。長時間立位のままにした後に撮影すれば、静脈のうっ滞により実際より太く映ることは言うまでもない。この誤差を少しでも緩和するために、診察室ではベッドに仰臥位にした後に問診を開始し、5 分以上経過した後に写真撮影を行うことをお勧めする。立位での撮影の場合は、仰臥位から起こしてすぐに撮影するのがよいであろう。

　最後に、撮影時期であるが、術前に保存療法を行っていればそのことと術前の状態を記録しておくことが望ましい。手術自体の効果を見るためには、この状態と術後を比較しなければ保存療法の影響を取り除くことができないからである。また、術後どれくらいの期間で撮影したかということも重要である。術後 1 週以内の撮影については、手術直後や入院中はベッド上にいる時間が長いため、浮腫は軽減しやすく、手術の効果以外の要因が大きく影響してしまう。患者が日常生活に戻ってからでなければより正確な比較はできないため、術後 1 ヵ月以上経過した後の撮影がよい。

2. 周径の測定

　周径の測定は、いつでも簡単に行うことができ、患者自身も理解しやすいため、重要な評価法である。さまざまな測定方法があるが、リンパ浮腫の病態を考慮すると、少なくとも足背、足関節、下腿、膝、大腿の 5 ヵ所における測定は必須と考える。絶対値ではなく、周径の増減を知ることが目的であるため、常に同じ体位で、同じ部位で、そして同じメジャーの強さで計測することが大切である。そのためには、最大径といった抽象的な表現ではなく、解剖学的にメルクマールとなる部位を基準にそこから○○cm といった目安を決めておくことをお勧めする。またストッキング装着の有無でかなり周径は違ってくるため、測定日は朝から外すかあるいは履いてくるかという条件も常に同じにすることを忘れてはならない。

3. エコーによる評価

　近年エコーの進化とともに、リンパ浮腫の分野でもエコーが積極的に使われ始めている。特に皮膚・皮下組織の肥厚、浮腫の状態の観察には優れており、同部位で術前術後を比較することで

肥厚部の性質の変化や浮腫部の水分量の変化など LVA 後の術後評価が可能である。また、エラストグラフィの機能を用いることで（Chap. 5-3「エコーによるリンパ管の同定とリンパ浮腫の評価」参照）「かたさ」を数値化し、術前術後の「かたさ」の変化を評価できることも、エコーの大きな特徴である。エコーによる評価は熟練した操作技能がまず大前提となるが、患者にとって侵襲性が低く、場所や時間を選ばないこと、そして何より real-time imaging であることから、エコーはリンパ浮腫の評価においては大変有用なツールであるといえる。

4. リンパ管シンチグラフィによる評価

リンパ管シンチグラフィ（99mTcDTPA-HSA）は、皮内に局注された核種がリンパ管に取り込まれ、リンパ流路を上行し静脈角に達し静脈に拡散するまでの画像を核医学的に評価する検査である。リンパ浮腫では、最終的にリンパ液がうっ滞して残った核種の分布と量により、黒色から灰色のびまん性の画像として表現される。

しかし、術後の評価を行うにはこの検査はいくつかの欠点を有している。検査により取り込まれた画像データはモニター上で明るさやコントラストなどをいくらでも調整可能であり、完成される画像には決まった条件や標準などがない。また、LVA を行うと静脈角に行く前にリンパ管から静脈への還流が起こり、手術後にはリンパ管の排泄経路そのものが変化している可能性があり、通常より早めに静脈系が染まり出す。そして同じ経過時間で撮影した画像であっても、術前と術後ではリンパ管系と静脈系の核種の分散比率が異なってきてしまう。そのため、脳や肺を基準にし画像条件を揃えてもリンパ管系の条件が揃わなくなり、正確な比較ができない。以上より、術前、術後の診断はそれぞれ可能であるが、両者を比較し手術後にどのように改善したかを評価するのは困難であると言わざるを得ない。

これらの欠点を補うには、まず LVA の特殊性を放射線科医に説明したうえで評価を行い、撮影条件を揃え、誰が見ても客観的に比較できる画像を撮影することが重要である。また、健側の大腿は、早期から静脈へ移行した核種の影響を受ける脳や肺、肝臓と異なり、末梢の組織であるため核種の影響を受けにくい。さらには、患肢と解剖学的に同一部位であり条件が近いことから、大腿を基準点にし、その同じ場所に相当する部位で条件を合わせ画像を調節することで、より正確な術前術後の比較・評価を行うことができる。

VI. Evaluation of postoperative course

LVA is a bypass operation. We know that lymphedema will improve postoperatively, but conservative treatment is still to continue. Therefore, continuous limb movement of patients is also an important part of the prognosis. This is also hoped to increase the effectiveness of future treatment, whether it is follow-up re-operation LVA or conservative treatment. The effect of good or bad will affect the decision to the next treatment strategy including keeping continue to conservative treatment, reduction, lymph node transfer and liposuction. If we know exactly the degree of improvement the lymphatic function after surgery by objective evaluation, we can plan the right treatment strategy. Here we introduce several objective evaluation methods and points.

1. **Photography** : It is the simplest evaluation method and most likely to let patients understand the surgical results. Photography must take into account many conditions, such as photography exposure time and photography angle.

The patient is standing or lying flat must be consistent when taking a photograph. Both ways can evaluate it well. But, the greater contact area of the limb and bed when lying down, the look is relatively soft. It should also be noted that the effect of LVA is not significant when taking a photograph from the top position, because of the background becomes smaller. In addition, the angle of the knee and ankle will also affect the result.

It may cause the patient's mental burden when the time of standing or taking pictures too long. When measuring an outpatient patient, it is necessary to consider whether the patient is waiting for a medical examination for too long time or for a long distance to get to the hospital. The results will be different. The patients stand for too long time will have venous congestion of lower limb and the photographs are looked will be relatively thick. When taking a picture in lying position, we recommend to waiting 5 minutes at least and it can reduce the error. When taking a picture in standing position, we recommend resting lying down 5 minutes at least. Then take a picture in standing position immediately.

Finally, it is talking about the opportunity to take pictures. Before taking conservative therapy pre-operatively, we have to take the pictures to be a record. This is because the effect of conservative therapy cannot be ruled out post-operatively. It is also important how long the period of taking pictures after the surgery. Taking the pictures within a week after surgery, because of the reduction in edema is due to the hospitalization with bed rest, it is not a surgical effect. After the operation more than 1 month, we take the photographs again and the patient has returned to the daily life at that time.

2. The measurement of the circumference : The measurement of limb circumference is easy and without time-limited. We ask patients to measure and record by themselves. The patients with lymphedema have to measure the foot, ankle, calf, knee and thigh these five parts at least. The patient must measure the leg circumference at the same postural, position, and strength. Whether to stockings wearing must also take into account. The stockings are worn throughout the day or only at night have to be recorded.

3. Evaluation using ultrasound : In recent years, postoperative ultrasound measurements have been used in lymphedema surgery. Changes in the thickness of the skin and subcutaneous tissue after LVA surgery were measured as well as changes in the volume of the edema limb. We also used ultrasound to measure functional elastography to compare preoperative and postoperative skin softness differences. Under the prerequisite of familiarity with operating ultrasound, it can provide a useful lymphedema assessment and a low-invasive, real-time image without having to select a location and time.

4. Evaluation by the lymphatic vessel scintigraphy : In nuclear medicine assessment, the radiation material injected into the dermis layer to observe the lymphatic vessels until the high way of angulus venosus. Lymphatic vessel scintigraphy (99mTcDTPA-HSA) can be used to distinguish lymphatic vessel and venous canal. The development of diffuse gray image is noted in patients with lymphatic edema because the relationship between lymph retention. This check may be erroneously evaluated after LVA surgery. The brightness of the image is related to the residual amount of the radiation material and is not a standard fixed final image. In LVA surgery the radiation material begins to flow into venules where the lymphatic pathways will be different.

The ratio of the nuclide in the lymphatic vessel to that in the blood vessel after LVA surgery was different from that before the operation, even if the interval of takin a photograph was the same. So cannot correctly show the lymph tract. Even if we control the brain and lungs at baseline still the same, the incorrect comparison is between preoperative and postoperative. Postoperative evaluation is also difficult to compare preoperative and postoperative limb amelioration is associated with LAV. In order to take a more objective image, we must explain with the nuclear medicine physician about the specificity of LVA. The healthy side of the thigh is less affected by radioactive substances because it is peripheral tissue. Unlike brain, lungs and liver the radiation substances will be discharged into the venous system in the early stage. This healthy limb of the nuclear medicine photography can be done the reference point of the affected limb because of the same anatomical structure and the same site.

Ⅶ 症 例

1. 症例1

　81歳、女性。30年前に子宮体癌に対し、婦人科にて子宮全摘・付属器切除術（リンパ節郭清術含む）施行。14年前より左下肢の浮腫を自覚するようになり、弾性ストッキングにて圧迫療法を開始した。しかし、浮腫は次第に増悪し、当科に紹介され手術となった。手術は局所麻酔下に、鼠径部・大腿部で1ヵ所、下腿部で2ヵ所、足背で1ヵ所の計5ヵ所でLVAを行った。術後2年の状態では、著明な改善を認めている（**Fig. 7-1-17**）。

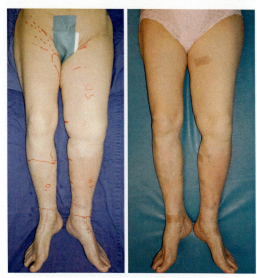

Fig. 7-1-17. 術前（左）と術後2年（右）
Pre-operative course (left) and post-operative course of 2 years (right)

2. 症例2

　68歳、男性。8年前に膀胱癌に対し、骨盤内リンパ節郭清術を含む膀胱全摘術を施行。3年前より左下肢の浮腫を自覚するようになり、弾性ストッキングにて圧迫療法を開始した。しかし、浮腫は次第に増悪し、1年前より右下肢の浮腫も自覚するようになり、当科に紹介され手術となった。手術は局所麻酔下に、左下肢の鼠径部・大腿部・下腿部・足首でそれぞれ1ヵ所の計4ヵ所、右下肢の鼠径部・大腿部・下腿部でそれぞれ1ヵ所の計3ヵ所でLVAを行った。術後8ヵ月の状態では、著明な改善を認めている（**Fig. 7-1-18**）。

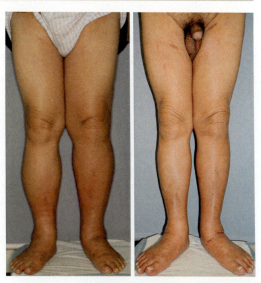

Fig. 7-1-18. 術前（左）と術後8ヵ月（右）
Pre-operative course (left) and post-operative course of 8 months (right)

3. 症例3

　65歳、女性。27年前に左母趾の爪を鉄の扉で挟み、その後左足背浮腫が出現。その後左下肢の蜂窩織炎を繰り返していた。25年前より左下腿全体まで浮腫が増悪し、8年前より弾性ストッキングにて圧迫療法を開始したが、さらに6年前より誘因なく右下腿の浮腫が出現するようになった。その後左右の蜂窩織炎を繰り返すようになり、当科に紹介され手術となった。手術は局所麻酔下に、左下肢の大腿部・下腿部・足首でそれぞれ1ヵ所の計3ヵ所、右下肢の大腿部・下腿部・足首でそれぞれ1ヵ所の計3ヵ所でLVAを行った。術後9ヵ月の状態では、著明な改善を認めている（**Fig. 7-1-19**）。

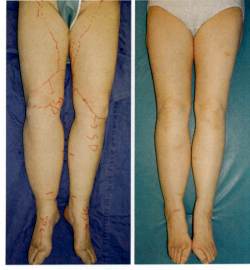

Fig. 7-1-19. 術前（左）と術後9ヵ月（右）
Pre-operative course (left) and post-operative course of 9 months (right)

4. 症例4

　60歳、男性。8年ほど前に誘因なく左下肢の浮腫が出現。その後浮腫は増悪し、右下肢と陰嚢にも浮腫が出現するようになった。2年前より圧迫療法を開始するも大きな改善を認めず、蜂窩織炎を繰り返し増悪傾向となったため、当科に紹介され手術となった。手術は局所麻酔下に、左下肢のより陰部に近い鼠径部・大腿部・下腿部・足首でそれぞれ1ヵ所の計4ヵ所、右下肢のより陰部に近い鼠径部・大腿部・下腿部・足背でそれぞれ1ヵ所の計4ヵ所でLVAを行った。術後2年6ヵ月の状態では、著明な改善を認めている（**Fig. 7-1-20, 21**）。

VII. Cases

　1. **Case 1**：An 81-year-old female received total hysterectomy and lymph node resection surgery 30 years ago because of endometrial tumors. She was suffered from left lower extremity edema 14 years ago and began to pressure therapy with elastic stockings. However, edema continued to progress so referral to our department. We arranged LVA in two locations one at dorsal foot and another in the inguinal region. After surgery for two years, there was marked improvement of swelling of left lower limb(**Fig. 7-1-17**).
　2. **Case 2**：A 68-year-old man underwent total cystectomy surgery and lymphadenectomy 8 years ago due to bladder cancer. He was found the left lower extremity edema and began pressure therapy with elastic stockings 3 years ago. However, edema continued severe and he was found that the right lower extremity edema a year ago, then he was referred to our department. We arranged LVA under local anesthesia for the left lower limb over inguinal region, femoral region, lower leg and ankle. In the right lower limb, we had LVA in the inguinal region, femoral region and lower leg. After surgery 8 months, the edema of lower limbs was significantly improved(**Fig. 7-1-18**).

7-1. リンパ管細静脈吻合術(LVA)

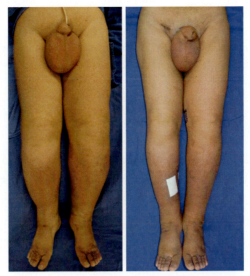

Fig. 7-1-20. 術前(左)と術後 2 年 6 ヵ月(右)
Pre-operative course (left) and post-operative course of 2 years and 6 months (right)

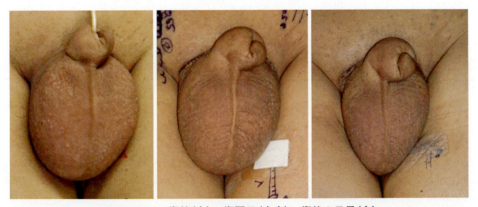

Fig. 7-1-21. 術前(左)、術翌日(中央)、術後 5 日目(右)
Pre-operative course (left), post-operative course of next day (center), post-operative course of 5 days (right)

3. **Case 3**: A 65-year-old woman received valgus surgery for left big toe 27 years ago, but edema was noted over left dorsal foot subsequently. Then she was suffered from cellulitis over left lower limb. The edema continued to deteriorate to the entire left leg since 25 years ago. She accepted pressure therapy with elastic stockings 8 years ago. However, the edema over right leg was found 6 years ago. Due to repeated cellulitis of lower limbs, she was referred to our hospital. We arranged LVA under local anesthesia for both lower limbs over femoral region, lower leg and ankle. After surgery 9 months, the edema of lower limbs was significantly improved (**Fig. 7-1-19**).

4. **Case 4**: A 60-year-old man was noted edema over left leg 8 years ago. The edema was increasingly serious later, and the edema also appeared over right lower extremity and scrotum. Because repeated

199

cellulitis and pressure therapy with elastic stockings for 2 years without improvement, she was referred to our hospital. We arranged LVA under local anesthesia for the left lower limb over pubic region, near inguinal region, femoral region, lower leg and dorsal foot. In the right lower limb, we had LVA in the inguinal region, femoral region, lower leg and ankle. After surgery 2 years and 6 months, the edema of lower limbs was significantly improved(**Fig. 7-1-20, 21**).

■おわりに

　LVA は、局所麻酔下に小さな皮膚切開から施行可能な低侵襲のリンパ浮腫外科治療である。しかし、「低侵襲」の意味をはき違えてはならない。LVA により低侵襲に確実な治療結果を出すには、リンパ浮腫治療における LVA の意義や戦略をしっかりと理解しておかなければならない。局所麻酔下に効率よく LVA を行うために計画を立てることも重要であるが、それ以上に、どのような症例にいつ LVA を行うかという治療戦略がさらに重要である。進行したリンパ浮腫の重症例においては LVA による治療効果は低く、その他のリンパ節移植や脂肪吸引、脂肪切除術が必要となることが多く、圧迫療法が不要になることはほとんどない。それに対し、リンパ浮腫の早期の段階において LVA を行うことができれば、治療効果も高く浮腫の進行を遅らせることができ、また圧迫療法を軽減あるいは不要にする確率は高くなる。ICG リンパ管造影を用いたリンパ動態・病態評価によりしっかり手術の適応を考えたうえで、解剖の知識や吻合の技術を駆使し手際よく手術を行うことで、真の意味での低侵襲の LVA が可能となるのである。

　そして、術後評価をしっかり行うことも忘れてはならない。定期的・継続的な評価を行うことで、LVA の追加やその他の術式の追加の必要性、弾性ストッキングの変更の必要性をタイミングを逃すことなく判断できる。定期的・継続的な評価・経過観察は、人生の長い期間浮腫と向き合わなければいけないリンパ浮腫患者にとって大きな利益につながるのである。

（林　明辰）

■Conclusion

　LVA is a low-invasive method for surgical treatment of lymphedema and it can be performed under local anesthesia in the small skin incision to finish this surgery. We must understand the LVA for the treatment of lymphedema can bring a certain degree of effect. LVA in the implementation is more effective under local anesthesia, but more important of all is that such a treatment strategy for what kind of patients. LVA treatment is less significant in patients with severe lymphedema, so Lymph node transplantation, liposuction and lipectomy may be necessary subsequently. The pressure therapy is rarely useless. If the LVA can be provided in the early stage of lymphedema, it is more effect and can slow down the progression of edema. Pressure therapy will also be a high effect. Using ICG lymphangiogram to do a good assessment, good anatomical dissection and anastomotic technique, and skilled operation, these are the real meaning of low-invasive LVA.

　Of course not forget the postoperative evaluation. Regular and continuous follow-up assessment is important. It is necessary to assess that additional LVA or additional surgery is required or not. Besides, assessing the compression force of elastic stockings to decide that stockings need to be changed or not. Periodic follow-up and evaluation are beneficial for patients with lymphedema so that it can combat long-term edema.

(*Akitatsu Hayashi*)

外科治療
Surgical treatment

CHAPTER 7

2. リンパ脂肪弁によるリンパ管移植法

Lymphadiposal flaps for severe leg edema functional reconstruction for lymph drainage system

■はじめに

　集合リンパ管を通したリンパ液の輸送には、平滑筋の収縮が大きく関係する。平滑筋は微細な毛細血管により栄養される。リンパ浮腫における集合リンパ管の変性は、平滑筋細胞の変性と関与することが、これまで報告されてきた。長年リンパ浮腫に対する外科的治療を行ってきたわれわれの経験から、保存的治療のみでは正常なリンパ管ドレナージ機能を再獲得することは難しいと考えられる。また頻回の蜂窩織炎はリンパ管の栄養血管を障害し、この阻血性変化によりリンパ管の線維化が促進されると考えられる[1)-5)]。

　リンパ浮腫の初期段階では、リンパ管細静脈吻合術(LVA)によりリンパ管はドレナージ機能を取り戻すことが可能である。しかしながら、重症リンパ浮腫では、非可逆的な平滑筋の変性が起こっており、LVA ではリンパ管のドレナージ機能は取り戻すことができない。

　重症四肢リンパ浮腫治療における LVA 治療の限界を乗り越えるために、機能的リンパ脂肪弁移植(リンパ管移植)が開発された。この方法では、正常なリンパ液ドレナージ機能をもったリンパ管または外側胸リンパ節を移植し、リンパ系の再構築を目指す。

■Introduction

　Collecting lymphatics have lymph-drainage function with contraction of smooth muscle cells. The smooth muscle cells are fed by a tiny capillary artery and vein on the lymphatic wall. Patients with edema have lost this drainage function due to degeneration of smooth muscle cells. We assumed that lymphatics in human lymphedema never regain normal drainage function with only physiotherapy(without bypass surgery). Also, repeated lymphangitis(cellulitis) damages feeding vessels on the lymphatic wall and this ischemia causes sclerotic change in the lymphatics(we named this change "lymph sclerosis")[1)-5)].

　Regarding the changes of collecting lymphatic channels in human lymphedema, in an initial stage just after lymphadenectomy, regeneration following degeneration of smooth muscle cells occurs with bypass surgery. Lymphaticovenular(LV) anastomosis salvages smooth muscle cells from reversible degeneration(mild edema), but muscle cells cannot be recovered from irreversible degeneration(severe edema). Therefore, in severe edema, LV anastomoses cannot reestablish the drainage function of the lymphatic system.

　To overcome this weakness of LV bypass methods for severe edema, new methods were instituted for repair of this missing drainage function using a lymphadiposal flap from the contralateral foot for hemilateral edema, or transfer of lateral thoracic lymph nodes for bilateral edema. Lymphadiposal flaps are transferred to reestablish normal lymph drainage function in legs with irreversible degeneration of lymphatic smooth muscle cells.

I 手術法

1. 第1趾間からのリンパ脂肪弁の挙上(Fig. 7-2-1)

　片側性の重症リンパ浮腫がこの方法のよい適応となる。全身麻酔の下、浮腫側の下肢の鼠径部に皮切が置かれ、浅腸骨回旋動静脈と皮下の静脈を露出する。浅腸骨回旋動脈の遠位の細い枝を移植床動脈として使用する。

　リンパ脂肪弁は反対側の正常な下肢の第1趾間からターニケットによる駆血下に採取する。パテントブルーまたはICGを第1趾または第2趾の皮下の層に注射する。正常な機能をもったリンパ管はパテントブルー注射後すぐによく染まる。注入したICGは近赤外線カメラによりよく描出される。通常1～3本のよく染まるリンパ管が第1趾間に同定される。こうして見つかったリンパ管はパテントブルーがすぐwash outされてしまうため、7-0ナイロンでマーキングしておく。これらのリンパ管と周囲の脂肪組織は第1中足骨動静脈から派生する穿通枝を付けて挙上する。知覚麻痺を防止するため深腓骨神経の本幹は温存する。最後に血管茎として第1中足骨動静脈と皮下静脈まで含めて皮弁を挙上しリンパ脂肪弁が得られる。

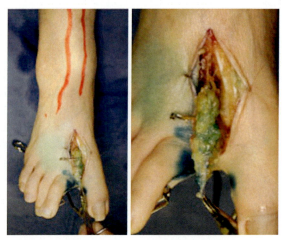

Fig. 7-2-1. 重症の片側性の浮腫に対して第1趾間からのリンパ脂肪弁移植
Lymphadiposal flap from the first web space, for severe edema of hemilateral leg
皮弁の血管は第1中足骨動脈の穿通枝と皮下静脈。深腓骨神経は温存し、パテントブルーを注射し機能的なリンパ管を染めた。
Pedicle of this flap is the first metatarsal artery perforator and cutaneous vein. The deep peroneal nerve is preserved and Patent Blue injection can stain functioning lymphatics.
(Koshima I, Narushima M, Mihara M, et al：Lymphadiposal flaps and lymphaticovenular anastomoses for severe leg edema；Functional reconstruction for lymph drainage system. J Reconstr Microsurg 32(1)：50-55, 2016 による)

2. 機能的外側胸リンパ節の挙上 (Fig. 7-2-2)

両側性の重症の浮腫に対しては、対側の第 1 趾間からのリンパ脂肪弁移植は不可能である。そのような症例に対しては、外側胸リンパ節を含めたリンパ脂肪弁を使用する。収縮可能な正常リンパ管とリンパ節が含まれることでリンパ液を静脈に貫流することができる。外側胸部にパテントブルーまたは ICG を皮下注射した後、数本の染められたリンパ管とリンパ節を、外側胸動静脈または胸背動静脈から派生する細い穿通枝を付けて挙上する。われわれは通常、腋窩リンパ節は温存し、場合によっては腋窩で LVA を行うことで、採取部のリンパ浮腫を予防している。

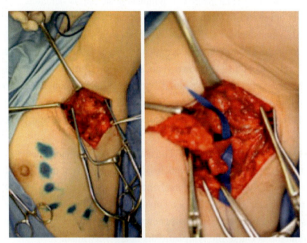

Fig. 7-2-2. 機能的外側胸リンパ節の挙上
Transfer of functioning lateral thoracic lymph nodes
重症の両側性の浮腫に対して外側胸部からリンパ節皮弁を挙上。皮弁は外側胸動脈もしくは胸背動脈からの穿通枝により栄養される。機能的なリンパ管がパテントブルーにより染色される。
Lymph node flap from lateral thoracic region is used for severe edema of bilateral legs (no contralateral normal leg to harvest from). Flap is nourished by perforators from the lateral thoracic or/and thoracodorsal system. Functioning lymphatics are stained by Patent Blue.
(Koshima I, Narushima M, Mihara M, et al：Lymphadiposal flaps and lymphaticovenular anastomoses for severe leg edema；Functional reconstruction for lymph drainage system. J Reconstr Microsurg 32 (1)：50-55, 2016 による)

3. 皮弁を鼠径部に移植する

採取された皮弁(またはリンパ節)は、鼠径部の皮下組織内に移植される。皮弁の栄養血管は、浅腸骨回旋動静脈の枝もしくは皮下静脈に吻合される。外側胸リンパ節もまた血管吻合により栄養される。移植された組織内のリンパ管と静脈の吻合が望ましいが、リンパ管が非常に細いため時に難しいこともある。

I. Operative techniques

1. **First web space lymphadipofascial flap** (**Fig. 7-2-1**)：Patient with severe unilateral edema are good candidates for this method. Under general anesthesia, an incision through the inguinal ligament of the

edematous leg is made to explore the superficial circumflex iliac artery and concomitant veins (SCIA and SCIV), and cutaneous vein. Small distal branches of this SCIA system are recipient vessels for lymphadiposal flap. The lymphadiposal flap is harvested from the first web space of the contralateral normal leg under tourniquet control. Patent Blue or indocyanine green (ICG) (0.1 mm) is injected into the subdermal layer of the first and second toes. Although nonfunctioning lymphatics show little staining, normal functioning lymphatics are well stained just after Patent Blue injection. Also injected ICG fluorescent dye can be visualized using a near-infrared camera system. One or three stained lymphatics are usually detected on the first web space. These stained lymphatics are marked with 7-0 nylon ligation because the dye soon disappears. These lymphatics involving surrounding adiposal tissue are dissected with several perforators arising from the first metatarsal vessel. The main trunk of the deep peroneal nerve is preserved to avoid the sensory loss of the first web space. Finally, after dissection for a short segment of the first metatarsal artery and dorsal cutaneous veins as vascular pedicle, a lymphadiposal flap is obtained.

  2. Transfer of functioning lateral thoracic lymph nodes (Fig. 7-2-2)：In cases with severe bilateral edema, a contralateral lymphadiposal flap from the first web space is impossible. For those cases, a lymphadiposal flap including the lateral thoracic lymph nodes is used, because contraction of lymph nodes can collect and transport lymphatic fluid to their own venous system. After subdermal injection of Patent Blue or ICG in the lateral thoracic region, a few stained lymphatics and lymph nodes are elevated with small perforators arising from the lateral thoracic vessels or/and the thoracodorsal system. We always preserve large axillary lymph nodes and also establish LVA in axillary region to prevent postoperative edema of the donor arm.

  3. Flap transfers to recipient groin region：The obtained flaps (or lymph nodes) are transferred into the subcutaneous layer in the groin region. The pedicle of the flap is anastomosed to the branch of SCIA and SCIV and/or cutaneous vein. The marked proximal ends of lymphatics of first web lymphadiposal flap were joined to the concomitant veins of the SCIV or cutaneous vein. The lateral thoracic lymph node is also vascularized with vascular anastomoses. LVA between the lymph-node flap and recipient vein is preferable, but sometimes it is difficult, because the lymphatic ducts are very small.

Ⅱ　症例提示

1.　症例 1：趾間からのリンパ脂肪弁移植 (Fig. 7-2-3)

　右下肢の原発性リンパ浮腫を患った 15 歳、男性。毎日の部活の練習のため（剣道）、圧迫療法を続けることができなかったため蜂窩織炎を頻繁に起こしていた。局所麻酔の下、右足首に LVA がなされたが、浮腫と蜂窩織炎はさらに悪化し、剣道の練習を続けることができなくなった。

　そのため、LVA を行った 2 年後、反対側の第 1 趾間からリンパ脂肪弁を挙上し右の鼠径部に移植を行った。皮弁の第 1 中足骨動脈と皮下静脈は、鼠径部の浅腸骨回旋動脈と皮下静脈に吻合された。皮弁内の 2 本のリンパ管は、浅腸骨回旋静脈に吻合された。また 2 ヵ所の LVA が足首と下腿の近位部に施行された。

　移植から 4 年後、術前術後の圧迫療法なく、下肢の浮腫は劇的な改善を示した。剣道を継続することができ、皮弁移植後 1 度も蜂窩織炎を起こさなくなった。

7-2．リンパ脂肪弁によるリンパ管移植法

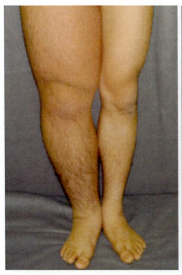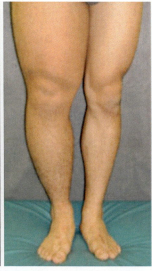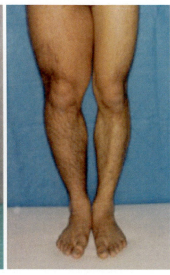

Fig. 7-2-3．症例1　Case 1
左：原発性の片側性浮腫の15歳、男性。毎日の部活のため圧迫療法ができず、頻回の蜂窩織炎を起こしている。足首にLVAを行ったが改善なし。
中：左側の第1趾間からのリンパ脂肪弁移植後7ヵ月。
右：移植後4年5ヵ月。圧迫療法なく蜂窩織炎も起こしていない。
Left：A 15-year-old boy with primary edema of right leg. No compression due to daily sport activity, frequent phlegmone. Worse after LV anastomosis at ankle. No compression.
Middle：7 months after lymphadiposal flap from the first web space on contralateral foot.
Right：4 years and 5 months after flap transfer. No compression and no phlegmone after flap transfer.
（Koshima I, Narushima M, Mihara M, et al：lymphadiposal flaps and lymphaticovenular anastomoses for severe leg edema；functional reconstruction for lymph drainage system. J Reconstr Microsurg 32（1）：50-55, 2016による）

2．症例2：趾間からのリンパ脂肪弁移植 (Fig. 7-2-4)

　左下肢の2年半にわたる原発性リンパ浮腫を患った20歳、女性。毎日の圧迫療法に耐え切れなくなり、2度蜂窩織炎のエピソードあり。そのため右足背からのリンパ脂肪弁移植を行った。
　皮弁内に3本のパテントブルーでよく染まるリンパ管を含めた。この3本のリンパ管と静脈の吻合を行い、第1中足骨動脈と皮下静脈は浅腸骨回旋動脈と皮下静脈に吻合された。
　手術から3年経過し、圧迫療法を継続しながら、浮腫は劇的に改善し、蜂窩織炎も起こさなくなった。長年履きたいと願っていたハイヒールを履くことができた。

3．症例3：外側胸リンパ節移植 (Fig. 7-2-5)

　11年にわたる両下肢の二次性リンパ浮腫を患った56歳、女性。子宮体癌による子宮摘出と術後の放射線治療が行われていた。圧迫療法が行われていたが蜂窩織炎を頻回に起こしていた。
　この重症の両側性浮腫に対して、リンパ節を含んだリンパ脂肪弁が左の外側胸部から採取され、右の鼠径部に移植された。皮弁の血管は浅腸骨回旋動静脈に吻合された。皮弁内の2本のリンパ管は、皮下静脈の枝に吻合された。追加のLVAが両下腿に行われた。
　術後4年が経過し、簡単な圧迫のみで立ち仕事を続けられている。両下肢の浮腫は劇的な改善

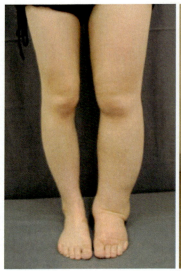
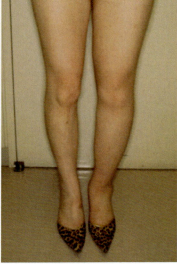

Fig. 7-2-4. 症例 2　Case 2
左：左下肢の原発性浮腫、20 歳、女性。頻回の蜂窩織炎を起こしている。
右：右足の第 1 趾間からのリンパ脂肪弁移植、LVA も施行。手術から 3 年後、ハイヒールを履くことができた。
Left：A 20-year-old woman, primary edema of left leg with frequent phlegmone.
Right：lymphadiposal flap from the contralateral foot was transferred as well as LVA. 3 years after surgery, she could wear a high heel.
(Koshima I, Narushima M, Mihara M, et al：lymphadiposal flaps and lymphaticovenular anastomoses for severe leg edema；functional reconstruction for lymph drainage system. J Reconstr Microsurg 32（1）：50-55, 2016 による)

を示し、蜂窩織炎は起こしていない。

II. Case reports

1. **Case 1：Lymphadiposal flap from web space（Fig. 7-2-3）**：A 15-year-old boy was suffered from primary edema of right leg. He could not continue with compression therapy because he wanted to practice "Kendo（a Japanese traditional sport using bamboo sword）" every day, but frequent cellulitis disturbed his sports life. Although LVA was established at the ankle region under local anesthesia, the edema and cellulitis became worse and the patient could not continue Kendo practice

Therefore, after he accepted LVA for 2 years, he agreed to transfer a lymphadiposal flap from the first web space of left foot to right groin region. The first metatarsal artery and cutaneous vein of the flap were anastomosed to the SCIA and cutaneous vein in right groin region. The proximal ends of two lymphatic ducts in the flap were joined to the concomitant veins of the SCIA, and additional two LV anastomosis were done at the ankle and proximal side of the left lower leg.

He did not need compression therapy after the flap transfer 4 years later, and the leg showed complete recovery (dramatic improvement without any postoperative compression therapy). He could continue "Kendo" practice daily. He had no episodes of cellulitis after the flap transfer.

2. **Case 2：Lymphadiposal flap from web space（Fig. 7-2-4）**：A 20-year-old woman suffered from primary edema in her left leg for 2 and a half years. She could not tolerate daily compression therapy and had two episodes of cellulitis. Therefore, a lymphadiposal flap was transferred from right foot.

The flap involved three well-stained lymphatics by Patent Blue injection. The first metatarsal artery and

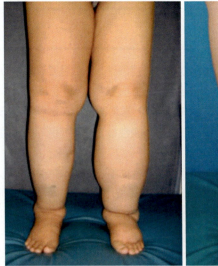
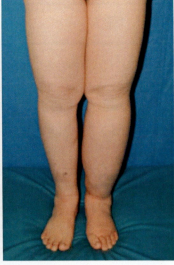

Fig. 7-2-5. 症例 3　Case 3

左：56 歳、女性、二次性リンパ浮腫、両側性、放射線治療後、頻回の蜂窩織炎を起こしている。

右：外側胸部からのリンパ脂肪弁が右の鼠径部に移植された。同時に LVA もなされた。手術から 4 年後、蜂窩織炎なく、軽度な圧迫療法のみである。

Left：A 56-year-old woman, secondary edema of bilateral legs, with radiated, frequent phlegmone.

Right：Lymphadiposal flap from the lateral thoracic region was transferred to the right groin. Simultaneous LVA was done. 4 years after the surgery without any phlegmone, with a slight compression.

(Koshima I, Narushima M, Mihara M, et al：lymphadiposal flaps and lymphaticovenular anastomoses for severe leg edema；functional reconstruction for lymph drainage system. J Reconstr Microsurg 32（1）：50-55, 2016 による)

cutaneous vein of the flap were anastomosed to the SCIA and cutaneous vein in left groin area. Besides, LVA was also established between the lymphatic ducts of flap and cutaneous veins.

After surgery, she accepted some compression therapy for 3 years, the leg showed dramatic improvement without any cellulitis. She could wear high heeled shoes which she had wanted to wear for a long time

3. Case 3：Lateral thoracic lymph node transfer（Fig. 7-2-5）：A 56-year-old woman had secondary lymphedema over bilateral lower extremities for 11 years. This lymphedema occurred after a hysterectomy for uterine cancer with postoperative radiation. In spite of extensive compression therapy, both legs developed frequent cellulitis.

For this severe bilateral edema, a lymphadiposal flap including lymph nodes was transferred from the left lateral thoracic region. The flap was transferred to the right groin which was the more severely affected side. The pedicle vessels of flap were anastomosed to the SCIA and SCIV. Two lymphatic ducts of the flap were anastomosed to two branches of the cutaneous vein over right groin region. Additional LVA was established in both legs.

After surgery for 4 years, she could continue her daily job with simple compression. The legs showed dramatic improvement without cellulitis.

III 考　察

　われわれのこれまでのリンパ浮腫治療の経験から、重症のリンパ浮腫では集合リンパ管のドレナージ機能は完全に失われ、リンパ管の平滑筋細胞が非可逆的な変性を起こしていることがわかっている。特に頻回の蜂窩織炎はリンパ管を破壊すると言える。LVA は軽症から中等症のリンパ浮腫に対して改善を示すが、リンパ管の平滑筋細胞が変性している症例では改善はあまり期待できない[1)3)−11)17)]。

　リンパ脂肪弁は、リンパ管平滑筋機能が非可逆的な変性に陥っている下肢に対して正常なドレナージ機能をもつリンパ管を再構築する。反対側の趾間からのリンパ脂肪弁は片側性の重症浮腫で、頻回の蜂窩織炎を起こし、LVA があまり効かないケースに対して用いられる。外側胸リンパ節移植は重症の両側性の浮腫に対して効果が認められる。

　これらの治療法は LVA 単独と比べて、よりよい結果が得られる。Chen HC と Becker C は動物や上肢のリンパ浮腫に対して LVA を行わずにリンパ節移植だけで浮腫を治療する方法を初めて行った[12)13)]。以後、諸家からリンパ節移植の有用性について報告されている[14)−16)]。リンパ脂肪弁は、重症の長期にわたる下肢のリンパ浮腫に対してよい適応であり、特に圧迫療法や LVA に抵抗性、頻回の蜂窩織炎を起こす方が適応と言える。

　ドナーサイトの選択に関して、鼠径部のリンパ節を使うことは、上肢のリンパ浮腫や片側性のリンパ浮腫に対して有効と考えられる[13)−16)]。しかしながら、わずかにドナーサイトのリンパ浮腫のリスクもある。そのため、巨大なリンパ管が存在し、ドナーサイトのリンパ浮腫のリスクがないため、第 1 趾間はよりよいドナーサイトと言える。

　両側性の重症の浮腫においては、下肢には有効なリンパ管が残っていないので、外側胸部からの正常なドレナージ機能をもったリンパ管移植は有効な治療法である。この周囲のリンパ管は足背部のリンパ管と比べ細いが、皮弁内や移植床との LVA は施行可能である。

　本方法の利点は、皮切が小さく皮弁も小さいため、侵襲が小さく、短時間で挙上可能で、合併症が少ない点である。技術的に難しい点は、0.8 mm 以下の脈管吻合をする supermicrosurgery の技術を必要とすることである。

（田代絢亮、光嶋　勲）

III. Discussion

　Based on our previous study for 23 years, it is assumed that in severe extremity edema, the dynamic drainage function of the collecting lymphatic ducts is completely lost, because of irreversible degeneration of smooth muscle cells within the lymphatic wall. Especially, frequent cellulitis resulting from lymphangitis, it destroys the lymphatic ducts completely of legs no matter proximal or distal part. LVA is performed for mild lymphedema with temporally degeneration of smooth muscle cells, and it shows some or dramatic improvement. However, LVA is used for lymphatic ducts with irreversible degeneration, and it shows little improvement (resisted LVA)[1)3) − 11)17)].

　Lymphadiposal flaps are transferred to reestablish the normal lymph drainage function in legs with irreversible degeneration of smooth muscle cells within the lymphatic wall. A lymphadiposal flap from the web space was used for cases with unilateral severe edema, frequent cellulitis, and resistance to LV anastomoses. Besides, performing the lateral thoracic lymph node transfer, severe lymphedema of lower extremities showed some improvement. These results are better than those of simple LV anastomoses, because these flaps and lymph nodes have normal lymphatic drainage function. Chen et al. and Becker et al. first advocated lymph nodes transfer without LV anastomosis for lymphedema in animals and human arms[12)13)]. Thereafter, some authors recently reported the usefulness of lymph nodes transfer from the groin region to establish drainage function of lymphatic system in arm[14)-16)]. Lymphadiposal flaps are considered for severe and long-term lymphedema of legs, particularly in patients who are resistant to compression therapy. Besides, it is also effective for the patients who received simple LVA but failure, or the patients who could not tolerated daily compression therapy. As for selection of donor site, it is considered that lymph nodes in the contralateral groin region may be suitable candidates for severe edema in the arm and unilateral leg[13)-16)]. However, there is a small risk of inducing edema in the donor legs. Therefore, it is believed that the first web space is a better site because there are larger lymphatic ducts compared with other sites. It is impossible for lymphedema occurrence below the donor site.

In the patients with severe bilateral lymphedema, all lymphatic ducts in the first web space, legs, and lower abdominal regions including lymph nodes in groin have lost their drainage function. Therefore, vascularized lymph nodes from the lateral thoracic region are obtained because they have normal drainage function. Although lymphatic ducts around nodes in this region are smaller than those of the first web space of foot, LVA still can be established between lymphatic ducts and venous system within flap or cutaneous veins of recipient site.

The advantages of these methods are less invasive surgery with small incisions, flap harvest taking a short time, and without complications. The disadvantages of these methods are applying super-microsurgical LVA, and small vascular anastomosis less than 0.8 mm.

(*Kensuke Tashiro, Isao Koshima/Shuhei Yoshida*)

1) Koshima I, Kawada S, Moriguchi T, et al : Ultrastructural observations of lymphatic vessels in lymphedema in human extremities. Plast Reconstr Surg 97(2) : 397-405, discussion 406-407, 1996.
2) Koshima I, Endo T : Experimental study of vascularized muscle ; multifactorial analysis of muscle regeneration following denervation. J Reconstr Microsurg 5(3) : 225-230, 1989.
3) Koshima I, Inagawa K, Urushibara K, et al : Supermicrosurgical lymphaticovenular anastomosis for the treatment of lymphedema in the upper extremities. J Reconstr Microsurg 16(6) : 437-442, 2000.
4) Koshima I, Nanba Y, Tsutsui T, et al : Long-term follow-up after lymphaticovenular anastomosis for lymphedema in the leg. J Reconstr Microsurg 19(4) : 209-215, 2003.
5) Koshima I, Nanba Y, Tsutsui T, et al : Minimal invasive lymphaticovenular anastomosis under local anesthesia for leg lymphedema ; is it effective for stage III and IV? Ann Plast Surg 53(3) : 261-266, 2004.
6) O'Brien BM, Chait LA, Hurwitz PJ : Microlymphatic surgery. Orthop Clin North Am 8(2) : 405-424, 1977.
7) O'Brien BM, Sykes P, Threlfall GN, et al : Microlymphaticovenous anastomoses for obstructive lymphedema. Plast Reconstr Surg 60(2) : 197-211, 1977.
8) O'Brien BM, Mellow CG, Khazanchi RK, et al : Long-termresults after microlymphaticovenous anastomoses for the treatment of obstructive lymphedema. Plast Reconstr Surg 85(4) : 562-572, 1990.
9) Huang GK, Hu RQ, Liu ZZ, et al : Microlymphaticovenous anastomosis in the treatment of lower limb obstructive lymphedema : analysis of 91 cases. Plast Reconstr Surg 76(5) : 671-685, 1985.
10) Campisi C : Use of autologous interposition vein graft in management of lymphedema ; preliminary experimental and clinical observations. Lymphology 24(2) : 71-76, 1991.
11) Campisi C, Boccardo F, Zilli A, et al : Long-term results after lymphatic-venous anastomoses for the treatment of obstructive lymphedema. Microsurgery 21(4) : 135-139, 2001.
12) Chen HC, O'Brien BM, Rogers IW, et al : Lymph node transfer for the treatment of obstructive

lymphoedema in the canine model. Br J Plast Surg 43(5) : 578-586, 1990.

13) Becker C, Assouad J, Riquet M, et al : Postmastectomy lymphedema : long-term results following microsurgical lymph node transplantation. Ann Surg 243(3) : 313-315, 2006.

14) Lin CH, Ali R, Chen SC, et al : Vascularized groin lymph node transfer using the wrist as a recipient site for management of postmastectomy upper extremity lymphedema. Plast Reconstr Surg 123 (4) : 1265-1275, 2009.

15) Gharb BB, Rampazzo A, Spanio di Spilimbergo S, et al : Vascularized lymph node transfer based on the hilar perforators improves the outcome in upper limb lymphedema. Ann Plast Surg 67(6) : 589-593, 2011.

16) Saaristo AM, Niemi TS, Viitanen TP, et al : Microvascular breast reconstruction and lymph node transfer for postmastectomy lymphedema patients. Ann Surg 255(3) : 468-473, 2012.

17) Koshima I, Narushima M, Mihara M, et al : Lymphadiposal flaps and lymphaticovenular anastomoses for severe leg edema : Functional reconstruction for lymph drainage system. J Reconstr Microsurg 32(1) : 50-55, 2016.

CHAPTER **7**

外科治療
Surgical treatment

3. リンパ節移植

Lymph node transfer

Ⅰ　総　論

　1979年に Shesol らが初めてラットで血管付きリンパ節移植を行ったことを報告して以来、リンパ節移植はリンパ浮腫に対する治療として徐々に広がってきた[1]。1990年にイヌでリンパ節移植を行ったことを報告した台湾の Hung-Chi Chen[2]、1991年にヒトに臨床応用したことを報告したフランスの Corinne Becker が[3]、現在でもリンパ節移植の第一人者として有名である。リンパ節移植とは、健常部位にあるリンパ節とその周囲の脂肪組織を栄養血管ごと採取し、リンパ浮腫の部位に移植し、顕微鏡下にリンパ節を栄養する動静脈と移植床の動静脈を吻合する術式である。移植床のリンパ管と移植したリンパ節のリンパ管は自然につながることが報告されており、リンパ管-リンパ管吻合は行わないのが一般的である。

　リンパ節移植がリンパ浮腫に対して効果をもつメカニズムには諸説ある。移植したリンパ節からリンパ管新生因子が放出されるため、新たなリンパ路が形成されてリンパ液うっ滞が改善するという説が1つである。また、リンパ節自体にポンプ作用があり、同時にリンパ節の中は生理的なリンパ管-静脈吻合があるため、この交通路を介してうっ滞したリンパ液が排出されるようになるという説もある。

　コンセンサスのとれたメカニズムが確立していない分、リンパ節移植の術式もいまだに多岐にわたっている。リンパ節の採取部位にもさまざまな報告があり、下肢リンパ浮腫に対して最も一般的なリンパ節採取部位は腋窩～側胸部である（**Fig. 7-3-1, 2**）。栄養血管として外側胸動静脈や胸背動静脈の枝が用いられる。腋窩から採取する方法もあるが、腋窩リンパ節を採取すると上肢のリンパ流が障害されることがあるため、腋窩を避けて側胸部から採取するとする報告もある。上肢リンパ浮腫に対して最も一般的な採取部位は鼠径部である。この場合の栄養血管は主に浅腸骨回旋動静脈が用いられる。下肢のリンパ流を妨げないよう、鼠径靱帯より中枢側で採取するという報告もある。その他にも、鎖骨上リンパ節（栄養血管は頸横動静脈の枝）や顎下リンパ節（栄養血管はオトガイ下動静脈）などを採取した報告も散見される。いずれの部位からリンパ節を採取するのがよいかについてはコンセンサスに至っていない。

　患肢のうちどこを移植床とすべきかについても、議論のあるところである。Becker らはリンパ浮腫のある肢の近位部にリンパ節を移植することが有用であると報告している。つまり、上肢リンパ浮腫であれば腋窩、下肢リンパ浮腫であれば鼠径部である（**Fig. 7-3-3**）。それらの部位には、がん治療の際に生じた瘢痕組織があることが多いため、その瘢痕組織を除去し、組織欠損部にリンパ節を含む十分量の脂肪組織を移植する。一方 Chen らは、重力によって一番リンパ液が貯留すると考えられる遠位にリンパ節を移植する方が有用であると報告し、手関節部や足関節部にリンパ節移植を行っている。膝関節、肘関節周囲に移植するという報告も、数は少ないながら存在

211

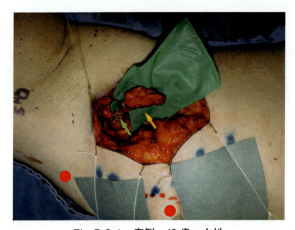

Fig. 7-3-1. 症例：48 歳、女性
Case：48-year-old woman

両下肢リンパ浮腫に対し、左側胸部から右鼠径部へリンパ節移植を行った。前胸部に ICG を注射し、前胸部からのリンパが流入するリンパ節を同定した。リンパ節の栄養血管として外側胸動静脈を用いた。
赤丸：ICG 注射部位、緑矢印：栄養血管、黄色矢印：リンパ節を含む脂肪弁。
For both lower limb lymphedema, lymph node transfer was performed from the left chest to the right inguinal region. Indocyanine green (ICG) was injected into the anterior chest, and the lymph nodes into which lymph flows from the anterior thorax were identified. An external thoracic vein was used as a nutrient vessel of lymph node.
Red circle：ICG injection site, green arrow：nourishing blood vessel, yellow arrow：fat valve including lymph node.

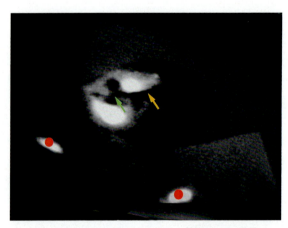

Fig. 7-3-2. Fig. 7-3-1 のリンパ節の ICG 所見
ICG findings of lymph nodes in Fig. 7-3-1

前胸部に注射した ICG が流入したリンパ節を採取した。
赤丸：ICG 注射部位、緑矢印：栄養血管、黄色矢印：ICG で造影されたリンパ節。
Lymph nodes with ICG injected into the anterior chest were collected.
Red circle：ICG injection site, green arrow：nourishing blood vessel, yellow arrow：ICG-enhanced lymph node.

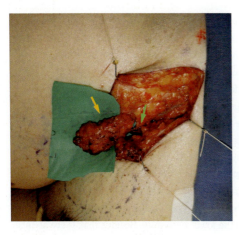

Fig. 7-3-3. Fig. 7-3-1 と同じ患者
The same patient as Fig. 7-3-1
右鼠径部にリンパ節を移植した。移植床血管として、浅腸骨回旋動静脈を用いた。
緑矢印：血管吻合部、黄色矢印：リンパ節を含む脂肪弁。
Lymph nodes were transplanted into the right inguinal region. As a transplanted floor vessel, a superficial iliac rotation artery was used.
Green arrow : vascular anastomosis, yellow arrow : fat valve including lymph node.

する。部位の違いによる効果の差については、今のところほとんど報告がない。また、どの部位に移植すればどの部位に効果が現れるのかについても、コンセンサスが得られていない。

移植した組織の血流モニタリングのために、リンパ節および周囲の脂肪組織に皮膚を付けて移植することもある。より確実な移植組織の生着が期待できるが、整容的に劣るため、一定期間を経た後に皮膚のみ切除することが多い。

リンパ節移植の効果については、79～98％の患者で術後になんらかの改善を認めたと報告がある。周径の減少のほか、蜂窩織炎の減少、患肢の重い感じや硬さの改善、リンパ浮腫部の疼痛の改善などが、リンパ節移植の効果として報告されている。リンパ節移植によりリンパ還流が改善されるため上記のような効果が得られると考えられるが、リンパ浮腫では脂肪増生が起こることが報告されており、リンパ移植のみで既に増生してしまった脂肪を減少させるのは困難と考えられる。このため、増生した脂肪を除去するために脂肪吸引術やCharles法を併用する施設もある。

リンパ節移植に関して、最も注意すべき合併症は、リンパ節採取部に新たに起こるリンパ浮腫である。腋窩リンパ節は上肢リンパ管の流路であるし、鼠径リンパ節は下肢リンパ管の流路である。これを採取することで、新たにリンパ浮腫が発症することがあり、既に何例か論文として報告されている。これを防ぐために後述するようなreverse lymphatic mappingなどの方法が開発されている。その他の合併症として、創部のリンパ漏、漿液腫、縫合不全、創部感染などがある。

I. General statement

Lymph node transfer has gradually spread as a treatment for lymphedema since Shesol et al. first reported in 1979 that he had performed vascularized lymph node transfer in rats[1]. Hung Chi Chen in Taiwan who reported to perform lymph node transfer in dogs in 1990[2], and Corinne Becker of France who reported clinical cases of lymph node transfer in 1991[3] are still famous as the forerunner of lymph node transfer. Lymph node transfer is a method in which lymph nodes at a healthy site and surrounding adipose tissue are collected together with nutrient blood vessels and transplanted to a site of lymphedema and arteriovenous anastomosis performed. It is reported that the lymphatic vessels of the transplanted floor and the lymphatic vessels of the transplanted lymph node are naturally connected, and lymphatic-lymphatic anastomosis is not generally performed.

There are various theories on mechanisms by which lymph node transplant has an effect on lymphedema.

One theory is that lymphatic neoplasia is released from the transplanted lymph node, and a new lymphatic pathway is formed to improve lymphatic stasis. In addition, there is a theory that the lymph nodes themselves have a pumping action and at the same time, the lymph nodes in the lymph nodes have physiological lymphatic-venous anastomosis, so that stagnant lymph fluids are discharged via this pathway.

There is still a wide variety of techniques for lymph node transfer, as no consensus mechanism has been established. There are various reports on the site of the collection of lymph nodes, and the most common lymph node sampling site for lower limb lymphedema is the axillary to the lateral chest (**Fig. 7-3-1, 2**). Outer thoracic vein and thoracic back vein branch are used as nutrient blood vessels. Although there is a method of sampling from the axilla, there are reports that it is collected from the lateral chest while avoiding the axilla, as the lymph flow of the upper limb may be hindered when the axillary lymph node is collected. The most common collection site for upper limb lymphedema is the groin. In this case, the superficial descending artery vein is mainly used as the nutrient blood vessel. There is also a report that it collects on the central side from the inguinal ligament so as not to disturb the lymph flow of the lower extremity. Besides that, there are also reports that collected supraclavicular lymph nodes (branches of the cervical transverse vein) and submandibular lymph nodes (nutrient vessels down artery and vein) etc. Consensus has not been reached as to which lymph nodes should be taken from which site.

There are arguments as to which part of the affected limb should be the recipient site. Becker and colleagues report that it is useful to implant lymph nodes in the proximal part of a limb with lymphedema. In other words, it is the axillary if it is upper limb lymphedema, and the groin if it is lower limb lymphedema (**Fig. 7-3-3**). Since there is often scar tissue generated at the time of cancer treatment at those sites, the scar tissue is removed and a sufficient amount of adipose tissue including the lymph nodes is transplanted to the tissue defect portion. Meanwhile, Chen and colleagues report that it is more useful to transplant lymph nodes to the distal region, which is thought to be most likely to reserve lymph fluid by gravity, and lymph node transfer is performed on the wrist joint and the ankle joint.

There are also reports that transplanting around the knee joint and the elbow joint, although there are few, it exists. There is almost no report on the difference in effects due to differences in parts at the moment. Also, the consensus has not been obtained on which part will be effective if it is transplanted to which part.

For blood flow monitoring of transplanted tissues, lymph nodes and surrounding adipose tissue may be transplanted with skin. More reliable engraftment of the transplanted tissue can be expected, but since it is cosmetically inferior, only the skin is frequently excised after a certain period of time.

Regarding the effect of lymph node transfer, it is reported that 79% to 98% of patients had some improvement after surgery. In addition to the reduction of circumflex, reduction of honey cell floss, improvement of heavy feel and hardness of affected limb, improvement of lymphedema pain, etc. are reported as effects of lymph node transfer. As lymph node refusal improves lymph node reflux, it is thought that the above effect will be obtained, but it is reported that fat multiplication occurs in lymphedema, and fat which has already increased by lymph transplant alone is considered to be difficult to reduce. For this reason, some facilities use liposuction or Charles method in combination to remove the increased fat.

Regarding lymph node transfer, the most notable complication is lymphedema newly occurring in the lymph node harvesting section. The axillary lymph node is the flow path of the upper limb lymphatic duct and the inguinal lymph node is the flow path of the lower limb lymph duct. By collecting this, new lymphedema may develop, and some cases have already been reported as articles. To prevent this, methods such as reverse lymphatic mapping as described later have been developed. Other complications include lymphorrhea of the wound, seroma, suture failure, wound infection and the like.

7-3. リンパ節移植

Ⅱ　リンパ節移植の適応

　リンパ節移植は、基本的にどのようなリンパ浮腫にも適応になる。しかし、リンパ節採取部に新たなリンパ浮腫が起こる可能性を考慮すると、良好なリンパ管機能が残存している部位にはリンパ管細静脈吻合術（LVA）も検討すべき選択肢となる。

　筆者らは、術中に認める集合リンパ管の性状を Normal Type、Ectasis Type、Contraction Type、Sclerosis Type の４つに分類し、NECST 分類（ネクスト分類）と名づけた[4]。さらにインドシアニングリーン（ICG）蛍光リンパ管造影法の所見と、NECST 分類の関連を報告した。ICG 検査で Linear pattern や Splash pattern といった軽症部位では機能良好なリンパ管を認めることが多いが、重症化して Diffuse pattern を示す部位では、硬化が進み機能の落ちたリンパ管を認めることが多い。このことから、ICG 検査で Diffuse を示す部位はリンパ節移植のよい適応と考える。

　Makoto Mihara らは、リンパシンチグラフィにてリンパ管機能が残存している部分とリンパ管機能が低下している部分がモザイク状になっている患者に対して、リンパ管機能が残存している部分に対して LVA を、リンパ管機能の低下している部分に対してリンパ節移植を行ったことを報告した[5]。

　Ming-Huei Cheng らは、リンパ節移植の適応を下記のように提唱している。①リンパシンチグラフィでリンパ管が完全閉塞しているもの、②国際リンパ学会の重症度分類で Stage 2 で蜂窩織炎を繰り返すもの、③蜂窩織炎急性期でないもの、④12ヵ月以上経過をみたもの、である。

　リンパ浮腫に対する治療の第一選択は複合的理学療法（CDT）とされており、CDT に抵抗性のリンパ浮腫が外科治療の適応といわれてきた。しかし、リンパ浮腫が長期間続くと次第にリンパ管が硬化し、機能を失っていく。そうなる前に、早期に外科的介入を行うべきであるとの意見もあり、リンパ節移植の適応については今後のエビデンス構築が待たれる。

Ⅱ. Indication of lymph node transfer

　Lymph node transfer is basically adaptable to any lymphedema. However, considering the possibility of donor site lymphedema, lymphaticovenous anastomosis (LVA) is also an option to consider for sites where good lymphatic function remains.

　The authors classified the properties of the collecting lymphatic vessels that are recognized during surgery into four types, Normal Type, Ectasis Type, Contraction Type, and Sclerosis Type, and named the NECST classification (Next Classification)[4]. In addition, the findings of indocyanine green (ICG) fluorescent lymphangiography and the association of NECST classification were reported. In ICG examination, lymphatic vessels with good function are often found in mild sites such as Linear pattern and Splash pattern, but in regions showing severity and Diffuse pattern, lymph ducts whose function has declined are often found. From this, we think that the site showing Diffuse by ICG examination is a good indication for lymph node transfer.

　Makoto Mihara and colleagues reported that in lymphatic scintigraphy patients with lymph duct function remain and those with lymphatic function declining are mosaic-shaped, in contrast, LVA was reported to have undergone transplantation of lymph nodes to parts of lymphatic vessels that are degraded[5].

　Ming-Huei Cheng and colleagues propose adaptation of lymph node transplant as follows. ①lymphatic scintigraphy in which lymphatic vessels are completely occluded, ②those that repeat the cellulitis in Stage 2 in the severity classification of the International Lymphological Society, ③those not in the acute phase of

215

cellulitis, ④12 months it is what has seen the passage of time.

The first choice of treatment for lymphedema is considered to be combined physical therapy (CDT), and lymphedema which is resistant to CDT has been said to be suitable for surgical treatment. However, as long as the lymphedema continues, the lymphatic vessels gradually harden and lose their function. There is also the opinion that surgical intervention should be done early before it becomes so, and future evidence building is awaited for adaptation of lymph node transfer.

Ⅲ Reverse lymphatic mapping

Joseph Dayan らは、より安全にリンパ節採取を行うため、reverse lymphatic mapping を報告した[6]。まずリンパ節採取部より遠位の末梢（鼠径部から採取する際は趾間部）にテクネシウムを皮下注射し、ガンマプローブにてその肢からのリンパが流入するリンパ節を同定し、このリンパ節は採取しないようにする。さらに近傍の体幹（鼠径部から採取する際は下腹部）に ICG を皮下注射し、赤外線カメラを用いて体幹からのリンパが流入するリンパ節を同定し、このリンパ節を採取するようにする。この手法によって、上下肢からのリンパ排出を障害することなくリンパ節を採取することが可能である。肢からのリンパと体幹からのリンパが同じリンパ節に流入する場合は、他の部位からリンパ節を採取するように変更する。

Ⅲ. Reverse lymphatic mapping

Joseph Dayan and colleagues reported reverse lymphatic mapping for safer lymph node collection[6]. First, technetium is injected subcutaneously into the distal region from the lymph node harvesting part (interdigital space when harvesting from inguinal part), and gamma probe identifies the lymph node into which lymph flows from the limb, and this lymph node will not be harvested. In addition, indocyanine green (ICG) is injected subcutaneously into the proximal trunk (lower abdomen when ingesting from inguinal part), lymph nodes into which lymph flows from the trunk are identified using infrared camera, this lymph node will be harvested. By this technique, it is possible to take lymph nodes without disturbing lymph drainage from the upper and lower limbs. If the lymph from the limb and the lymph from the trunk flow into the same lymph node, alter lymph nodes from other parts.

Ⅳ 乳房再建とリンパ節移植

上肢リンパ浮腫患者では、乳癌に対して乳腺切除術を受けていることが多い。Anne Saaristo らは、そのような患者に対して深下腹壁動脈穿通枝皮弁（DIEP flap）や腹直筋皮弁による乳房再建を行う際に、皮弁に鼠径リンパ節を含めることで乳房再建とリンパ節移植を同時に行うことを報告した。場合によってはリンパ節の血流を確保するために、皮弁の栄養血管と別に浅腸骨回旋動静脈が必要となることがある。乳房再建の移植床血管としては内胸動静脈が用いられることが多く、リンパ節は腋窩に配置する必要があるため、深下腹壁動静脈を内胸動静脈と吻合し、浅腸骨回旋動静脈を外側胸動静脈または胸背動静脈と吻合するなど工夫が施される。

IV．Breast reconstruction and lymph node transfer

In upper limb lymphedema patients, breast cancer is often subjected to mastectomy. Anne Saaristo and colleagues reported that by including inguinal lymph nodes in the deep inferior epigastric artery perforator (DIEP) flap or a rectus abdominis flap, breast reconstruction and lymph node transfer are performed at the same time. In some cases it may be necessary to include the superficial circumflex iliac artery and vein in addition to the blood vessels of the flap to ensure blood flow in the lymph nodes. Since the internal mammary vessels are often used as a recipient vessel of breast reconstruction and the lymph nodes are required to be placed in the axilla, the deep inferior epigastric vessels are anastomosed with the internal mammary vessels, and the superficial circumflex iliac vessels are anastomosed to lateral thoracic vessels or thoracodorsal vessels.

Ⅴ　リンパ節移植の応用

Mihara らは、中咽頭癌患者に対して浅腸骨回旋動脈穿通枝皮弁による再建を行う際に、皮弁に鼠径リンパ節を含めて採取して移植することで、センチネルリンパ節再建を行ったことを報告した[7]。これによりがんが局所再発した場合の全身転移予防、早期発見ができる可能性がある。

Saaristo らのグループは、リンパ節移植の際に VEGF-C をエンコードしたウイルスベクターを注入すると、移植されたリンパ節の構造が保たれ、リンパ管新生が効率的に起こることを基礎実験のデータをもとに報告した[8]。移植したリンパ節と移植床のリンパ管の自発的な結合も、VEGF-C 存在下の方が良好であった。VEGF-C は悪性腫瘍の転移を助長する可能性があるため、がん術後のリンパ浮腫患者に対しては適応を慎重に検討する必要があるが、今後の展開が期待される方法である。

V．Application of lymph node transfer

Mihara and colleagues reported to perform sentinel lymph node reconstruction by harvesting and transplanting inguinal lymph nodes in the flap when transferring the superficial circumflex iliac artery perforator flap for the reconstruction of oropharyngeal carcinoma[7]. There is a possibility that prevention and early detection of systemic metastasis in the case where cancer recurs locally.

The group of Saaristo and colleagues reported that when implanting a VEGF-C encoded viral vector at the time of lymph node transfer, the structure of the transplanted lymph node was maintained and lymphangiogenesis occurred efficiently[8]. Spontaneous binding of transplanted lymph nodes to the lymphatic vessels of the transplanted floor was also better in the presence of VEGF-C. Because VEGF-C may promote the metastasis of malignant tumors, adaptation needs to be carefully examined for lymphedema patients after cancer surgery, but it is a method expected to develop in the future.

■おわりに

本章では、さまざまな文献からリンパ節移植についての現状を述べた。一般的なマイクロサージャリーの技術で施行できるため、世界的には LVA よりもリンパ節移植の方が広く行われている。リンパ節移植を行うにあたり、最も注意が必要なのはリンパ節採取部のリンパ浮腫である。Reverse lymphatic mapping などを活用し、細心の注意を払う必要がある。術前に患肢のリン

パ管機能を評価し、適応を十分に検討したうえで施行するのがよいと考えられる。現在、リンパ節移植には多種多彩な術式が乱立している状況であり、今後エビデンスの構築に伴い、より安全に、確実なリンパ節移植が行われることを期待する。

（原　尚子）

■Conclusion

In this section, the current situation of lymph node transfer was described from various documents. Lymph node transfer is widely carried out worldwide than LVA because it can be performed using general microsurgery techniques. In lymph node transfer, the most important thing to notice is the donor site lymphedema. Reverse lymphatic mapping may be helpful to prevent donor site lymphedema. It is considered better to evaluate the lymphatic function of the affected limb prior to surgery and to enforce it after fully considering the indication. Currently, lymph node transfer is a situation where a wide variety of surgical procedures are muzzled, and we expect that more safe and reliable lymph node transfer will be carried out as evidence is constructed in the future.

(*Hisako Hara*)

1) Shesol BF, Nakashima R, Alavi A, et al：Successful lymph node transplantation in rats, with restoration of lymphatic function. Plast Reconstr Surg 63(6)：817-823, 1979.
2) Chen HC, O'Brien BM, Rogers IW, et al：Lymph node transfer for the treatment of obstructive lymphoedema in the canine model. Br J Plast Surg 43(5)：578-586, 1990.
3) Becker C, Hidden G, Godart S, et al：Free lymphatic transplant. Eur J Lymphol Relat Probl 6：25-77, 1991.
4) Hara H, Mihara M, Seki Y, et al：Comparison of indocyanine green lymphographic findings with the conditions of collecting lymphatic vessels of limbs in patients with lymphedema. Plast Reconstr Surg 132(6)：1612-1618, 2013.
5) Mihara M, Zhou HP, Hara H, et al：Case report：a new hybrid surgical approach for treating mosaic pattern secondary lymphedema in the lower extremities. Ann Vasc Surg 28(7)：1798.e1-1798.e6, 2014.
6) Dayan JH, Dayan E, Smith ML：Reverse lymphatic mapping；a new technique for maximizing safety in vascularized lymph node transfer. Plast Reconstr Surg 135(1)：277-285, 2015.
7) Mihara M, Iida T, Hara H, et al：Autologus groin lymph node transfer for "sentinel lymph network" reconstruction after head-and-neck cancer resection and neck lymph node dissection；a case report. Microsurgery 32(2)：153-157, 2012.
8) Hartiala P, Saaristo AM：Growth factor therapy and autologous lymph node transfer in lymphedema. Trends Cardiovasc Med 20(8)：249-253, 2010.

Important Reference

■ リンパ学に残された不思議 ─ リンパ系と脂肪とのかかわり ─

The mysteries in lymphology ─ Relationships between the lymphatic system and the fat ─

■はじめに

リンパ浮腫は慢性化するとわずかな傷害でも蜂窩織炎を起こしやすく、炎症組織周囲の線維化や脂肪化（脂肪浮腫）が進むとともに組織変化が非可逆的になり、最終的には皮膚の過角化を伴った象皮症をきたす。では、なぜリンパ浮腫が次第に脂肪浮腫や象皮症と呼ばれるような病態となるのであろうか？　実は、その疑問を紐解くヒントになるかも知れない、古くから知られるいくつかの事実が存在する。つまり、リンパ系と脂肪との間には切っても切れない不思議な関係がある[1]。本稿では、若い外科医の皆さんにもより身近で現実に即した現象論に近いレベルでの話題に絞って取りあげ、難題であるリンパ浮腫に対する治療のために少しでもお役に立てれば幸いである。

リンパと脂肪とのかかわりについては、現代病ともいわれる肥満や代謝性疾患についての関心の高まりとともに、分子レベル・遺伝子レベルでの研究も盛んになってきている。ここでは私自身がリンパ系と脂肪の関係について以前から不思議に感じてきたいくつかの事実を挙げてみたい。かなり断片的な話題となるが、若い外科医の皆さんにも一緒に考えて頂きたい。

■ Introduction

When lymphedema progresses to the chronic stage, even minor injuries are likely to result in cellulitis. When fibrosis and lipedema are inflated, the histopathological changes will be irreversible and the final skin will exhibit elephantiasis symptom because of hyperkeratosis. Why does lymphedema cause lipedema and elephantiasis symptom? In fact, there have been some clues to answer this question for a long time. In other words, the lymphatic system and fat have a close and mysterious relationship[1]. In this session, I would like to assist young surgeons and scientists in the treatment of lymphedema with using practical aspects to render these various phenomena.

At the molecular and genetic level, many studies on the relationships between lymph and fat are progressing with increasing concerns about modern diseases, such as obesity and metabolic diseases. Here, I want to raise some facts that I feel mysterious relationships between lymphatic system and fat. I hope that young surgeons can share the interest and think about them together.

1 リンパ組織と脂肪組織は共に細網組織を基本構築としている

リンパ節をはじめとするリンパ組織と脂肪組織とは緊密な関係をもっている。もともと両者はいわゆる細網線維（主にⅢ型膠原線維から成る）が豊富な組織、つまり細網組織に属する。細網組織とは、間葉系の細網細胞（線維芽細胞の特殊型）とその細胞が産生する細網線維のネットワークで構成されていて、組織液や細胞・物質の移動が盛んな場を提供する特殊な結合組織であり、特に造血組織やリンパ組織、さらに脂肪組織に特によく発達している。つまり、すべてのリンパ組織および造血組織は、この細網組織を基本骨格としており、そこに居候である血球系の細胞が移住したものである。また、脂肪組織でも脂肪細胞の周囲が細網線維で包まれていて、盛んな代謝が行われていることから、細網組織の一種であることに間違いはない。さらに、リンパ節は通常は身体の屈曲部（腋窩、鼠径、膝窩など）、つまり脂肪組織中に存在することもご承知のとおりである。したがって、正常状態でリンパ節を触診することは難しく、感染時など炎症が起こって初めて触知可能となる。このときのリンパ節の腫大は 2、3 倍〜10 倍以上にも及ぶことがある。そのためにも脂肪組織中に普段から埋もれていることで免疫応答の自由度を残していると考えられている。

ところで、全身の末梢組織には血管やリンパ管のような管状の構造のない部位でも組織液や物質、細胞が移動しやすい経路が存在する。木原（1956）はこれを「脈管外通液路」と呼び、特に血管の周囲やリンパ管の周囲を中心としてその存在を証明している。そこには特に細網線維が豊富に分布しており、組織液をリンパ管系へと排導する有力な誘導路であることが明らかである。同時に、いざリンパや脂肪がうっ滞する場合にも、ここが現場となるであろう。

以上のことからも、細網組織の構成要素こそがリンパ系と脂肪組織の両者の不思議な関係を解き明かすための重要な"鍵"の 1 つである。

1. Both lymphatic and fat tissues primarily consist of the reticular tissue

There are close relationships between the lymphoid tissue and the adipose tissue. Originally both belong to the reticular tissue that is rich in reticular fibers (mainly consisting of type Ⅲ collagen fibers). The reticular tissue is actually composed of reticular cells (a special type of fibroblasts) of mesenchymal origin and a network of reticular fibers produced by these cells. It is a special type of the connective tissue providing the place where the movement of tissue fluids, cells and various substances is prosperous. Therefore, the hematopoietic tissue, the lymphoid tissue, and the adipose tissue all develop in the reticular tissue in proper. In other words all lymphoid tissues and hematopoietic tissues provide this reticular tissue as a special microenvironment (*i. e.*, landlords/landladies) for immigrating immature blood cells to develop (*i. e.*, tenants). In addition, it is sure that the adipose tissue is a kind of the reticular tissue because the abundant reticular fibers envelop each fat cell and provide the cells with a special microenvironment for their active metabolism. Furthermore, lymph nodes usually exist in the sites of flexion (*e. g.*, axillary, inguinal, and popliteal regions) in the body, where are actually the adipose tissues. Therefore, it is difficult to palpate lymph nodes in a normal state and they become palpable only after the inflammation. The swelling of lymph nodes during the inflammation may be more than 2 or 3〜more than 10 times of their normal size. Therefore it is thought that the lymph nodes can leave ample flexibility of their immune responses by being always surrounded by the adipose tissue.

By the way, there exist special routes through which various tissue fluids, substances and cells can easily pass at the periphery of the body, even if without the tubular structures such as blood vessels and lymphatic vessels. Kihara (1956) regarded these structures as "the extravascular fluid pathways" and proved their existence mainly around blood vessels and lymphatic vessels. The fluid pathways are abundant in reticular fibers, and it is convincing that they are the major draining routes for the tissue fluid into the local lymphatic vessel system. At the same time, here will become the spot of the lymph and fat congest.

Altogether, component of the reticular tissue is one of the important "keys" to solve the mysterious relations of both lymphatic system and the adipose tissue.

2 油でリンパ管腫が誘導される

1970年代にミネラル油や腹水誘導用の pristane など油性の物質を腹腔内に投与すると、種々のリンパ系細胞の腫瘍（骨髄腫、B細胞系腫瘍など）が発症することが知られていた[2]。実は、同時に腹腔表面には別の種類の腫瘍が発症していた。当時はほとんど注目を集めていなかったが、それから20年以上も後に Mancardi ら[3]によって同じ油性のアジュバント油を用いて良性のリンパ管腫が誘導できることが報告された。彼らは、病理学的にリンパ管腫と診断したが、われわれの経験からは、実はこの腫瘍は腹膜を構成する中皮細胞の腫瘍、つまり中皮腫の一種である。つまり、アジュバントを腹腔内に投与後1週間以内にこの腫瘍は腹膜表面の至るところから発症するが、その原因として中皮細胞がアジュバントによってなんらかの刺激を受けて、異物であるアジュバント油をいったん取り込みながら腫瘍化したものだと言える。さらに油を溜め込んだ腫瘍細胞同士で融合することによって、最終的に腹腔内から油を排導するため（？）に新たにリンパ管様の管を形成することを発見した。面白いことに、"栄養素としての一般の脂肪はリンパ管からしか吸収されない"こととともどうやらなんらかの関係がありそうだ。

面白いのはそれだけではない。実は、腹腔内の特定部位、つまり横隔膜表面に存在する篩状斑では、腹膜の中皮細胞とリンパ管内皮細胞同士が連続性に直接接している。したがって、両者が互いに移行し合える（中皮-内皮間形質転換）非常に緊密な関係にあると言える。そこで、われわれは上記のアジュバント誘導性のリンパ管腫の成立には、アジュバントという異物（油）を中皮細胞が摂取して取り込み、自らそれらを腹腔外へ排導するために、互いに融合して管状に連なり、ついには長く伸びたリンパ管様の排導路を形成するのではないかと考えている。つまりは、「中皮-脂肪摂取細胞-リンパ管内皮同士の形質転換」が起こっている可能性を報告[4]している。このことは、最近特に注目を集めているリンパ管新生のメカニズムを解明するうえで極めて重要な問題でもある。

中皮細胞とリンパ管内皮との移行を制御できれば、慢性リンパ浮腫や腹膜透析患者が抱える腹膜硬化症などの治療への応用にもなんらかの手がかりが得られるかも知れない。実際にその基礎的段階として、われわれはマウスにこの腫瘍を誘導し、その腫瘍を大量のリンパ管内皮を含む免疫原としてラットを免疫することによって、マウスのリンパ管内皮に対するモノクローナル抗体を作製することに成功した[5]。それまで、マウスから大量のリンパ管内皮を採取する術がなかったのだが、この"油によるリンパ管腫"がその難題を1つ解決した。

2. Oil induces lymphangiomas

In the 1970s, it was known that an intraperitoneal injection of mineral oil or some oily materials including pristane induced tumors of various kinds of lymphoid cells (*e.g.*, myelomas, B-cell tumors) in the abdominal cavity[2]. In fact, it developed simultaneously different types of tumor on the surface of the abdominal cavity. It hardly be attracted attention at that time, but then it was reported more than 20 years later by Mancardi et

221

al.[3] that adjuvant oil induced benign lymphangiomas. They diagnosed the tumor as a lymphangioma pathologically, but in fact, from our experience, this tumor is mesothelioma, a kind of tumors of mesothelial cells constituting the peritoneum. In other words, this tumor can develop from anywhere of the peritoneal surface within one week after the adjuvant injection into the abdominal cavity. As the cause, mesothelial cells catch some kind of stimulation by adjuvant, and they became tumors by taking in the adjuvant oil, an alien substance. Furthermore, I found that these cells newly formed lymphatic vessel-like tubular structures by fusing each other as if for exhausting the oil from the abdominal cavity. Interestingly enough, it seems to have some kind of relation to "the general fat as the nutrient being absorbed only from the lymphatic vessel". Furthermore, there are very special sites in the abdominal cavity, the Macula cribriformis, where the mesothelial cells and lymphatic vessel endothelial cells contact directly with continuity. Therefore, it may be said that both cell types have a close relation that they can be changed to each other (the transformation between the mesothelium and the endothelium). We think that the mesothelial cells take in the alien adjuvant and fuse each other to form tubular structures like lymphatic vessels, so that they can drain the adjuvant out of the peritoneal cavity. In other words, we report here the possibility of "the transformation between the mesothelial cell- fat intake cell- lymphatic vessel endothelial cell"[4]. This is is an extremely important topic in elucidating the mechanism of lymphangiogenesis, which is now attracting much attention.

Some clues may be provided for application to the treatments for such as chronic lymphedema and the peritoneal sclerosis that peritoneal dialysis patients have, if they can control mesothelium cells to change to the lymphatic vessel endothelial cells. In fact, we have successfully produced a rat monoclonal antibody against mouse lymphatic vessel endothelial cells by immunizing rats with this tumor as a source of immunogens for the mouse lymphatic vessels with a large quantity in the tumor[5]. It was very difficult to obtain a large quantity of lymphatic vessel endothelial cells from a normal mouse, but this "lymphangioma indued by the oil" actually solved the difficult problem till then.

3 　リンパ組織は加齢とともに脂肪化（加齢退縮）をきたす

　先に述べたとおり、リンパ組織と脂肪組織は同じ起源をもつと言っても不思議ではない。現に、リンパ組織や造血組織は、加齢とともに居候である血球系が居なくなると、最終的には脂肪組織でほぼ完全に置き換わってしまうことからも理解できる。両者は発生学的に同じ間葉系細胞に由来し、細網線維をつくる細網細胞が分化したものと考えられる。つまり、リンパ組織（造血組織）とは細網細胞の形成する物質移動や代謝の盛んな微小環境下に一度は血球系が移住してきて居を構えたものの、加齢とともに造血能力が落ちてくると、居候である血球が居なくなるため、後に残った細網細胞は豊富な栄養源や蓄積物を貯め込むために脂肪細胞へと移行するのかも知れない。これも一種の形質転換と言ってもよかろう。長澤ら[6]は骨髄の細網細胞が、造血幹細胞に対する微小環境（niche）としての役割を果たすと同時に、この細胞自身が脂肪細胞または骨芽細胞へと分化することを報告している。しかし、これらの細胞間の相互分化を促すメカニズムはいまだ明らかではない。また、リンパ組織の加齢による退縮・脂肪化が、そこに在住する細網細胞が直接脂肪細胞に変化することによって起こるのか、それともそれ以外の細胞が脂肪細胞として変化を遂げていくのか、現時点では結論は出ていない。

　しかし、骨髄線維症などに特徴的な骨髄が脂肪化や線維化を招くような疾患・病態の解明のためにも、そのメカニズムを研究することは極めて重要であると言える。慢性化したリンパ浮腫における脂肪浮腫化・線維化についても、ある意味ではリンパ組織の加齢退縮（脂肪化）と大変類似していることから、この方面でも研究の進展を期待したい。

3. Lymphoid tissues cause involution with fat deposition with age (aging regression)

As mentioned above, it is not surprising to say that both lymphatic tissues and adipose tissues derived from the same origin. It is easy to understand from the fact that the lymphoid tissue and the hematopoietic tissue are eventually replaced almost completely by adipose tissues when their tenant blood cells disappear with age. Both are considered to be derived from embryologically the same mesenchymal cells, differentiating to reticular cells that produce reticular fibers in these tissues. In other words, lymphoid tissues (or hematopoietic tissues) first form a microenvironment for immigrating blood cells, where reticular cells provide a good flow and metabolism of various nutrients. As its hematopoietic activity decreases and blood cells disappear from these tissues with age, the remaining reticular cells may change into fat cells to store the excessive nutrients left by the lost blood cells. It may as well say that this is also a kind of the transformation. Nagasawa et al[6] have reported that reticular cells of the bone marrow, at the same time play a role as a microenvironment (niche) for hematopoietic stem cells, differentiate into fat cells, or osteoblasts. However, the mechanism to promote mutual differentiation between these cells has yet to be clear. In addition, no conclusion has been reached for the questions whether the aging regression & fat deposition of lymphoid tissues is caused by the resident reticular cells changing directly to fat cells, or whether other type of cells rather than reticular cells are changing to fat cells.

However, it is very important to study its mechanism for understanding the diseases and symptoms of the bone marrow specifically causing fat deposition or fibrosis, such as myelofibrosis. I hope investigations on the lipedema & fibrosis due to chronic lymphedema are making more progress in this direction, because in a sense, these are very much like the aging regression (with fat deposition) of lymphoid tissues.

4 リンパ組織はステロイドホルモンの影響を受けやすい

強力な免疫抑制薬として副腎皮質ステロイド薬が治療に使用されているとおり、リンパ球自体が糖質ステロイドホルモンに対する受容体をもつことは明らかである。これに対して、先に述べたリンパ組織の加齢退縮には思春期頃から始まる二次性徴に伴う性ホルモンの影響を強く受けることもよく知られている。面白いことに、性ホルモン自体も脂質性のステロイドホルモンの一種であり、ここでもリンパ組織と脂肪との関係は切り離せない。思春期に入って性ホルモンの産生が高まってくると、胸腺はじめリンパ組織のほとんどがその影響を受け、退縮の引き金が引かれる。ヒトでは思春期を過ぎると胸腺はその免疫学的な役割をほとんど終え、退縮の一途をたどり、後に残った細網組織のほとんどが脂肪化してしまう。

ここで興味深いのは、後に残った細網細胞をはじめとするストローマ細胞自体もステロイドホルモンに対する受容体をもつのか否かという問題である。春木ら[7]によると、胸腺におけるエストロジェン受容体をもつ主体は胸腺リンパ球ではなく、むしろ細網性ストローマ細胞である。このことは、胸腺の退縮と脂肪化が一元的に起こっているのではなく、性ホルモンの影響が胸腺のリンパ球にも微小環境にも多元的に起こる可能性を示唆している。

4. Lymphoid tissues are susceptible to steroid hormones

As adrenocortical steroids are used for various clinical treatments as potent immunosuppressive agents, it is clear that lymphocytes themselves have receptors for glucocorticoid steroid hormones. In contrast, it is also well known that the aging regression of lymphoid tissues mentioned earlier is induced by sex hormones in a close association with the secondary sex characteristics starting from puberty. Interestingly, even sex hormones themselves are a kind of lipid as steroids, and again there is an inseparable relationship between the lymphoid tissue and fat. As the production of sex hormones starts increasing in puberty, thymus and most of lymphoid tissues are affected and triggered to cause involution. In humans, the thymus stops its immunological functions after puberty, causing involution, and then the remaining reticular tissues are replaced mostly by the adipose tissue.

Another interesting point here is whether or not the stromal cells themselves including the remaining reticular cells have receptors for steroid hormones. According to Haruki et al.[7], the major cell population having the estrogen receptor in the thymus is not the lymphocytes, but the reticular stromal cells. This means that the thymic involution with fat deposition does not occur in a unified pattern and suggests the possibility that the effects of sex hormones occur multiply on both lymphocytes and microenvironment of the thymus.

5 慢性リンパ浮腫や自己免疫病は女性に多い

慢性リンパ浮腫（特に一次性）や自己免疫病の多くになぜ性差（**Table 1**）があるのか、本当に不思議である。もともと、免疫応答自体も女性の方が男性よりも反応性が高いのだが、Ansar Ahmed ら[8]によるとこれらの性ホルモンの効果はほとんどが胸腺由来の細胞、つまりT細胞を介して働くという。しかも、末梢での免疫応答では免疫調節性T細胞が性ホルモンに対する感受性が最も高い。

われわれの実験ではマウスの胸腺重量に対する影響で判断すると、副腎皮質ステロイドホルモンが最も退縮効果が強く、それに続いて女性ホルモン（エストロジェン）、最も効果の弱かったのが男性ホルモン（テストステロン）であった。しかし、これらのホルモンがもつ実際の標的はどう

Table 1. **女性に多い自己免疫疾患** Autoimmune diseases common in women

主な疾患 Major disorder	女性の発症頻度（対男性比：倍）* Incidence ratio in female (compared with male) *
全身性エリテマトーデス SLE	9〜10
高安病（大動脈炎） Takayasu arteritis	10
シェーグレン症候群 Sjögren syndrome	14
線維筋痛症候群 Fibromyalgia syndrome	7
全身性強皮症 Systemic sclerosis	3〜9
関節リウマチ Rheumatoid arthritis	5
多発性筋炎・皮膚筋炎 Polymyositis／Dermatomyositis	2.5
バセドウ病 Basedow disease	4〜7
橋本病 Hashimoto's thyroiditis	10〜20
重症筋無力症 Myasthenia gravis	2

*参考：内科学第8版，朝倉書店，東京，2003 ほか
*References：Internal Medicine 8th edition, Asakura-Shoten, Tokyo, 2003, etc.

も異なっているらしい。まず、副腎皮質ステロイドホルモンは容赦なく末梢の成熟リンパ球はもちろん胸腺リンパ球そのものにも致命的打撃を与える。しかし、エストロジェンは胸腺リンパ球を直接殺すのではなく、むしろ胸腺外に叩き出すことにより胸腺退縮をもたらすことがわかった。エストロジェンの中でも私が特に関心をもったのは女性ホルモンとしては最も生理活性の低いエストリオール（E3）であった。E3 はエストラジオール（E2）やエストロン（E1）に比べると、女性ホルモンとしての作用は極めて弱いが、リンパ組織に対しては、両者に決して劣らないか、または両者がもたない別の作用[9]ももっている。E3 はすべての性ホルモンの最終産物でもあるだけに、その作用は侮れない。特に、妊娠後期には E3 が正常時の数百倍以上にも増加し、胎盤を介する"妊婦と胎児の助け合い（母児相関）"に一役買っていることを忘れてはならない。これに対して、男性ホルモンは幼若な B 細胞に対して作用する[10]。ニワトリ卵をテストステロン液に漬けることによって誘導される B 細胞欠損（chemical bursectomy）動物モデルは有名である。

　リンパ系以外にも、エストロジェンは生体内でさまざまな細胞や組織に影響を与えると考えられる（**Table 2**）。このようなエストロジェンの作用は、ほかのステロイドホルモンはもちろん、ビタミン A やビタミン D などの脂溶性ビタミンや甲状腺ホルモンなどと同様に、核内受容体に結合し活性化させることによって、極めて多くの遺伝子転写を調節しているため、生体にとって強い効果をもたらすと考えられる。このようにみていくと、免疫疾患だけでなく、慢性リンパ浮腫における性差の問題もエストロジェンによる影響の幅広さを垣間見ることによって見えてくるような気がする。今後ますます、性ホルモンとリンパ浮腫との直接的な関係が解明されることを心から期待したい。

5.　Chronic lymphedema and autoimmune diseases are more common in women

　It is really strange that attack rate of chronic lymphedema (especially primary lymphedema) and many autoimmune diseases have a clear sex difference (**Table 1**). Basically, females are immunologically more reactive than males. According to Ansar Ahmed et al[8], these effects of sex hormones are mediated mostly by thymus-derived cells, in other words T cells. Moreover, immunoregulatory T cells have the highest sensitivity to sex hormones in the immune responses in the periphery.

　In our experiments, judged by the effect on the thymus weight in mice, adrenocortical steroid hormones have the strongest involuting effect, followed by female hormones (estrogen), and the weakest is male hormones (testosterone). However, the actual targets of these hormones seem somehow different. First, adrenocortical steroid hormones mercilessly give a fatal blow not only to mature lymphocytes in the periphery, but also to thymic lymphocytes. However, we have found that estrogen does not kill thymic lymphocytes directly, but drive them out of the thymus resulting in the thymic involution[1]. The estrogen that I have been especially interested in is estriol (E3) having the lowest bioactivity as the female hormone. Compared with estradiol (E2) and estrone (E1), E3 acts very weak as a female hormone, however for the lymphoid tissues, it is not inferior in any way to other two estrogens, but even has another action that both don't have[9]. Because E3 is the end product of all of the sex hormones, its action is to be reckoned with. Don't forget that E3 increases in late pregnancy to several hundred times higher than in normal state, being responsible to "the relationship between pregnant mother and fetus (the feto-maternal relationship)" through the placenta. In contrast, male hormones affect immature B cells[10]. The B cell-deficient animal model in the chicken induced by soaking eggs in testosterone solution (as the chemical bursectomy) is well-known.

　Besides on the lymphatic system, estrogen is thought to have many effects on various cells and tissues *in vivo* (**Table 2**). Likewise various fat-soluble vitamins, such as vitamin A and vitamin D, and thyroid

Table 2. 想定されるエストロジェンの生体内での標的への影響
Possible effects of estrogen on various targets *in vivo*

標的　Target	作用・効果* 　Action・Effect*
生殖器官：本来の標的 Reproductive organs：（original targets）	増殖・成熟促進（機能促進） ⇧：growth and maturation（promote function）
リンパ組織系　Lymphoid tissues	
・胸腺　thymus	退縮（胸腺細胞の末梢への排出） involution（driving thymocytes out of thymus）
・造血器官（骨髄）　hematopoietic tissues （*e. g.* bone marrow）	造血促進（EPO、GM-CSF 産生） 血小板因子産生促進 ⇧：hematopoiesis（production of EPO, GM-CSF） ⇧：production of platelet-derived factors
結合組織系　Connective tissues	
・線維芽細胞　fibroblast	基質（ヒアルロン酸など）合成促進 線維合成抑制 ⇧：synthesis of extracellular matrix（hyaluronic acid etc...） ⇩：synthesis of fiber
・血管内皮細胞　vascular endothelial cell	増殖促進、透過性亢進 ⇧：vascular growth and permeablity
・マクロファージ　macrophage	RES 系細胞の貪食活性促進 組織内 MMP-9 など上昇 ⇧：phagocytic activity of RES cells ⇧：tissue MMP-9
・NK 細胞　natural killer cell	活性化 ⇧：killer function
・肥満細胞　mast cell	脱顆粒（ヒスタミン・セロトニン） ⇧：degranulation（histamine・serotonin）
代謝系　Metabolic system	
・骨代謝　bone metabolism	Osteoclast 抑制、Osteoblast 活性化 ⇩：Osteoclasts/⇧：Osteoblasts
・脂質代謝　lipid metabolism	血中 Cholesterol・TG 低下 LDL 酸化抑制 → 動脈硬化防止 ⇩：blood cholesterol & TG ⇩：oxidation of LDL→prevent arteriosclerosis
・肝細胞　hepatocyte	増殖・alphafetoprotein 合成促進、albumin 合成低下（肝細胞の幼若化？） ⇧：proliferatipon（dedifferentiation of hepatocytes?） ⇧：synthesis of alpha-fetoprotein ⇩：synthesis of albumin
・顎下腺　submandibular gland	導管上皮細胞：EGF 産生抑制 ⇩：production of EGF by duct cells
中枢神経系　Central nervous system	脳の性分化促進 アミロイド産生抑制（アルツハイマー病の抑制） ⇧：sexual differentiation of the brain ⇩：synthesis of amyroid（protection from Alzheimer disease）

*われわれのデータならびに一般的教科書による

*According to our data and general textbooks

hormones, not to speak of other steroid hormones, these effects of estrogen may be induced by controlling enormous gene transcriptions by binding and activating its nuclear receptors, and then estrogen powerfully acts in a living body. It might be easily appreciable that the wide range of effects by estrogen can also cause the sex difference in chronic lymphedema as well as in autoimmune diseases. I really hope that the direct relationship between sex hormones and lymphedema is much more clearly elucidated in the future.

■おわりに

　リンパ学は、この十数年の間に急速な展開を遂げてきている。1つには、それまで確定の難しかったリンパ管内皮の特異的マーカーの発見、さらにリンパ管に対するさまざまな増殖因子の発見による基礎医学研究の進歩とさらに臨床では外科的治療の開発であろう。これらを今後さらに支えていくには、特に、わが国のリンパ学研究の流れをベテラン研究者からこれから研究を始めようとする若手研究者に至るまで、脈々と継承していくことが重要である。正に、"温故知新"である。今回紹介したいくつかの"不思議"もそのほんの一部であって、やがてなんの問題もなくすっきりと解明されることを心から願っている。ただし、どんなに些細なことでもそれらの話題に興味をもってくれる人材の確保が何よりも重要である。こんな話にでも、1人でも、1ヵ所でも面白いと思って頂けると幸いである。

（江﨑太一）

■ Conclusion

　Lymphology has made a very rapid progress in the last two decades. This was achieved by the discovery of specific markers for the lymphatic vessel endothelium which has been very difficult to identify till then, and by the discovery of various growth factors for lymphatic vessels in the basic research, and was also brought about by the development of surgical techniques in the clinical treatments. In order to support this progress further for the future, it is especially important to keep handing down our knowledges of lymphology in this country from professional researchers to young researchers who are starting their investigation. This is actually "Learning history's lessons". The "mysteries in lymphology" that I introduced in this session are just some examples and I really hope that these will be clarified without any problem soon. For this aim, it is extremely important to secure and bring up young scientists who are interested in any small pieces of issue about these topics. I would be very happy even if only one scientist finds any interest in even one part of this session.

(*Taichi Ezaki*)

1) 江﨑太一：リンパ学に残された謎をめぐって；リンパと脂肪の関わり．リンパ学 37(1)：4-9, 2014.
 Ezaki T：Some remaining mysteries in lymphology；Relationships between lymph and fat. Jap J Lymphol 37(1)：4-9, 2014.
2) Cancro M, Potter M：The requirement of an adherent cell substratum for the growth of developing plasmacytoma cells *in vivo*. J Exp Med 144(6)：1554-1567, 1976.
3) Mancardi S, Stanta G, et al：Lymphatic endothelial tumors induced by intraperitoneal injection of incomplete Freund's adjuvant. Exp Cell Res 246(2)：368-375, 1999.
4) 江﨑太一，出崎順三：アジュバント誘導性リンパ管腫モデルにおけるリンパ管の形成機構．リンパ学 35(1)：14-17, 2012.
 Ezaki T, Desaki J：Lymphangiogenic responses in an ajuvant-induced lymphangioma model. Jap J Lymphol 35(1)：14-17, 2012.

5) Ezaki T, Kuwahara K, et al : Production of two novel monoclonal antibodies that distinguish mouse lymphatic and blood vascular endothelial cells. Anat Embryol 211(5) : 379-393, 2006.

6) Nagasawa T, Omatsu Y, et al : Control of hematopoietic stem cells by the bone marrow stromal niche : the role of reticular cells. Trends Immunol 32(7) : 315-320, 2011.

7) Haruki Y, Seiki K, et al : Estrogen receptor in the "non-lymphocytes" in the thymus of the ovariectomized rat. Tokai J Exp Clin Med 8(1) : 31-39, 1983.

8) Ansar Ahmed S, Penhale WJ : Sex hormones, immune responses, and autoimmune diseases. Mechanisms of sex hormone action. Am J Pathol 121(3) : 531-551, 1985.

9) 小谷正彦, 名和行文, ほか：肝臓に対するエストロジェンの新しい作用. 肝胆膵 8(3) : 339-343, 1984. Kotani M, Nawa Y, et al : A novel effect of estrogen on the liver. Liver, Gall bladder, Pancreas 8(3) : 339-343, 1984.

10) Fujii H, Nawa Y, et al : Effect of a single administration of testosterone on the immune response and lymphoid tissues in mice. Cell Immunol 20(2) : 315-326, 1975.

CHAPTER 7

外科治療
Surgical treatment

4. Brorson 法
Brorson's method

■はじめに

　リンパ浮腫の治療は、外科的治療と保存療法に分けられる。外科治療は大きく2つに分けられ、リンパ流路の再建を目的とするもの（LVA、リンパ節移植など）と、余剰組織の除去を目的とするものがある。余剰組織の除去を目的とする手術の中で、脂肪吸引術は近年その有用性が確立しつつあり、その第一人者として有名なのがスウェーデンの Brorson である。本章では Brorson による脂肪吸引術を紹介する。

　1987 年に乳癌術後の上肢リンパ浮腫患者に対して脂肪吸引術を行って以来、Brorson らはリンパ浮腫における余剰脂肪組織に着目してきた。従来、リンパ浮腫の患肢にはリンパ液が貯留しており、それに伴って線維組織が形成されるのみと考えられていたが、十分な保存療法により浮腫に圧痕を伴わない状態になったとしても、つまりリンパ液の貯留をほぼ完全に解消したとしても、左右対称性を得ることは困難である。これは、リンパ浮腫の患肢にはリンパ液以外のものが沈着しているということを示しており、それが脂肪であると考えられるようになった。最近ではCT や MRI を用いて、リンパ浮腫の患肢における脂肪組織増生が確認されている。リンパ浮腫における脂肪増生の分子細胞学的メカニズムはいまだ不明であり、血流に対してリンパ液排出量が少ないために脂肪の排出も滞り、マクロファージに貪食された脂肪がそのまま沈着するという説や、貯留したリンパ液から脂肪細胞の増殖を促進するようなサイトカインが放出されているという説など諸説あるが、リンパ浮腫で脂肪組織が増生するということだけは確かなようである。

■Introduction

　Treatment of lymphedema is divided into surgical treatment and conservative therapy. Surgical treatment is roughly divided into two, there are those aimed at the reconstruction of the lymphatic pathway [lymphatico-venous anastomosis (LVA), lymph node transfer etc.] and some aiming to remove surplus tissue. In surgery aimed at removing surplus tissue, liposuction is becoming established in its usefulness in recent years, and Brorson in Sweden is famous as its leading expert. This section introduces liposuction by Brorson.

　Brorson and colleagues have focused on surplus adipose tissue in lymphedema since liposuction surgery was performed on upper limb lymphedema patients after breast cancer surgery in 1987. Conventionally, lymph fluid was accumulated in the affected limbs of lymphedema, and it was thought that only fibrous tissue was formed in association therewith. Even if sufficient conservative therapy caused the edema not to be accompanied by indentation, it is difficult to obtain bilateral symmetry even if reservoir of lymph fluid is almost completely eliminated. This indicates that lymphedema affected limbs are deposited other than lymph, which is considered to be fat. Recently, CT and MRI have been used to confirm adipose tissue proliferation in lymphedema affected limbs. The molecular cytological mechanism of adipogenesis in lymphedema is still unknown, the discharge of fat is stagnant due to the lymph fluid discharge to the blood flow, the fat that phagocytosed by macrophages is deposited as it is, and the theory that retention. There are various theories that the cytokine that promotes the proliferation of adipocytes is released from the lymph fluid that is done, but it seems to be certain that only adipose tissue is increased by lymphedema.

Ⅰ　手術手技

　手術は全身麻酔、脊髄麻酔、または硬膜外麻酔で行う。ターニケットを用いて"dry technique"を行うため、麻酔薬やエピネフリンの局所注入は行わない。患肢において3mmの皮膚切開を20〜40ヵ所に入れる。吸引器を用いて0.9気圧の陰圧で脂肪吸引を行う。通常、美容を目的とした脂肪吸引では太さ3mm以下の吸引管を用いることが多いが、リンパ浮腫の脂肪吸引では太さ3〜6mmの吸引管を使っており、吸引管の側孔も美容手術で用いるものよりも大きくなっている。これは、リンパ浮腫に伴って沈着した線維組織も効率的に吸引除去するためである。吸引器は通常の脂肪吸引器を用いている。これらを用いて、過剰に沈着した脂肪組織をできるだけすべて吸引する（上肢で1,000〜3,800mL程度）。皮膚切開部は縫い閉じず、ドレナージ孔として開放しておく。術後の出血や浮腫を予防するため、術直後から、上肢には弾性包帯または弾性スリーブを、下肢には弾性ストッキングを着用し、2日間そのままにする。手術時間は平均2時間で、術後1日は抗生剤を点滴で投与し、その後2週間抗生剤を内服させる。

Ⅰ. Surgical techniques

　Surgery is performed under general anesthesia, spinal anesthesia, or epidural anesthesia. Because "dry technique" is performed using tourniquet, local injection of anesthetic and epinephrine is not performed. Place skin incision of 3 mm in 20 to 40 places in affected limbs. Liposuction is carried out with a negative pressure of 0.9 atm using an aspirator. Normally, suction pipes with a thickness of 3 mm or less are often used for cosmetic liposuction, but suction pipes with a diameter of 3 to 6 mm are used for liposuction of lymphedema, and the side holes of the aspiration tube are larger than those used in usual liposuction. This is to efficiently aspirate and remove the fibrous tissue deposited with lymphedema. The aspirator uses a normal liposuction device. Use these to aspirate as much as possible of excessively deposited adipose tissue (1,000 to 3,800 mL in upper limbs). Do not sew the skin incision, leave it open as a drainage hole. In order to prevent postoperative bleeding and edema, wear elastic bandages or elastic sleeves for upper limbs and elastic stockings for lower limbs from immediately after surgery and leave them for 2 days. The operation time is 2 hours on average. One day after surgery, antibiotics are administered by drip infusion and antibiotics are administered orally for 2 weeks thereafter.

Ⅱ　術後の圧迫療法

　術後の圧迫療法は非常に重要で、入浴時を除く常時、弾性着衣を着用するよう指導する。術直後にオーダーメイドの弾性着衣を作成し、初めの3ヵ月は、患肢のボリューム減少に応じて外来受診の度に弾性着衣をミシンで縫ってサイズダウンしていく。その後も定期的に弾性着衣を買い換え、結果的に術後1年間で3〜4回買い換えることとなる。この controlled compression therapy（CCT）を行うことができないと予想される場合は、脂肪吸引術の適応外となる。

Ⅱ. Postoperative compression therapy

　Compression therapy after surgery is very important and it is instructed to the patients to wear elastic wear at all times except when bathing. Made-to-ordered elastic wearing is created immediately after surgery, and in the first 3 months, elastic wearing is sewn with a sewing machine and downsized in size each time an outpatient visit is made according to the volume decrease of the affected limb. Even after that, they regularly replace elastic wear and, as a result, will be replaced three to four times in a year after surgery. If it is anticipated that you cannot do this controlled compression therapy（CCT）, it will be contraindication for liposuction.

Ⅲ　合併症

Brorson らは、脂肪吸引の術後に大きな合併症はないと報告している。皮膚の知覚低下は避けられないが半年以内に改善することが多い。超音波式脂肪吸引器を用いる際は、カニューレから熱が発せられ、熱傷による皮膚壊死が起こる可能性があるため、注意が必要である。ターニケットを使わずに 2,000 mL 以上の脂肪吸引を行う際には輸血が必要になることがある。その他に生じた合併症としては、軽度な表皮剥離、肺炎、呼吸困難などが挙げられている。

Ⅲ. Complications
Brorson and colleagues report that there is no major complication after liposuction surgery. Decline in skin perception is inevitable, but it often improves within half a year. When using an ultrasonic liposuction device, caution should be exercised because heat is emitted from the cannula and skin necrosis due to burns may occur. Transfusion may be necessary when liposuction of 2,000 mL or more is done without using a tourniquet. Other complications that have occurred include mild epidermolysis, pneumonia, dyspnea and the like.

Ⅳ　長期経過

Brorson らは、48 人の片側上肢リンパ浮腫患者に対して脂肪吸引術を行った結果を報告している。術前の平均浮腫ボリュームは 1,890 mL で、平均脂肪吸引量は 2,140 mL であった。術前の浮腫ボリュームに対する、術後のボリューム減少率は、術後 6ヵ月で 98%（n＝41）、術後 1 年で 104%（n＝35）、術後 4 年で 106%（n＝12）であり、術後長期において安定した結果が得られた。

Ⅳ. Long term outcome
Brorson and colleagues report the results of liposuction for 48 unilateral upper limb lymphedema patients. The mean edema volume before surgery was 1,890 mL and the average liposuction volume was 2,140 mL. 98%（n＝41）in the 6 months after surgery, 104%（n＝35）in 1 year after surgery, 106%（n＝12）, and stable results were obtained in the postoperative long-term.

Ⅴ　脂肪吸引術後の患肢の血流

Brorson らは、12 人の片側上肢リンパ浮腫患者に対して、脂肪吸引術前後の患肢において皮

膚血流をレーザードプラ(laser Doppler imaging;LDI)で調べ、健側との比をLDI indexとして報告した。術前には手、前腕、上腕におけるLDI indexはそれぞれ1.01、0.90、0.92であり、皮膚表層への血流は低下していた。術後3ヵ月では手、前腕、上腕においてそれぞれ1.03、1.01、1.15、術後6ヵ月ではそれぞれ1.06、1.05、1.07であり、術後には健側と同程度にまで皮膚血流が増加していた。

V. Postoperative blood flow of the affected limb

　　Brorson and colleagues examined the skin blood flow in the affected limbs before and after liposuction with laser doppler imaging(LDI) for 12 unilateral upper limb lymphedema patients and reported the ratio to the healthy side as LDI index did. Prior to surgery, the LDI index in the hands, forearms, and upper arm was 1.01, 0.90, 0.92, respectively, and blood flow to the skin surface layer was decreased. 1.03, 1.01, 1.15 in the hands, forearms, and upper arm, respectively, 1.06, 1.05, 1.07 in the 6 months after surgery at 3 months postoperatively, and the skin blood flow increased to the same extent as the healthy side.

■VI■　脂肪吸引術とリンパ管機能

　　Brorsonらは、20人の片側上肢リンパ浮腫患者に対して、脂肪吸引術前後のリンパ管機能を調べる前向き研究を行った。仰臥位で第2、3指間に放射性同位体(^{99m}Tc)を皮下注射し、経時的にリンパシンチグラフィを撮影した。リンパ浮腫の患肢では、脂肪吸引術前にはリンパ管があまり描出されず、放射性同位体は腋窩まで到達しなかった。この所見は術後にも変化なく、既に障害されたリンパ管機能は、脂肪吸引術後にも悪化していないことが示された。

VI. Postoperative lymphatic function

　　Brorson and colleagues conducted a prospective study to investigate the function of lymphatic vessels before and after liposuction for 20 unilateral upper limb lymphedema patients. Radiant isotope(^{99m}Tc) was injected subcutaneously between the 2nd and 3rd fingers in the supine position, and lymphoscintigraphy was taken with time. In the limbs of lymphedema, the lymphatic vessels were not much depicted before liposuction, and the radioactive isotope did not reach the axilla. This finding did not change even after surgery, indicating that already impaired lymphatic function has not deteriorated even after liposuction surgery.

■VII■　考　察

　　本章ではBrorsonによる脂肪吸引術についてまとめたが、脂肪吸引術は、慢性化したリンパ浮腫において増生した脂肪組織を除去する方法である。既に増大してしまった患肢のボリュームを縮小するためには、現存する外科的治療の中で一番確実な方法の1つであろう。古くから行われてきた単純切除法やCharles法と比較すると術後瘢痕は小さく、審美的にも優れた方法であるといえる。

　　Brorsonは脂肪吸引術の際にターニケットを使用しており、出血量を減少させ輸血を避ける

7-4. Brorson 法

ためには重要な手順と思われる。リンパ浮腫の患肢では、ターニケットを装着した直後には術野が虚血状態になっていても、時間経過とともにターニケットで圧迫された部分の浮腫が軽減することにより、相対的にターニケットが緩み、術野の虚血状態が保たれなくなることがある。したがって、経時的に数回ターニケットを巻き直すことが必要と考えられる。

　脂肪吸引術は、LVAやリンパ節移植などと異なり、リンパ流路を再建する術式ではない。また、脂肪吸引術により、残存するリンパ管がダメージを受ける可能性は否定できない。Brorsonの報告によれば、慢性期リンパ浮腫で既にリンパ管機能が低下していた患者では、脂肪吸引術を行ってもそれ以上リンパ管機能が悪化することはなかったということである。より安全に脂肪吸引術を行うためには、ICG検査やリンパシンチグラフィなどを術前に行い、機能良好なリンパ管が残存する部位は避けて脂肪吸引を行うなどの工夫が必要と考える。

　現在美容外科の分野では、単純脂肪吸引器や、超音波式、レーザー式、ウォータージェット式など、さまざまなタイプの脂肪吸引器が用いられている。リンパ浮腫の患肢では硬い線維組織が増生しているため、脂肪吸引を行う際には通常の皮下組織に対する脂肪吸引よりも労を要する。どのようなタイプの脂肪吸引器を用いればより簡便で安全に効率よく脂肪吸引を行えるのか、今後も検討が必要なところである。さらに、リンパ浮腫に対する脂肪吸引術では、通常の美容外科における脂肪吸引よりも多量の脂肪吸引を行うことが多く、深部静脈血栓症（DVT）、肺塞栓など術後の合併症にも注意が必要である。

　脂肪吸引術は、確実に皮下脂肪量を減らすことができる一方で、リンパ管損傷の危険性も孕んだ術式である。また、脂肪吸引術の術後には入浴時を除く常時の徹底した弾性着衣着用が必要になること、術中の神経損傷などにより疼痛が長期間持続する可能性があることなども考慮し、適応の選択に際しては慎重を期すべきである。

（原　尚子）

VII. Discussions

This section summarizes the liposuction procedure by Brorson. Liposuction is a method of removing adipose tissue which has increased in chronic lymphedema. It would be one of the most reliable methods of existing surgical treatment to reduce the volume of the affected limb which had already increased. Compared to the simple resection method or Charles method which has been done since a long time, the postoperative scar is small, and it can be said that it is an aesthetic superior method.

Brorson uses a tourniquet during liposuction and it seems to be an important procedure to reduce blood loss and to avoid transfusions. In the affected limbs of lymphedema, immediately after wearing the tourniquet, even if the operative field is in an ischemic state, edema in the part pressed by the tourniquet is reduced with the lapse of time, the tourniquet is relaxed relatively, and the ischemic state of the operative field may not be maintained. Therefore, it is considered necessary to rewind the tourniquet several times over time.

Unlike LVA and lymph node transfer, liposuction is not a technique to reconstruct lymphatic channels. Also, it is undeniable that the remaining lymphatic vessels will be damaged by liposuction. According to Brorson's report, in patients with chronic phase lymphedema already lymph node function declines, lymph duct function did not worsen anymore even with lipoaspiration. In order to carry out liposuction more safely, it is thought that ingenuity such as indocyanine green (ICG) examination and lymphoscintigraphy is performed before surgery, and a part with good functioning lymphatic vessels is avoided and liposuction is performed.

Currently in the field of cosmetic surgery, various types of liposuction devices such as simple liposuction devices, ultrasonic type, laser type, water jet type, etc. are used. As lymphedema affected limbs, hard fibrous

233

tissues are increasing, so it takes more labor to perform liposuction than liposuction for a normal subcutaneous tissue. Whether liposuction can be performed more easily, safely and efficiently by using what type of liposuction device, it is still necessary to investigate. Furthermore, in liposuction surgery against lymphedema, a lot of liposuction is performed more often than liposuction in normal cosmetic surgery, attention must also be paid to postoperative complications such as DVT and pulmonary embolism.

Liposuction is a surgical procedure that can definitely reduce the amount of subcutaneous fat but also has the risk of lymphatic vessel damage. Also, after surgery for liposuction surgery, regular thorough elastic wear except for bathing is required, and it is also possible that pain may last for a long period of time due to intraoperative nerve damage, the indication of liposuction should be thought carefully.

(Hisako Hara)

1) Brorson H : Liposuction in arm lymphedema treatment. Scand J Surg 92(4) : 287-295, Review, 2003.
2) Brorson H : Liposuction gives complete reduction of chronic large arm lymphedema after breast cancer. Acta Oncol 39(3) : 407-420, Review, 2000.
3) Brorson H, Svensson H, Norrgren K, et al : Liposuction reduces arm lymphedema without significantly altering the already impaired lymph transport. Lymphology 31(4) : 156-172, 1998.
4) Wojnikow S, Malm J, Brorson H : Use of a tourniquet with and without adrenaline reduces blood loss during liposuction for lymphoedema of the arm. Scand J Plast Reconstr Surg Hand Surg 41(5) : 243-249, 2007.
5) Brorson H, Ohlin K, Olsson G, et al : Controlled compression and liposuction treatment for lower extremity lymphedema. Lymphology 41(2) : 52-63, 2008.

CHAPTER 7

外科治療
Surgical treatment

5. 合併外科治療

Treatment of surgery for a complication

■ **はじめに**

リンパ浮腫はリンパ流不全を起因とする患部の増大病変であるが、その病変はリンパ液の貯留によるものだけではない。

まず、リンパ浮腫部では樹状細胞などがリンパ管を通ってリンパ節で抗原提示を行う獲得免疫系反応が破綻した状態であり局所的な免疫不全状態になっていることが考えられ[1,2]、免疫不全状態はリンパ浮腫患肢に蜂窩織炎などの感染性病変をきたす原因になっている。

また、リンパ浮腫組織内ではヘルパーT細胞2(Th2)や2型マクロファージ(M2)などが優位で2型免疫反応に傾き慢性炎症状態になっているといわれている[3]。2型免疫反応は組織修復的な反応傾向も示し、特にリンパ浮腫患部では脂肪細胞の分化を制御する転写因子のPPARγやCEBPファミリーが優位に発現している[4]。この機序を通してリンパ浮腫患肢では異常な脂肪増生が進行していくことが推測される。

加えて脂肪組織ではTNF-α(tumor necrosisfactor-α)やMCP-1(monocyte chemoat-tractant protein-1)などに代表される炎症性サイトカインやケモカインが過剰に産生され、これに対して、アディポネクチンに代表される抗炎症性サイトカインの産生は減少する。このようなアディポサイトカイン産生調節の破綻により脂肪組織を起点に、アディポサイトカインを介して全身に慢性炎症が波及する[5,6]。

このようなリンパ浮腫における免疫不全状態を起点とする脂肪増生と慢性炎症、感染のサイクルの繰り返しはリンパ管の硬化性病変を進行させる。こうした悪循環にリンパ浮腫患者は陥っていて組織増大も進行していく。

リンパ管細静脈吻合(LVA)やリンパ管移植によりリンパ流を改善させることでこの増悪のサイクルを断ち切ることが重要であるが、残念ながら今のところリンパ流改善で増生した脂肪組織を減少させる効果は、少なくとも進行したリンパ浮腫症例では確認されていない。

増生した脂肪組織はリンパ浮腫患者のQOLを低下させる大きな要因であり、リンパ浮腫の進行例では脂肪減量術を組み合わせた合併外科治療が必要となる。

■ **Introduction**

Although one of the symptom about lymphedema is increasing the volume of affected part, lymphatic fluid accumulation is not the only cause of this symptom.

In lymphedema, the acquired immune response, which is initiated by dendritic cell, is assumed to fall into disorder, because the route for dendritic cells to lymph node is obstructed[1,2]. This immune deficient status is one of the cause of cellulitis.

In addition, the differentiation into M2 macrophages and Th2 inflammatory response is dominant and causing chronic inflammatory status in lymphedema[3]. Th2 inflammatory response tends to have the features of tissue remodeling, too. Especially, in affected part of lymphedema, proteins regulating adipose differentiation including CCAAT/enhancer-binding protein-α and peroxisome proliferator-activated

235

receptor-γ, were markedly up-regulated in response to lymphatic fluid stasis[4].

These mechanism is assumed to be the factors that promote fat deposition and fibrosis.

Adipose tissue excessively produce inflammatory cytokine and chemokine, such as tumor necrosisfactor-α and monocyte chemoattractant protein-1, on the other hand produce insufficiently anti-inflammatory cytokine, such as adiponectin.

The chronic inflammation which is triggered by the rapture of adipocytokine control affects whole area by adipocytokine emitted from adipose tissue[5][6].

The cycle of adipogenesis, chronic inflammatory, and infection, which is triggered by immune deficiency caused by lymphedema, deteriorate sclerotic changes in lymphatic duct.

The lymphedema patients are in the status of this vicious circle, and suffering from the increasing volume.

It is important to arrest this vicious circle by LVA or lymphatic transfer, however there has been no observation that conventional lymphatic therapy decreased adipogenesis at least in advanced cases so far.

Combined surgical treatment including liposuction or adipose excision is necessary for severe leg lymphedema to reduce the limbs volume, since increased adipose tissue is main factor to lower living standard with lymphedema patients.

■ I ■ 術前評価・適応

ICG 局注による PDE 観察で患肢全長広範囲にわたり Diffuse あるいは Stardust pattern が観察される重症のリンパ浮腫患者で、かつ高度な脂肪増生を片側性あるいは両側性に認めるリンパ浮腫患者が適応となる。

あるいは以前にリンパ管静脈吻合やリンパ管移植術を行ったが、十分な患肢の周径減量が得られていない患者にも適応可能である。

I. Preoperative assessment/operability

The patients who has operability for the combined surgical treatment are the advanced and severe cases who show diffuse or stardust pattern all along lower limbs through PDE observation and have the high fat deposition hemi or bilaterally. And the patients who have undergone lymphatic transfer or LVA before and have insufficient reducing volume, also have the operability for this treatment.

■ II ■ 手術手技

全身麻酔下で施行している。

LVA とリンパ管移植術、脂肪減量術を併用する。脂肪減量術と LVA あるいはリンパ管移植術は症例に応じ同時あるいは複次的に行う。

1. リンパ管移植

外側胸リンパ節を含めずに血管柄付リンパ脂肪弁を使用する。収縮可能な正常リンパ管が含まれることでリンパ液を静脈に貫流することができる。

7-5. 合併外科治療

　乳輪周囲にパテントブルーまたはICGを皮下注射した後、数本の染められたリンパ管を外側胸動静脈または胸背動静脈から派生する細い穿通枝を付けて挙上する。外側胸動静脈を使用することが多い。

　われわれは通常、腋窩リンパ節は温存し、場合によっては腋窩でLVAを行うことで、採取部のリンパ浮腫を予防している。モニター皮弁は付けても付けなくてもよい。

　術前にエコーで大胸筋などにマーキングを行うとよい。腋窩の側胸部大胸筋縁に、エコーで大胸筋表層近くに拍動する外側胸動脈穿通枝が確認できる。通常浅枝と深枝の2本が確認でき、この枝を使用して複数の血管柄付きリンパ脂肪弁が挙上可能である（**Fig. 7-5-1～4**）。

　採取された皮弁は、鼠径部あるいは大腿基部の皮下組織内、または下腿に血管柄付リンパ管組織弁として移植する。2つ以上リンパ管弁が用意できればこれら複数ヵ所へ移植する。1つしか用意できない場合はレシピエントの血管の状態を見極め、一番状態のよい場所へ移植する。われわれは術前にレシピエント部もエコーを施行し血流を評価して優先順位を決めている。

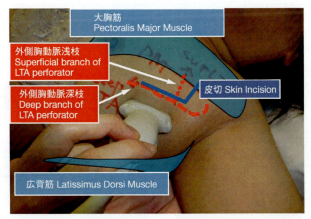

Fig. 7-5-1. 術前エコー　Preoperative ultrasonography
術前にエコーで大胸筋マーキングを行うとよい。腋窩の側胸部大胸筋縁にエコーで大胸筋表層近くに拍動する外側胸動脈穿通枝が確認できる。通常穿枝と深枝の2本が確認できる。
Preoperative marking by using ultrasonography is useful. Lateral thoracic artery perforator is detectable at the lateral edge of pectoralis major surface with ultrasonography. Deep and superficial brunch are usually detectable.

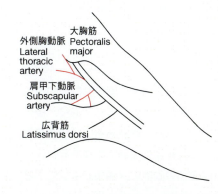

Fig. 7-5-2. 外側胸動脈シェーマ
Schema of lateral thoracic artery
外側胸動静脈または肩甲下・胸背動静脈から派生する細い穿通枝を血管柄付リンパ脂肪弁の栄養血管系とする。外側胸動静脈を使用することが多い。
The nutrient vessels for the lymphatic adipose tissue flap are lateral thoracic artery perforator or infrascapular/thoracodorsal artery perforator. We usually use lateral thoracic artery perforator.

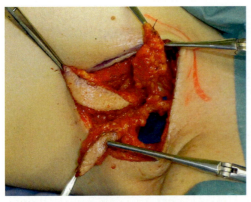

Fig. 7-5-3. 血管柄付リンパ脂肪弁の挙上
Harvesting vascularized lymphatic adipose flaps
腋窩リンパ節は温存し、浅枝と深枝の2本およびこれらの枝を使用して複数の血管柄付リンパ脂肪弁が挙上可能である。図では3つの脂肪弁を挙上している。
Axillary lymph nodes are not included in this lymphatic adipose flap system. Several flaps can be harvested by superficial and deep branch. Three flaps are harvested in the photograph.

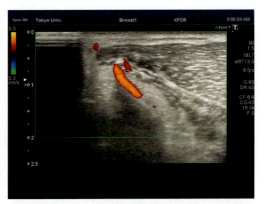

Fig. 7-5-4. 外側胸動脈穿通枝のエコー画面
Ultrasonographical image of lateral thoracic perforator
大胸筋表層近くに拍動する外側胸動脈穿通枝が確認できる。
Pulsatile lateral thoracic artery perforator is detected on the surface of pectoralis major muscle.

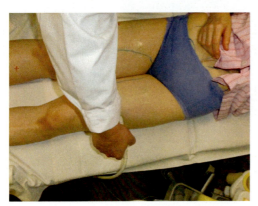

Fig. 7-5-5. レシピエント穿通枝の術前確認
Preoperative ultrasonographic examination of recipient perforator
移植レシピエント部位の動静脈は術前にエコーで確認しマーキング。起始部の動脈が何であるかは特にこだわらない。
Recipient vessels are detected and marked on the surface preoperatively with ultrasonography. It is not important which artery is the origin of the perforator.

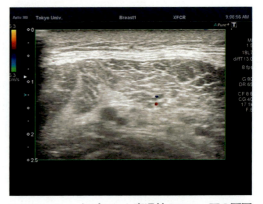

Fig. 7-5-6. レシピエント穿通枝のエコー下の画面
Ultrasonographical image of recipient perforator
エコー所見での血管径や血流などを参考にレシピエントの優先順位をあらかじめ決めておく。
The priority of recipient vessels should be decided preoperatively regarding the diameter and flow.

浮腫側の下肢の鼠径部あるいは大腿部あるいは下腿に皮切が置かれ、浅腸骨回旋動静脈の遠位の細い枝あるいは外側大腿回旋動脈下行枝穿通枝あるいは内側大腿回旋動脈下行枝穿通枝、後頸骨動脈穿通枝、これらの伴走静脈と皮下の静脈を露出する。下腿では皮下静脈あるいは伏在静脈の枝を移植床に使用する。皮弁の栄養血管は、大腿部であれば浅腸骨回旋動静脈の枝あるいは大腿部の各種穿通枝動脈や皮下静脈に吻合される。下腿であれば後頸骨動脈の穿通枝および皮下静

7-5. 合併外科治療

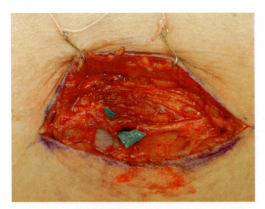

Fig. 7-5-7. 実際の穿通枝　Dissected perforator

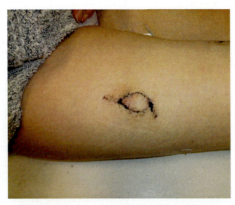

Fig. 7-5-8. モニター皮弁　Monitoring flap
モニター皮弁を置いたときの状態。置かなくてもよい。切除してもしなくてもよい。
The status of lymphatic flap attached monitoring flap. Monitoring flap is not always necessary.

脈が選択されることが多い。しかしながら実際の手術においては移植予定部付近にエコーで確認できた穿通枝を使用することになり、起始がどの動脈であるかまでは考慮することは少ない（Fig. 7-5-5〜8）。

　LVA は大伏在静脈に沿い 1 回の手術で 3〜8 カ所施行する。

　術前に PDE による観察で Linear pattern が観察されないような症例においても、手術中顕微鏡下に 0.3〜0.8 mm の十分吻合可能な集合リンパ管が伏在静脈に沿う 3〜4 cm 以内の範囲の皮下脂肪層に通常発見されるので、ほぼ全症例で LVA も施行できる（Fig. 7-5-9）。

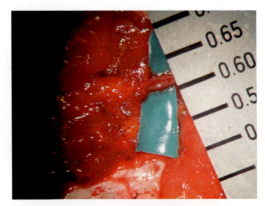

Fig. 7-5-9. リンパ管細静脈吻合　LVA
術前の PDE で Linear pattern が確認できなくても吻合可能な集合リンパ管を術中に顕微鏡下に見い出せる。
Collecting lymphatic vessels which can be anastomosed are detectable under microscope during surgery, even if Linear pattern was not observed preoperatively by PDE.

2. 脂肪切除

　脂肪吸引、あるいは小切開からの脂肪組織切除を大腿内側部、臀部、下腹部、恥骨部に行う。大腿内側部での脂肪組織除去は集合リンパ管の経路を避けるように配置する。あるいは脂肪切除部位が集合リンパ管の走行位置と重なるときは、脂肪切除部位とリンパ管静脈吻合部位を長軸方向に分節的に交互に配置する。

　脂肪組織除去に際し除去予定範囲の皮下脂肪層に止血目的で 1% エピネフリン入りキシロカイン®を 30 倍に希釈して浸潤させる。脂肪吸引が使える場合は脂肪吸引器を使用する。

　脂肪吸引器が使えない場合、小切開からメスの刃で脂肪組織を掻き出すように行うとよい。そ

の場合メスの刃を小刻みに動かし掻爬すると掻き出しやすい。伏在静脈などを損傷すると出血が多くなる。力を込めず小刻みに行うのがコツである。出血が多い場合は術中包帯で数十分強く圧迫していれば十分である。脂肪切除後は皮下を生食で洗浄し弾力絆創膏などで圧迫する。

II. Operative Procedure

The adipose excision and lymphatic transfer are performed under general anesthesia.

The treatments are performed with the combination simultaneously or secondary depending on the cases.

1. Lymphatic transfer : Vascularized lymphadiposal flap excluding the lateral thoracic lymph nodes is harvested. Contraction of lymph vessels can collect and transport lymphatic fluid to their own venous system.

After subdermal injection of Patent Blue or ICG in the lateral thoracic region, a few stained lymphatics are elevated with small perforators arising from the lateral thoracic vessels or/and the thoracodorsal system. We always preserve large axillary lymph nodes and also establish LVA in axillary region to prevent postoperative edema of the donor arm. Monitoring flaps are not always necessary.

Preoperative marking by using ultrasonography is useful. Lateral thoracic artery perforator is detectable at the lateral edge of pectoralis major surface with ultrasonography. Deep and superficial brunch are usually detectable, and several vascularized lymphadiposal flaps can be harvested including these branches(**Fig. 7-5-1 to 4**).

Harvested flaps are transferred to inguinal or proximal thigh subdermal region, or lower leg region.

When you can harvest more than two flaps, you transfer to multiple regions. When it is only one flap, you have to judge the most appropriate region by considering about the status of recipient vessels.

We decide preoperatively the priority with detecting recipient vessels by using ultrasound sonography. Each recipient vessels are the branch of SCIA and SCIV and/or cutaneous vein, the descending brunch perforator of lateral circumflex femoral artery and vein and/or cutaneous vein, the descending brunch perforator of medial circumflex femoral artery and vein and/or cutaneous vein, the perforator of posterior tibial artery and vein and/or cutaneous vein. However, we don't actually care about which perforator it is. We just care about if there is appropriate perforators and veins the diameter and flow of which are good enough to anastomose in the transfer region(**Fig. 7-5-5 to 8**).

LVAs are performed along the great saphenous vein from 3 to 8 at one time.

LVA can be performed even in the case no linear pattern is observed, since 0.3-0.8 mm lymphatic vessels which are large enough for anastomosis can be detected under microscope along the great saphenous vein within 3-4 cm range in almost all cases(**Fig. 7-5-9**).

2. Adipose excision : Liposuction or adipose excision through small skin incision are performed in medial thigh, buttock, lower abdominal and pubic region. The regions are placed with avoiding the collecting lymphatic route. When the region have to be overlapped with lymphatic route, for example medial side of knee, they are placed alternately in the longitudinal direction.

Tumescent technique is applied before adipose excision.

When we can't use liposuction, we scrape out adipose tissue by using scalpel through small skin incision. We should care not to damage great saphenous vein.

When you damage great saphenous vein, pressure hemostasis with bandage during operation is good enough.

Washing in the excisional area with saline and placing penrose drain are the final step of adipose excision.

7-5. 合併外科治療

Ⅲ　周術期評価・管理

　リンパ移植後のルーチンとしては、POD1までベッド上安静とし、POD2〜トイレ処置歩行可としている（金曜術日の場合は週末ベッド上、月曜〜トイレ処置歩行）。患者の状態に応じ徐々に安静度解除を拡大していく。

　リンパ管移植部、リンパ管静脈吻合部の圧迫は術後1ヵ月から。

　LVA、リンパ管移植に対しては、

- 当日帰室時：タンデトロン®3V/メイロン®1A20mL/ソルデム®3A200mLを2時間で点滴注射（div）している。
- 翌日〜POD6：「タンデトロン®3V/メイロン®1A20mL/ソルデム®3A200mLを2時間でdiv」を1日2回行っている。

脂肪切除を行った際も投与している。

Ⅲ.　Postoperative management and assessment

　Compression on the adipose excision area with elastic tape if oozing continue.

　Postoperative management is bed rest on the first postoperative day, starting to walk from the second postoperative day, allowing compression therapy postoperatively in about one month.

　For LVA, lymphatic transfer

- ・On the day of surgery, After returning to ward,
  prostaglandin E_1 20 μg 3 V + sodium bicarbonate 8.4% 1 A 20 mL + maintenance infusion 200 mL
  Drip intravenous infusion in 2 hours
- ・Postoperative day 1〜6：
  prostaglandin E_1 20 μg 3 V + sodium bicarbonate 8.4% 1 A 20 mL + maintenance infusion 200 mL
  Drip intravenous infusion in 2 hours, twice a day.

Ⅳ　術後評価

　LVA部脂肪切除部位では、蜂窩織炎の再発、創部の創傷治癒遅延、リンパ漏、脂肪切除部位のリンパ嚢胞形成が起こることがあり注意を要する。

　リンパ浮腫の圧迫療法は術後1ヵ月後より許可している。

Ⅳ.　Postoperative evaluation

　Recurrence of cellulitis, protracted wound healing, lymphorrhea, lymphocele, should be cared postoperatively.

　We allow compression therapy in one month postoperatively after LVA or lymphatic transfer.

■おわりに

　リンパ浮腫では既に他章でも述べられているとおりリンパ管静脈吻合が低侵襲でかつ効果的である。進行例においてもリンパ管移植を行うことでリンパ浮腫改善が得られる。

　しかしながらリンパ浮腫の患部の増大はリンパ不全による組織間液貯留のみならず脂肪組織増大による部分も大きい。特に進行例ではリンパ管静脈吻合とリンパ管組織移植によるリンパ改善のみでは十分な減量が得られないこともある。

　そのような症例では脂肪切除などの組織減量術が効果的である。しかしながら安易な脂肪減量術は大変危険である。当然組織減量術はリンパを傷害する危険性をもつ治療法である。

　一見進行したように見える症例で PDE で Linear image が確認できないような症例でも顕微鏡下に LVA を施行すると吻合可能なリンパ管を見い出すことは多い。またリンパ浮腫は患部の組織増大が最も感知しやすい自覚および他覚所見であるが原因はリンパ不全にあり、組織減量術はリンパ管静脈吻合やリンパ管移植と併用して初めてリンパ浮腫治療法として意味をなす。

（吉田周平）

■Conclusion

　LVA is less invasive and effective in lymphedema. Lymphatic transfer is applied to severe lymphedema cases.

　The Symptom of increasing volume in lymphedema is not only attributed to pooling lymphatic fluid but also adipogenesis. Especially in advanced cases, the improvement regarding only lymphatic flow by LVA and lymphatic transfer can't always accomplish satisfactory volume reduction.

　The surgical volume reduction by using adipose excision is effective in such cases. However, we can't apply adipose reduction surgery carelessly. Needless to say, adipose reduction surgery is the treatment which contain the risk to injure the lymphatic flow.

　As we described previously, even in the severe case where no Linear pattern is observed through PDE, there are collecting lymphatic vessels the lymphatic flow of which is good enough to anastomose under microscope. The adipose excision will be applied to these patients after treatment of lymphedema with LVA and/or lymph transfer. These patients with multiple lymphedema are caused by lymphatic obstruction and lead to the increase in limb volume and easy to infection.

（*Shuhei Yoshida*）

1) Ruocco V, Schwartz RA, Ruocco E：Lymphedema；an immunologically vulnerable site for development of neoplasms. J Am Acad Dermatol 47：124-127, 2002.
2) Lambert PB, Frank HA, Bellman S, et al：The role of the lymph trunks in the response to allogeneicskin transplamts. Transplantation 3：62-73, 1965.
3) Ghanta S, Cuzzone DA, Torrisi JS, et al：Regulation of inflammation and fibrosis by macrophages in lymphedema. Am J Physiol Heart Circ Physiol 308(9)：H1065-H1077, 2015.
4) Aschen S, Zampell JC, Elhadad S, et al：Regulation of Adipogenesis by Lymphatic fluid Stasis Part II；Expression of Adipose Differentiation Genes. Plast Reconstr Surg 129(4)：838-847, 2012.
5) Hotamisligil GS：Inflammation and metabolic disorders. Nature 444：860-867, 2006.
6) Suganami T, Ogawa Y：Adipose tissue macrophages；their role in adipose tissue remodeling. J Leuko Biol 88：33-39, 2010.

| CHAPTER 7 |

外科治療
Surgical treatment

6. 症例提示
Case presentation

Ⅰ　リンパ管細静脈吻合術[1)-4)]

筆者らが行っている各種外科的治療法について詳述する。

リンパ管細静脈吻合術は、最近は世界的に LVA と略されることが多い。

リンパ液を静脈系に返し、最終的には心臓に還流させる方法が以前から報告されている。これがリンパ管静脈吻合術であるが、過去の吻合術は肉眼下の吻合術であった。筆者らは縫合糸は 50 ミクロンの針を用い、顕微鏡下に約 20～30 倍に拡大した視野でリンパ管細静脈吻合術（超微小血管吻合術）を行ってきた。従来の顕微鏡下リンパ管静脈吻合術（O'Brien, 1977）[5)-7)] と異なる点は、還流させる皮静脈を真皮直下または脂肪層浅層の細い静脈に吻合することである。原則として、手術施行最低 6 ヵ月前から徹底した持続圧迫とマッサージによる保存的治療（外来通院を主とする）を行ったうえで LVA を行う。

浮腫発生後早期のものであれば、本術式でかなりの効果が期待できる。リンパ浮腫が発生する前のリンパ管の平滑筋細胞が機能している時期であれば、1 本のみの吻合であってもリンパ浮腫が予防できる症例もある。長期経過し、平滑筋細胞の機能が失われたリンパ浮腫例でもリンパ管と静脈を吻合すれば、機能不全は術後のストッキングで他動的なリンパ管の収縮が得られるために、リンパ液は正常ほどではないが還流されると思われる。吻合後は蜂窩織炎の頻度減少、術前に比べ四肢のボリュームの著明な減少、周径の著減が起こることが多い。これまでの結果から、ほとんどすべてのリンパ浮腫例に対してこの治療法は適応があると思われる。

Ⅰ. Lymphaticovenular anastomosis[1)-4)]

The following are detailed descriptions of various surgical methods used by the authors.

Lymphaticovenular anastomosis is recently abbreviated more frequently as LVA in the world.

Drainage of lymphatic fluid first to venous circulation and then ultimately to the heart has been previously reported as a surgical treatment of lymphedema. This is the lymphatic venous anastomosis, and the previous anastomoses were performed under naked eyes. The authors perform lymphaticovenular anastomosis using suturing thread with the needle of 50 microns in diameter and under a microscope at a magnification of 20 to 30 times. The differences from conventional microscopic lymphaticovenous anastomosies (O'Brien, 1977)[5)-7)] is that lymphatic vessels are anastomosed to cutaneous venules in the subdermal or superficial subcutaneous fat tissue layers. As a general rule, conservative treatment by means of continuous application of compression and thorough massage should be carried out (as an outpatient treatment) at least 6 months in advance of the LVA surgery.

In cases for which treatment is performed soon after initial lymphedema, this technique is expected to be highly effective. There have been cases for which one anastomosis per patient can also play a role in the prevention of lymphedema, when treatment is conducted before the development of lymphedema, while the smooth muscle cells surrounding the lymphatic vessels are still functioning. Even in cases with long-term lymphedema and loss of lymphatic smooth muscle cells, if the lymphatic vessels are surgically anastomosed to the venules, lymphatic dysfunction can be hindered and lymphatic flow could be partially restored by postoperative compressive stockings, which promote passive constriction of lymphatic vessels. Postoperative changes after anastomosis include decrease in the frequency of cellulitis and significant reduction in both of the volume and circumference of the extremities. Based on these past results, this therapy seemed to be adapting for almost all of lymphedema cases.

Ⅱ 顕微鏡下リンパ管細静脈吻合術

手術に先立ち0.5 mm前後の超微小血管吻合技術に精通しておくべきである。ラットの下腹壁動静脈吻合を用いた遊離鼠径皮弁移植に成功する程度の吻合技術があるのが理想である。また、臨床例で指尖部の再接着に成功する程度の吻合技術をもつことが望ましい。

1．超微小血管吻合に必要な器具 (Fig. 7-6-1)

携帯用ドプラ聴診器、手術用ルーペ（USA デザインビュー社製）、マイクロサージャリー手術セット、超微小血管剥離子、血管クリップ、超微小血管吻合手術セット、マイクロ吻合針（8-0～12-0　30-65 ミクロン縫合針）など。

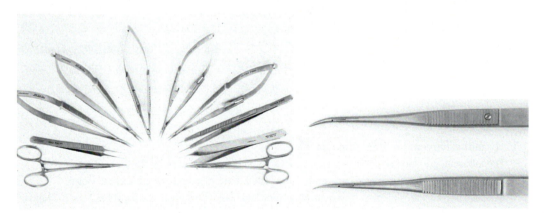

Fig. 7-6-1. 超微小外科に用いられる手術器具セット　Instruments for super-microsurgery
左：スーパーマイクロセット。右は持針器先端を示す。上：通常のマイクロ持針器、下：スーパーマイクロ持針器
Left : Instruments for super-microsurgery. Right : Tip of needle holder. Upper : Needle holder for usual microsurgery, Lower : Needle holder for super-microsurgery.

2．手術手技

全麻下または局麻（キシロカイン® E 局注）下に、患肢の内側と外側に（この部にはリンパ管が多く、主な皮静脈があるためその枝である細い静脈が得られやすい）数ヵ所の皮膚小切開（3～5 cm）を加える。

3．リンパ管と静脈の選択

　リンパ管とその近傍の真皮直下、または脂肪層浅層の細静脈（直径0.6～1.0 mm）を露出剥離する。同一切開部にリンパ管と静脈の両方が存在すれば、血管テープまたは3-0ナイロンなどでマークする。そうしないと、その後のspasmで視野から消えることがある。症例によっては10切開部のうち2部程度でのみリンパ管がみられるものや、まったく存在しないものも稀にある。筆者らは、通常の微小血管吻合術と同様に、ヘパリン加生食の局所洗浄で術野の凝血を防ぎ、リンパ管と細静脈の拡張に塩酸パパベリン10倍希釈液を使用している。

4．Patency test

　リンパ管と静脈のそれぞれの中枢と末梢側（リンパ液と血液の流れる方向）を確認し、リンパ流が順行性に流れるように両者を切断吻合する。静脈はpatency testで両方向に血行がみられ、方向性がはっきりしないことがある。皮膚直下の静脈は、浅層から深層に向かって流れているので、その3次元的な分布を参考にして血流方向を決める。静脈の切断の際には、末梢側を切断前にバイポーラーで焼灼止血した後に切断する。止血なしで放置すると、術後出血で再手術が必要となることもある。リンパ管を切断すると、多くの場合リンパ液の漏出は不良である。時に漏出が良好な場合は、1本の吻合のみでも術後著明な改善が得られることが多い。弁閉鎖不全があると、逆行性のリンパ流がみられることもある。重症型の先天性リンパ浮腫では、逆行性乳びリンパがみられることがある。広範な弁閉鎖不全のためであろう。

5．リンパ管と静脈の吻合 (Fig. 7-6-2～4)

　顕微鏡下にリンパ管と同径の細い真皮直下の静脈との端々吻合を行う。われわれは11-0または12-0ナイロン（針の直径50ミクロン）を用いた約6～8針のinterrupted sutureで吻合して

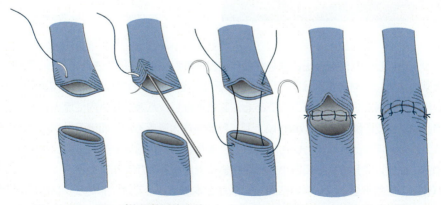

Fig. 7-6-2．リンパ管細静脈吻合法　Lymphaticovenular anastomosis (LVA)
30～50ミクロンの針を用い鑷子をリンパ管内に入れずに縫合針をかける。
30-50 micron needle is used to do the anastomosis without inserting the forceps into the lymphatic vessels.

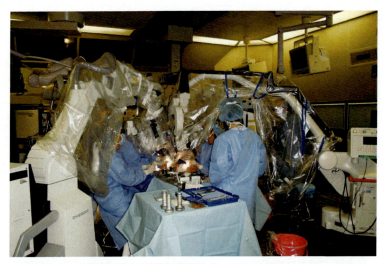

Fig. 7-6-3. 局麻下のリンパ管細静脈吻合　LVA under local anesthesia
下肢リンパ浮腫に対しての吻合術は、通常4人の術者が4台の顕微鏡を用いて3時間前後の手術を行う。上肢では2名の術者が2台の顕微鏡を用いる。
The anastomoses for lymphedema of lower extremities are usually performed by four operators with four microscopes within about three hours. The anastomoses for lymphedema of upper extremities are usually performed by two operators with two microscopes.

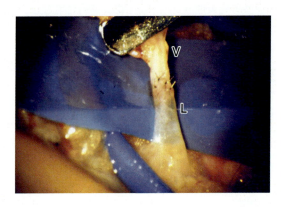

Fig. 7-6-4. 顕微鏡下リンパ管細静脈吻合術の実際
Established LVA under microscope
術直後よりリンパ管(L)から細静脈(V)内へのリンパ液の還流がみられる。
Immediately after operation, lymphatic flow can be seen from lymphatic vessel(L) to venule(V).

いる。リンパ管はリンパ液を漏出させながら(内腔が開存した状態にできるので)、顕微鏡下の視野を最大限に拡大して吻合する。針をリンパ管に通すときには手のブレによる壁の断裂が生じる。その防止には、呼吸を止めるのがコツである。吻合後はリンパ液が静脈内に流入するのが確認できる。吻合静脈が皮静脈など1.5mm以上で、静脈径が太過ぎると、血液のリンパ管内への逆流が起こり、術後の浮腫改善は難しいと思われる。また、吻合技術はやや高度のレベルが必要であろう。吻合には最近開発された超微小外科手術器具を用いるのが有利である。

- **リンパ管弁の閉鎖不全**：同一視野に還流静脈が2本ある場合では、1本のリンパ管を切断すれば2ヵ所のリンパ管断端ができるので、順行性と逆行性に2吻合するのがよい(一石二鳥吻合法)。リンパ管の切断中枢端からリンパ流の逆流がみられることが多い。その理由としては、中枢側リンパ管の弁の閉鎖不全があるように思う。

6．術後の血液のリンパ系への逆流

　吻合した静脈が逆行性であると血液がリンパ系に流入し、術後5時間頃より突然吻合部の近位側全域に皮下出血様の変化が起こる。足関節部で吻合した例では、下肢全体の蜂窩織炎が発生したようにみえる。患肢の痛み、熱発などの炎症症状はないのが特徴である。そのまま自然放置で経過を観察しても、4〜5日で自然消失するようである。

7．立位と臥位の差

　術中にリンパ管から静脈に良好な還流が得られる例では浮腫は改善することが多いが、術中はあくまでも臥位であり重力の影響がない状況である。立位ではリンパ液に重力がかかるので還流されにくい。そこで、術後は圧迫治療を併用する必要がある。

8．術後治療

　術後は吻合部狭窄を予防するため、プロスタグランディンE₁（PGE₁）の持続点滴を約5日間続け、その後数週間は経口でPGE₁を服用する。局所麻酔下の吻合後では術直後から手術された上肢の使用は可能である。下肢例でも術直後から歩行は可能である。術後1週で退院となり退院後は軽度の圧迫とし、1ヵ月以後強い持続圧迫治療を再開している。浮腫発生後、早期吻合ができた例など著明な減少が得られる。このような例では術後6ヵ月より圧迫を試験的、断続的に解除し始め、漸次保存療法を中止してゆく。

II．Lymphaticovenular anastomosis (under the microscope)

　Before performing this operation, the surgeon should be familiar with the super-microvascular anastomosis techniques involving vessels as small as about 0.5 mm in diameter. It is ideal that mastering the inferior epigastric arteriovenous anastomosis techniques to successfully transfer the free groin flap of a rat. In addition, it is desirable for the surgeon to have had experience in successful finger-tip replantation of clinical cases.

　1．Necessary instruments for super-microvascular anastomosis (Fig. 7-6-1)：Portable Doppler stethoscope, surgical loupe (USA Designs For Vision, Inc), microsurgery set, super-fine blood vessel stripper, vascular clip, super-fine vascular anastomosis surgery set, micro-anastomosis needle (8-0 to 12-0 suture line with 30 to 65 micron suture needle), etc.

　2．Surgical technique：Under general anesthesia or local anesthesia (xylocaine E local injection), several skin incisions 3-5 cm in length are created in the medial and lateral side of the affected limbs where there are many lymphatic vessels and thin venous branches can be easily obtained because of the existence of many main cutaneous veins.

　3．Selection of appropriate lymphatic vessels and veins：The surgeon should dissect and expose the lymphatic vessels and the surrounding venules (diameter 0.6-1.0 mm) in subdermal or subcutaneous superficial fat layer. If there are both lymphatic vessels and veins in the same incision site, the vascular band or 3-0 nylon should be used to label them separately. Otherwise, some lymphatic vessels or venules may disappear from the field of vision due to spasms during the subsequent procedure. In some cases, lymphatic vessels may only be seen in 2 out of 10 incisions, or, in rare cases, no lymphatic vessels were found. While doing the conventional microvascular anastomosis, the authors irrigate the tissue with heparin solution (2000

U in 50 ml saline) in order to prevent the blood coagulation in the operative field and additionally use a 10-fold dilution of papaverine hydrochloride solution to dilate the lymphatic vessels and venules.

4. Patency test : The proximal and distal ends of lymphatic vessels and venules (the direction of lymphatic fluid and blood flow) should be confirmed, so that the cut ends of both can be anastomosed to make the lymphatic flow along the anterograde direction. As venous circulation can be observed in both directions during the patency test, directionality is often not entirely clear. Because subcutaneous venous circulation flows from superficial to deep layers, it is necessary to use the 3-dimensional distribution of exposed venous vasculature as a reference to determine the direction of blood flow. When severing the vein, it is best to cauterize the distal end of the vessel with bipolar coagulator for hemostasis. If the distal end is left without hemostasis, it is possible that a repeat surgery will be needed due to postoperative bleeding. When lymphatic vessels are cut, lymphatic fluid leakage is insufficient in most instances. Occasionally, in the case that lymphatic fluid leakage is sufficient, significant improvement will be obtained with only one anastomosis. In case of valve insufficiency, retrograde lymphatic flow could be seen sometimes. In severe congenital lymphedema cases, retrograde chylothorax can be seen. It may be caused by extensive valve insufficiency.

5. Anastomosis of lymphatic vessels and venules (Fig. 7-6-2 to 4) : Under the microscope, the lymphatic vessels are anastomosed with the venules of the same diameter beneath the dermis by end-to-end technique. We performed 6 to 8 stitches of interrupted sutures using 11-0 or 12-0 nylon (needle of 50 microns in diameter). Upon the lymphatic leakage from open cavity, the lymphatic vessels are anastomosed at the maximum magnification of the visual field under the microscope. When the needle passes through the lymphatic vessel, rupturing of the wall occurs due to shaking of the hand. Holding breath is a key point in preventing this. After anastomosis, we can confirm that lymphatic fluid flows into the vein. If anastomosed veins including cutaneous veins are over 1.5 mm in diameter which may cause retrograde flow of blood into the lymphatic vessels, it is difficult to improve lymphedema after surgery. In addition, a moderately high level of skill with anastomosis is required. Recently developed supermicrosurgical instruments are advantageously used for anastomosis.

Lymphatic valve insufficiency : in the event of two circumfluent veins existing in the same field of vision, because there will be two ends if one lymphatic vessel is cut, it is better to conduct both anterograde and retrograde anastomoses (killing two birds with one stone). Reflux of lymph flow from the central cut-off end of lymphatic vessel is often observed. The reason might be the insufficient lymphatic valve closure on the central side.

6. Reflux of the blood into the lymphatic system following surgery : If the blood flows retrogradely into the lymphatic system through the anastomosed veins, erythema may suddenly occur at the proximal anastomosis site from 5 hours after operation. For the case in which we conduct anastomosis in the ankle joint area, it appears as if cellulitis has occurred throughout the entire lower limb. This is characterized by none of inflammatory symptoms such as pain in the affected limb, fever or other inflammatory symptoms. It will spontaneously disappear in 4 to 5 days even if without special treatment.

7. Difference between erect stance and recumbent positions : In the recumbent position with no effect of gravity, lymphedema is often improved in cases with good drainage from the lymphatic vessel to the vein during surgery. In the erect stance, the drainage of lymphatic fluid will be difficult due to gravitation. Therefore, compressive treatment must be combined after surgery.

8. Post-surgical treatment : In order to prevent anastomotic stenosis after surgery, prostaglandin E_1 is continuously infused for about five days, after which PGE_1 is orally taken for the next several weeks. Following anastomosis under local anesthesia, usage of the upper extremities is possible soon after surgery. In the cases of the lower extremities, walking is possible immediately after surgery. Patients are discharged from hospital one week after surgery and undergo mild compressive treatment after discharge, restarting continuous high level compressive treatment one month later. Once lymphedema occurs, significant decrease can be obtained for cases in which early anastomosis are performed. In such cases, we experimentally start intermittent compressive treatment from six months after surgery and gradually stop conservative treatment.

Ⅲ 症 例

1．上肢リンパ浮腫手術結果（Fig. 7-6-5〜7）

　LVA 開始初期の頃、18 人の患者（36〜73 歳）に対し上肢のリンパ管静脈吻合術を行った。これらの患者はリンパ浮腫発症から平均 7.2 年（11ヵ月〜22 年）経過しており、術前の前腕（肘から 10 cm 遠位）の平均余剰周径は 14.8（4〜18.5）cm であった。術後平均 2.6 年（1ヵ月〜10 年）の経過観察にて平均 4.5（0〜8.5）cm の減少が得られた。平均減少率は 45.2（0〜85）％であった[2]。

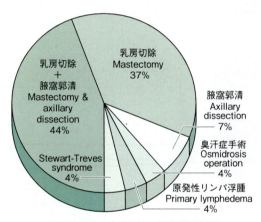

Fig. 7-6-5．上肢リンパ浮腫の内訳
Summary of upper extremities lymphedema
（Koshima I, Inagawa K, Urushibara K, et al：Supermicrosurgical lymphaticovenularanastomosis for the treatment of lymphedema in the upper extremities. J Reconstr Microsurg 16：437-442, 2000 による）

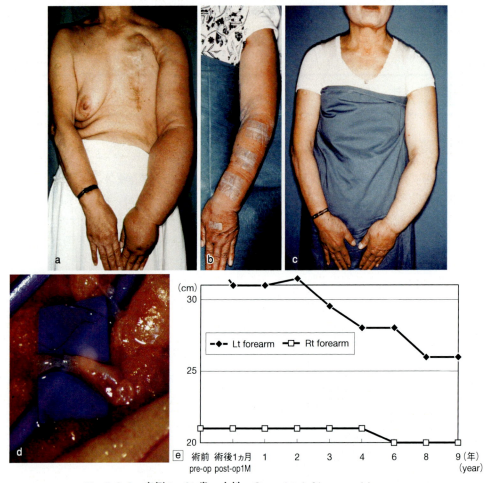

Fig. 7-6-6. 症例 1：61 歳、女性　Case 1：A 61-year-old woman

a：放射線照射後 15 年で浮腫発生。
b：浮腫発生後 11 年で 7 本の LVA がなされた。術後は圧迫療法併用で浮腫は著減。術後 6 日目。
c：術後 6 年目。
d：吻合したリンパ管と細静脈。
e：術後の前腕周径の変化。1 回の LVA で術後 9 年まで減少し続けている。
a：Lymphedema occurred 15 years after radiotherapy.
b：7 LVAs were performed 11 years after the occurrence of lymphedema. The edema improved obviously with compressive therapy after the operation. 6 days post operation.
c：6 years post operation.
d：Established LVA.
e：The change of forearm circumference after operation. The circumference has been continuously reduced until 9 years after once LVA.
(Koshima I, Kawada S, Moriguchi T, et al：Ultrastructural observation of lymphatic vessels in lymphedema in human extremities. Plast Reconstr Surg 97：397-405, 1996 による)

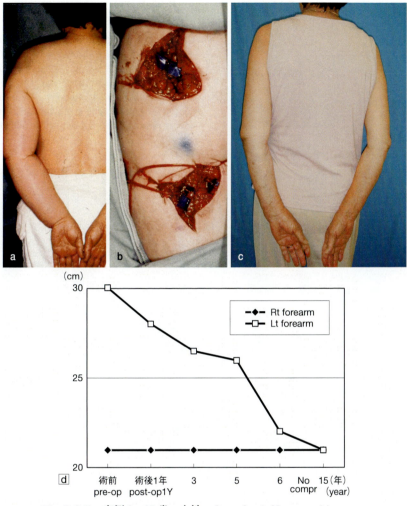

Fig. 7-6-7. 症例2：65歳、女性　Case 2 : A 65-year-old woman

a：放射線照射後26年で浮腫が発生。
b：浮腫発生後11ヵ月目に6吻合。
c：術後はストッキングによる圧迫を数年行った。術後15年。完治。術後数年で圧迫は不要となった。
d：術後の前腕周径の変化。吻合術は1回のみで術後6年で正常化した。

a : Lymphedema occurred 26 years after radiotherapy.
b : 6 anastomoses were performed 11 months after initial lymphedema.
c : Compressive therapy with stockings was conducted for several years after operation. The patient was cured and no need of compression a few years after operation.
d : Postoperative changes of forearm circumference after the operation. It returned to normal 6 years after once LVA.

2．下肢のリンパ浮腫に対する治療結果 (Fig. 7-6-8〜13)

1）圧迫療法

　筆者が吻合術を開始し始めた1990年頃、下肢の片側性または両側性リンパ浮腫患者のうち12名に外来通院でストッキング圧迫を主とする保存療法のみを行った。これらの患者の浮腫は発生後平均5.2年経過しており、術前の下腿（膝から10 cm遠位部）の平均過剰周径は7.1 cmであっ

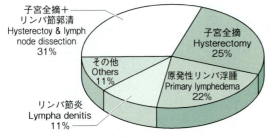

Fig. 7-6-8. 下肢のリンパ浮腫の原因
Causes of lymphedema of the lower extremities
一次性（特発性）よりも二次性が多い。子宮癌切除またはその後の放射線併用療法が原因となることが多い。
There are more cases of secondary lymphedema than primary (idiopathic) lymphedema. The main cause of secondary lymphedema is the combination of uterine cancer resection and subsequent radiotherapy.

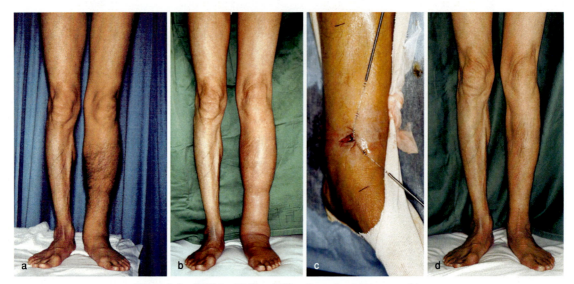

Fig. 7-6-9. 症例3：57歳、男性　Case 3：A 57-year-old man
a：睾丸腫瘍切除後6年で発生したリンパ浮腫。放射線照射なし。浮腫発生後7年目から弾性包帯による圧迫を開始。
b：7年間毎日圧迫したが、最近浮腫が増強した。
c：局麻下に足関節部で1本LVAを行った（入院1日）。
d：術後5ヵ月。術前と同程度のストッキング圧迫で浮腫は著減した。
a：Lymphedema occurred 6 years after testicular cancer resection without radiotherapy. Compressive therapy was started 7 years after the occurrence of edema.
b：The lymphedema aggravated in spite of daily compressive therapy for 7 years.
c：One LVA at ankle joint under local anesthesia was performed (hospitalization day1).
d：5 months post operation. The lymphedema significantly improved by the same stocking compression as the preoperative degree.

たが、平均1.5年の保存療法で平均0.6 cm減少した。4 cm以上著明に周径が減少した例は2例（16.7%）であった[3]。

2）手術療法（全麻下の下肢リンパ管細静脈吻合術）

　1990年頃、これまでの他施設または当科での圧迫療法が無効な16名に入院したうえで全麻下に複数のリンパ管細静脈吻合術と退院後の圧迫療法を行った。これらの患者の術前の過剰周径は平均9.8 cmで、発生後平均8.9年経過していた。術後平均3.3年の経過で平均2.7 cmの減少が得られた。4 cm以上の周径減少がみられたのは8例（50%）であった[3]。以上の結果から、手術を行ったうえで圧迫療法を続ける併用療法が優れていることがわかる。

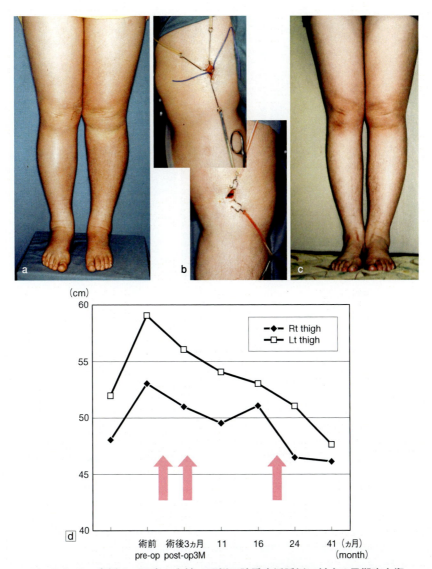

Fig. 7-6-10.　症例 4：35 歳、女性。両側下肢重度浮腫例に対する早期吻合術
Case 4：A 35-year-old woman. Early anastomosis for severe lymphedema of both lower extremities

a：子宮癌切除と放射線照射直後から両下肢の浮腫発生。
b：浮腫発生後 3 ヵ月で局麻下に右膝内側 1 本吻合。4 ヵ月で局麻下に左膝内側で 1 本吻合。
c：術後 2 年。圧迫療法のみで浮腫は予防できている。
d：術後の大腿部膝上 10 cm 部の周径の経時的変化。増悪する度に追加吻合（2 回、局麻）がなされ減少傾向にある。

a：Lymphedema of bilateral lower extremities occurred immediately after the uterine cancer resection and radiotherapy.
b：3 months after the occurrence of lymphedema, one LVA was performed under local anesthesia in the medial aspect of right thigh. 4 months after the occurrence of lymphedema, one LVA was performed under local anesthesia in the medial aspect of left thigh.
c：2 years post operation, lymphedema was prevented only by compressive therapy.
d：Changes in circumference of thigh at 10 cm above knee occurred over time after the operation. Because of aggravation, supplementary anastomoses (2 times, under local anesthesia) were performed and the lymphedema showed reduction tendency.

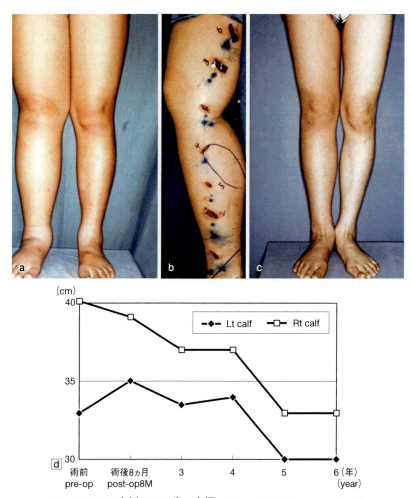

Fig. 7-6-11. 症例5：12歳、女児　Case 5：A 12-year-old girl

a：特発性浮腫。2年前から浮腫が続き、積極的に圧迫療法を継続している。ある程度の改善が得られたがそれ以上の改善は得られない。
b：全麻下に患肢の大腿部2ヵ所、下腿部2ヵ所、足背1ヵ所で合計5吻合行った。
c：術後6年。
d：術後の経過。術後5年までさらなる改善がみられ、以後改善状態を維持している。

a：Idiopathic lymphedema. The patient had been treated with continuous compressive therapy for 2 years since the lymphedema started to progress. Although some extent of improvement was achieved, no further improvement was seen.
b：Total 5 LVAs were performed under general anesthesia, including 2 LVAs at thigh, 2 LVAs at lower leg, and 1 LVA at dorsum of foot.
c：6 years after LVA.
d：Postoperative follow-up. Further improvements were seen up to 5 years after surgery, and the improvement status has been maintained since then.

7-6. 症例提示

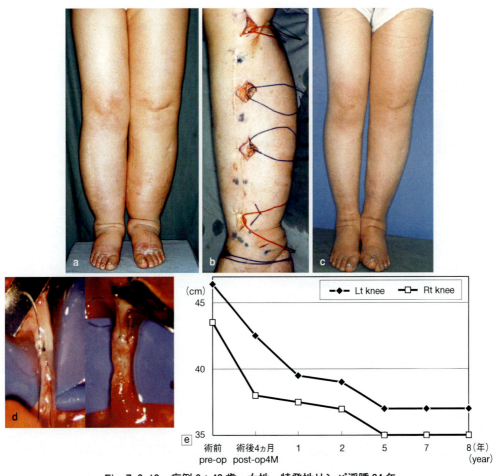

Fig. 7-6-12. 症例6：42歳、女性。特発性リンパ浮腫24年
Case 6：A 42-year-old woman. Idiopathic lymphedema for 24 years

a：24年前に明らかな誘因なく両下腿の浮腫が発生し、既に他医で積極的な持続圧迫療法と数回の組織切除術手術がなされた。浮腫の改善はみられず増大傾向がみられ、頻回の蜂窩織炎を繰り返していた。
b：右下腿内側の5ヵ所の皮切部で1吻合ずつ、合計5吻合行った。左下肢ではリンパ管が認められず、左鼠径部からの脂肪筋膜弁を大腿前面の皮下に移行した。
c：術後9年。右下腿周径で−13.5cm、左下腿で−11cmと高度の改善が得られた。蜂窩織炎は術後ほとんど発生しておらず毎日の作業(ミシンによる製縫)が可能となっている。
d：吻合したリンパ管と細静脈。リンパ管硬化症がみられる。
e：吻合術後9年までの経過。両下肢とも経時的に浮腫は改善傾向を示し、患者は仕事に復帰した。

a：Lymphedema of bilateral lower extremities occurred 24 years ago without obvious inducement, and tissue resection had been performed several times by other doctors together with continuous compressive therapy. However, the lymphedema progressed and the patient suffered repeated cellulitis.
b：5 LVAs were performed at 5 skin incisions in medial side of right leg. No lymph duct was found at left leg, then we transferred adipofascial flap from left groin to subcutaneous area of anterior thigh.
c：A remarkable reduction in the circumference(−13.5 cm at the right leg and −11 cm at the left leg) was achieved 9 years after operation. Cellulitis hardly occurred after the operation and she is able to do daily work(sewing by machine).
d：Established LVA and lymphangiosclerosis can be seen.
e：9 year follow-up showed the gradual improvement of bilateral lower limbs lymphedema, and the patient went back to work.

(Koshima I, Kawada S, Moriguchi T, et al：Ultrastructural observation of lymphatic vessels in lymphedema in human extremities. Plast Reconstr Surg 97：397-405, 1996 による)

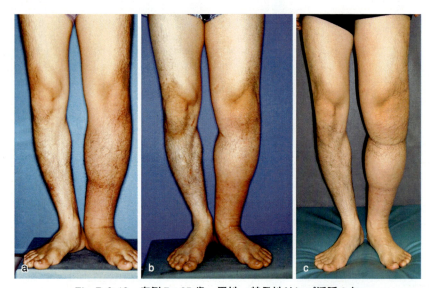

Fig. 7-6-13. 症例7：25歳、男性。特発性リンパ浮腫6年
Case 7：A 25-year-old man. Idiopathic lymphedema for 6 years

a：特発性浮腫で蜂窩織炎頻発例。浮腫発生後6年目に吻合術を行った。左下肢2吻合、右下肢予防的に2吻合。
b：術後4年目。
c：術後8年。改善がみられる。健側は浮腫発生が予防されている。
a：Idiopathic lymphedema with frequent cellulitis. LVAs were performed 6 years after the occurrence of lymphedema, including 2 LVAs at left lower limb and 2 prophylactic LVAs at right lower limb.
b：4 years post operation.
c：8 years post operation. Improvement can be seen and the occurrence of right side lymphedema was prevented.

3．局麻下の下肢リンパ管細静脈吻合術（追加治験）(Fig. 7-6-8〜13)

　1990年代に、外来受診した下肢のリンパ浮腫症例のうち33症例に対して局麻下に本術式を行った。これらの症例は両側性が7例で、片側性26例であった。平均年齢は54.6歳（10〜78歳）で、一次性浮腫6例（家族性4例）であった。子宮癌などの術後の二次性浮腫は27例で、術後平均3.7年で浮腫が発生しており吻合術まで平均5.1年間浮腫が続きこの間保存的療法が無効なものが多かった。術前の下腿の過剰周径は平均5.4 cmで、ほとんどの症例が手術回数は1〜2回で平均1.5吻合（1〜5吻合）行われた。その結果術後平均13.5ヵ月の経過観察で、浮腫が軽度進行した例が4例（術前周径の17〜21％増大）、不変であったもの2例であった。浮腫の改善がみられたものは27例（全体の82％）で多くは吻合部周辺の周径減少がみられた。これらの周径減少は1〜6 cm（過剰周径の平均57.7％の減少）であった[3]。この時点の分析結果では、全麻と局麻いずれの例でも浮腫の原因、術前の重症度、浮腫の期間、吻合数などと明らかな相関関係はないように思われた。最近では術式が向上し、複数の術者で複数の顕微鏡を用いて3〜4時間で1人の患者を治療することが可能となった。このため吻合数が10本前後と多くなり、過去の結果よりも良好な結果が出始めている。ストッキングの不要な完治例も出つつある。今後はさらに改善度が増すであろう。

7-6. 症例提示

III. Cases

1. Surgical results for lymphedema in the upper extremities (Fig. 7-6-5 to 7): In the initial stages of LVA, 18 patients (range, 36 to 73 years old) received lymphaticovenular anastomosis of the upper extremities. These patients suffered lymphedema for an average of 7.2 years (range, 11 months to 22 years), and the average excess circumference of the preoperative forearm (10 cm distal from the elbow) was 14.8 cm (range, 4 to 18.5 cm). The perimeter was reduced by 4.5 cm on average (range, 0 to 8.5 cm) according to the postoperative follow-up for an average of 2.6 years (range, 1 month to 10 years). The average decrease rate was 45.2% (range, 0 to 85%)[2].

2. Surgical results for lymphedema in the lower extremities (Fig. 7-6-8 to 13):

1) Compressive treatment: Around 1990 when the author first started performing lymphaticovenular anastomosis 12 outpatients with unilateral or bilateral lymphedema of the lower limbs received only conservative treatment mainly using elastic stockings. With lymphedema on average of 5.2 years' duration, the average excess circumference of the lower leg (10 cm distal from the knee) prior to treatment was 7.1 cm, and reduced by 0.6 cm after the conservative treatment over an average of 1.5 years. There were two cases (16.7%) in which the circumference substantially decreased more than 4 cm[3].

2) Surgical treatment: Lymphaticovenular anastomosis of the lower limbs under general anesthesia Around 1990, 16 patients with ineffective preoperative compressive treatment in other institutions or our department received multiple lymphaticovenular anastomoses under general anesthesia and compressive treatment after discharge. The average excess circumference of these patients was 9.8 cm prior to surgery, with an average duration of 8.9 years. An average decrease of 2.7 cm was observed over an average course of 3.3 years after surgery. Eight cases (50%) achieved a decrease in circumference of more than 4 cm[3]. Based on the above results, combined treatment of surgery and continuous compressive treatment after operation can achieve excellent efficacy.

3. Lymphaticovenular anastomosis of the lower extremities under local anesthesia (additional clinical trial) (Fig. 7-6-8 to 13): In the 1990's, 33 cases of outpatients with lymphedema of the lower extremities were operated upon with lymphaticovenular anastomoses under local anesthesia. These cases included 7 bilateral lymphedema patients and 26 unilateral lymphedema patients. The average age was 54.6 years old (range, 10 to 78 years old), with 6 cases of primary edema (4 cases of familial edema). There were 27 cases of secondary lymphedema that occurred within 3.7 years on average following surgery for uterine cancer, and the compressive treatment for most of patients showed inefficacy during the average duration of 5.1 years. The average preoperative excess circumference of the lower legs was 5.4 cm, and the average number of anastomosis in each patient was 1.5 (range, 1 to 5 anastomoses) in most cases within once or twice operations. As a result, according to 13.5-month follow-up on average, lymphedema was slightly aggravated in 4 cases by 17-21% increase of the preoperative circumference and remained constant in 2 cases. Improvement of the edema was observed in 27 cases (82% of the total), with decrease in circumference around the anastomotic region in most cases. The decrease in circumference was 1 to 6 cm (mean 57.7% decrease of excess circumference)[3]. An analysis of the results at this point revealed no clear correlation among the cause of edema, the degree of severity prior to surgery, edema stage, number of anastomoses, etc. in cases under either general or local anesthesia. Recently, with the improvement of the operative manner, it has become capable to perform multiple LVAs for one patient within 3 to 4 hours by a group of surgeons using multiple microscopes. Consequently, the number of anastomoses has increased to around ten and better results than previous operations have begun to appear. There have been cases of complete recovery with no need of elastic stockings. Further improvement will be obtained in the future.

Ⅳ　外科療法と圧迫療法の併用

　このように、手術と圧迫治療を併用すると圧迫または手術のみの単独治療に比べ有効性は高い。入院したうえで連日の徹底したマッサージ療法を主体とした複合的理学療法（Földi 法）の有効性もこれまでに報告されている[8)9)]。しかし、それのみでは退院後はもとに戻るとか進行する例も多い。理学療法のみでは根本的なリンパ還流システムの回復は困難であろう。われわれの治療の原則は、既に浮腫が発生している症例に対しては、手術によってリンパ系の還流ルートを再建し、術後のストッキングによる圧迫療法でその還流能を少しでも増強させるという2本立ての治療方針である。このLVAを主とする併用療法の効果は、徹底した複合的理学療法でなくとも簡単な圧迫療法を追加することで長期間の改善が得られる。特に上肢に有効例が多く完治例も多く出ている。これは吻合リンパ管のリンパ還流能（平滑筋細胞）がまだ保たれていることによると思われるが、理学療法のみに比べて極めて有効である。下肢でも半数で有効であることが判明した。蜂窩織炎頻発例では吻合術の効果は極めて大で、多くの患者が熱発から救われる。無効例の術中所見では、肉眼的に既にリンパ管の硬化、中膜肥厚、閉鎖、または消失している例が多かった。また、無効例のリンパ管の生検結果ではリンパ管中膜の平滑筋細胞数が著減または小型化しているものがほとんどであった[1)-4)]（**Fig. 1-10**、22頁参照）。このことは、たとえ吻合し得たとしてもリンパ流の還流機能障害によってリンパ液の静脈系への十分な還流が得られていない可能性があるので、追加吻合によってさらなる還流系を確立する。

1．浮腫発生後長期経過した例

　一般的に吻合術後の著効例は少ない。しかし、手術用顕微鏡下でリンパ管硬化がみられたり、皮下の線維化が著明な長期経過例でも術後の圧迫療法を行えば、長期的にみればなんらかの効果が得られることが多い。この併用療法の効果は、保存療法のみに比べて上肢では極めて有効である。下肢でも外見的な著効は得られずとも約半数で有効であった。特に、蜂窩織炎頻発例では吻合術後に蜂窩織炎の発生数が著減し、その効果は大きい[1)-4)]。時に、機能的なリンパ管が吻合された場合には、術前に比べ著明なボリュームの減少が得られることもある。

2．重度浮腫例に対する血管柄付きリンパ管（リンパ節）移植（Fig. 7-6-14）

　LVA無効例で長期経過した進行性の重症リンパ浮腫例は最も治療が難しい。このような例に対して、2005年、筆者は健側から正常なリンパ管に栄養血管を付けたまま採取して、患肢に移植する遊離血管柄付きリンパ管移植を行った。これは正常な平滑筋機能をもつリンパ管の移植によってリンパ液を静脈系に誘導するという方法である。片側下肢例では、対側の第1趾間部の還流機能をもつリンパ管を患肢の鼠径部に移植する。両側下肢の浮腫例では腋窩部からリンパ管を採取し、鼠径部に移植する。血管柄付きリンパ管移植片の平滑筋が生きたまま移植されるため、リンパ管のポンプ機能が復活しリンパ系の還流効果が期待される。機能する平滑筋移植ともいえる。これまでに重度リンパ浮腫の複数例に用いているが、完治例も出始めている。

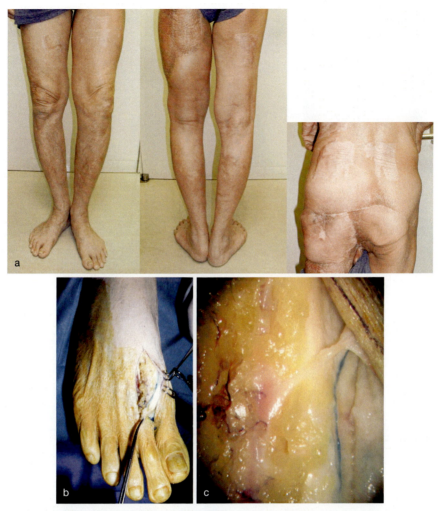

Fig. 7-6-14. 症例8：70歳、男性　Case 8：A 70-year-old man

a：左臀部扁平上皮癌切除・鼠径リンパ郭清後1ヵ月。左下肢浮腫と蜂窩織炎が発生。
b：右第1趾間部から血管柄付きリンパ管移植片を採取。
c：パテントブルーでリンパ管が染まっている。

a：Lymphedema and cellulitis of left lower limb occurred 1 month after the resection of squamous cell carcinoma in left buttock and lymphadenectomy of left groin.
b：Vascularized lymphatic graft was harvested from right first web space of toe.
c：Lymphatic vessels were stained with patent blue.

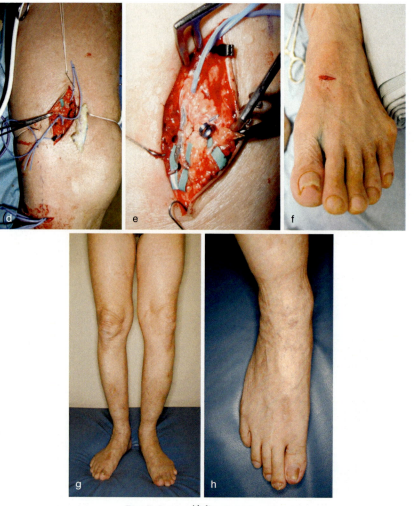

Fig. 7-6-14. 続き Continued

d：移植片を左大腿遠位内側に移植。
e：栄養血管を伏在動静脈に吻合し、LVA を追加した。
f：左足背でも LVA 追加。
g：術後 3 年。浮腫は消失。圧迫不要となっている。
h：ドナーの後遺症はない。

d：Lymphatic graft was transferred to distal part of the medial side in left thigh.
e：The pedicle vessels were anastomosed to saphenous vein and saphenous branch of descending genicular artery with added LVA.
f：LVA was also added at dorsal side of left foot.
g：3 years post operation. Lymphedema disappeared and no need of compression.
h：No complication in donor site.

3．骨盤内リンパ嚢胞に対するLVA

　子宮癌術直後に骨盤内リンパ嚢胞が発生する例がある。多くの症例では自然消滅するようであるが、難治例となる例もある。このような例に対しては、リンパ嚢胞の持続ドレナージがなされ、ブレオマイシンなどの炎症誘発物質注入による嚢胞癒着が試みられている。しかし、短期間に消

失しない例も多いようである。このような例は、下肢からのリンパ還流が骨盤内に貯留されているため、その後の経過で重症の下肢リンパ浮腫が発生することが多いとされている。大島ら（東京大学形成外科）の報告によると、このような例では、ICG造影法を行うと既にStage 0の下肢リンパ浮腫（肉眼的な浮腫はみられない）が発生していることが多い。筆者らは、局麻下に両鼠径部や下肢で複数のLVAを行っているが、嚢胞内のリンパ液が静脈系に還流され数週間で嚢胞が消失することが多い。この治療法は下肢リンパ浮腫の予防的治療法となり、リンパ嚢胞のみでなく下肢浮腫の発生も予防できる可能性がある。

4．乳び腹胸水に対するLVA

筆者らは特発性または先天性乳び腹水（胸水）例に対してLVAを行っているが、多くの例で完治、または改善が得られつつある。これらの例はこれまで治療法がなかっただけに、今後が期待できる。

5．浮腫早期例に対するLVAの効果

われわれの経験では、局麻下のLVAは浮腫発生後9ヵ月以内であれば、それ以後の手術例に比べて概して改善効果が大であった。その原因としてリンパ管還流機能の回復（平滑筋細胞の再生）が考えられる。筆者らの集計では、発生後9ヵ月まで（平均2.3ヵ月）の下肢の早期浮腫35症例に対して局麻下に1～3吻合（平均1.4吻合）を行い、術後6年（平均31.7ヵ月）までの経過観察を行った。その結果、全症例の88.5%が有効で11.5%は改善が得られなかった。この結果から、上・下肢ともまだ軽症の浮腫であっても、9ヵ月以内の早期LVAを行いたい。

6．術後の圧迫療法不要例の検討

LVA術後、数ヵ月または数年間の簡単な圧迫で、リンパ管還流機能が回復する例がある。過去に吻合術を行った約200例の上・下肢の浮腫のうち、上肢4例下肢6例で術後圧迫なしでも術前の進行が止まっている。その内訳は、術後経過観察期間は2ヵ月から15年で、上肢3例では浮腫発生後1年以内の軽症例と重症例であったが、11年の重症1例でも回復例があった。下肢例でも1年以内の軽症例と重症例が有効であったが、11年の軽症例でも有効であった。以上の結果から、リンパ管の平滑筋の再生は部位や症状によって個人差があり、術後の圧迫が不要になった症例では吻合術によって、未分化な再生平滑筋がさらに分化し、リンパ還流機能が回復するのではないかと思われる。

7．吻合術無効例と対策

早期例でも約10%で吻合術が無効であった。これらの例は主に下肢であり、術後の圧迫療法が中止されたり、高度の皮下組織の線維化があり、手術所見でリンパ管が硬化、閉塞または発見できなかった例であった。このような例では、たとえ吻合し得たとしてもリンパ液の静脈系への十

分な還流が得られていない可能性がある。血管柄付きリンパ管移植などのリンパ系機能再建術が必要であろう。

8. 進行性浮腫増悪例に対する治療

術後圧迫を継続していても、突然増悪するものもある。対策としては、圧迫を続けるとともに追加吻合によってさらなる還流系を確立して還流機能の再生を促す必要がある。進行する度に吻合術と術後圧迫両方を繰り返す必要がある。

IV. Combination of surgical treatment and compressive therapy

When surgery and compressive treatment are concomitantly used, the efficacy is higher than monotherapy involving only surgery or compression. The effectiveness of complete decongestive therapy (Földi method) mainly involving daily thorough massage therapy following hospitalization has been reported[8)9)]. However, with this treatment alone, many cases show recurrence or progress after discharge. Recovery of the fundamental lymphatic drainage system is difficult with physical therapy alone. The principle of our treatment, in the event an edema has already developed, is a two-stage treatment strategy to surgically rebuild the drainage route of the lymphatic system and reinforce the drainage ability as much as possible by compressive treatment using elastic stockings following surgery. The effect of combined therapy primarily involving lymphaticovenular anastomosis is the potential achievement of long-term improvement by adding simple compressive treatment rather than thorough complex physical therapy. In particular, many effective cases and complete recoveries have been observed in the upper limbs. It is believed that this is because the lymphatic drainage capacity of the anastomosed lymphatic vessels (smooth muscle cells) is still maintained and it is much more effective compared with physical therapy alone. Even in half the number of lower limb cases, the effectiveness has been proven. In cases with frequent cellulitis, the effect of anastomosis is substantially significant, with many patients saved from fever. Among the intraoperative findings of ineffective cases, sclerosis, thickening of the tunica media, and closure or disappearance of the lymphatic vessels were macroscopically observed in many cases. In addition, the pathologic findings of lymphatic vessels in ineffective cases revealed that smooth muscle cells in tunica media remarkably decreased or were mostly miniaturized (see **Fig. 1-10**)[1-4)]. This means that further drainage system should be established by additional anastomoses because drainage of the lymphatic fluid to the venous system may potentially not sufficient due to drainage dysfunction of the lymphatic vessels even if it can be anastomosed.

1. Cases with long duration since the occurrence of lymphedema： In general, there have been few significantly effective cases after anastomosis. However, even in cases of long duration, including those in which sclerosis of the lymphatic vessels was found under microscope or subcutaneous fibrosis was prominent, if postoperative compressive treatment was performed, some sort of effects were often observed over the long term. The effect of this concomitant therapy in the upper limbs was significantly greater than conservative treatment alone. Moreover, for cases involving the lower limbs, effectiveness was achieved in approximately half of the cases, although remarkable effectiveness was not observed. In particular, in cases with recurrent cellulitis, the frequency of cellulitis after anastomosis significantly decreased and the effect was great[1-4)]. Sometimes, when a functional lymphatic vessel is anastomosed, a significant decrease in volume could be observed compared with preoperative volume.

2. Transfer of vascularized lymphatic vessels (lymph nodes) for cases with severe edema (Fig. 7-6-14)： The long-term progressive severe cases of lymphedema with ineffective LVA are the most difficult to treat. For such cases, in 2005, the author harvested vascularized lymphatic vessels with isolated free vascular pedicle from the healthy side and transferred them to the affected extremities. This method involves

inducing lymphatic fluid into the venous system by transferring lymphatic vessels with normal functional smooth muscle cells. In the cases with unilateral lower limb lymphedema, the lymphatic vessels with drainage capacity which is harvested from the opposite first web space of toe are transferred into the groin region of the affected limb. In the cases of lymphedema in bilateral lower extremities, the lymphatic vessels are harvested from the axillary region and transferred to the groin region. Since the alive smooth muscle cells of the vascularized lymphatic vessel graft is transferred, the pump function of the lymphatic vessel revives and the drainage effect of the lymphatic system is anticipated. It can be termed as the functional smooth muscle cells transfer. So far, this method has been used for multiple cases with severe lymphedema and cases of complete recovery are beginning to appear.

3. LVA for pelvic lymphocyst : Some cases may develop pelvic lymphocyst immediately after the uterine cancer operation. Although it seems to spontaneously disappear in many cases, some can become refractory. For these cases, continuous drainage of the lymphocyst is carried out and cystic adhesion by injection of inflammatory inducible substances such as bleomycin is attempted. However, in many cases, the symptom does not disappear in a short period of time. In such cases, because lymph drainage from the lower limbs is retained in the pelvis, severe lymphedema in the lower limbs often seem to occur in the subsequent course. According to the report by Oshima et al.(Plastic Surgery Department, University of Tokyo Hospital), in many of these cases, Stage 0 lymphedema in the lower limbs(although no visible edema was observed) had already occurred found by ICG angiography. After the author performed multiple LVA in bilateral groin regions and the lower limbs under local anesthesia, cysts often disappeared in several weeks due to drainage of the lymph fluid in the cyst to the venous system. This treatment is a prophylactic therapy for lymphedema in the lower extremities and can prevent not only lymphocysts but also the occurrence of edema in the lower limbs.

4. LVA for chylothorax and chyloperitoneum : The authors performed LVA for cases of idiopathic or congenital chylothorax or chyloperitoneum, and many cases obtained complete recovery or improvement. As there is no available treatment so far for these cases, this therapy can be expected in the future.

5. Effect of LVA for early stage lymphedema : In our experience, LVA under local anesthesia within nine months since the occurrence of lymphedema in generally showed greater improvement compared with surgical cases treated over nine months after the presence of lymphedema. The recovery of the lymph drainage capacity by regeneration of smooth muscle cells can be considered as the reason. Total of 35 cases of early lower extremity lymphedema within nine months(2.3 months on average) were operated upon with 1 to 3 anastomoses(1.4 anastomoses on average) under local anesthesia and were followed until six years after surgery(31.7 months on average). As a result, 88.5% of all cases were effective 11.5% of all cases were ineffective. According to this result, even if the edema is still mild in either upper or lower extremities, we would like to perform lymphaticovenular anastomosis in the early stage within nine months.

6. Consideration of cases with no need of postoperative compressive treatment : In some cases, the drainage function of the lymphatic vessels recovers by several months' or years' simple compressive treatment after LVA surgery. Among approximately 200 patients with lymphedema of the upper or lower extremities who have been treated with lymphaticovenular anastomosis, progress in 4 cases with edema of the upper limbs and 6 cases with edema of the lower limbs have been controlled without postoperative compression compared to their preoperative situation. Among the 4 cases mentioned before with edema of the upper limbs, during the postoperative follow-up of 2 months to 15 years, 3 mild or severe cases within one year duration and one severe case for 11 years totally recovered. In addition, in the lower limb cases, it was effective for mild and severe cases within one year, and effectiveness was also observed even in the mild case with duration of 11 years. Based on the above results, it is believed that there are individual differences in the regeneration of smooth muscle cells of the lymphatic vessels depending on the site and symptoms among cases in which postoperative compression was rendered unnecessary. Meanwhile the regeneration and differentiation of undifferentiated smooth muscle cells, which was caused by anastomosis, resulted in the

recovery of the lymphatic drainage function.

7. Cases with ineffective lymphaticovenular anastomosis and strategy for them：Even in early cases, approximately 10% of anastomoses were ineffective. These cases mainly involved the lower limbs and patients with discontinous compressive treatment following surgery or were revealed through surgical findings that the lymphatic vessels were hardening, obstructed or could not be found due to extensive fibrosis of subcutaneous tissues. In such cases, despite being able to anastomose the lymphatic vessels with the venoules, it was possible that sufficient drainage of the lymphatic fluid to the venous system could not be obtained. Functional reconstruction of the lymphatic system by such as vascularized lymphatic vessel transfer is necessary.

8. Treatment for exacerbated cases of progressive lymphedema：Even if postoperative compressive treatment is continuousely applied, some cases was suddenly exacerbated. As a countermeasure, it is necessary to promote restoration of the drainage function by conducting additional anastomoses while continuing the compressive therapy. It is necessary to repeat both anastomosis and the application of postoperative pressure compressive treatment as symptoms progress.

Ⅴ　両側性下肢リンパ浮腫の頻度と予防

　　われわれの下肢リンパ浮腫 356 例の集計では、特発性は比較的少なく、子宮癌や泌尿器悪性腫瘍切除後の続発性リンパ浮腫が極めて多かった(87.4%)。特発性の浮腫は両側性浮腫が 44%で、それらの半数以上が初発時から両側性浮腫であったが、片側であっても両側性となる可能性があり、その時期は 9 年前後であった。続発性浮腫に関しては 26%が両側性で、手術直後から両側性であるものは約 26%で少なく、片側性から両側性になるものが約 69%と多い。平均すると術後 4 年半で片側に発生し、術後 7 年前後で対側にも発生し両側性となることが多い。このことから、片側のリンパ浮腫であっても 26%の確率で両側性となる可能性がある。われわれも手術前の圧迫療法中に片側下肢の浮腫例が両側性に移行し、急速に増悪した例を経験した[10]。片側性であっても健側下肢が浮腫を免れるとは言えない。

Ⅴ. Frequency and prevention of lymphedema of the bilateral lower extremities

In our summary of 356 cases of lower limb lymphedema, versus relatively few idiopathic cases, there were numerous cases of secondary lymphedema following resection of uterine cancer or urological malignant tumors(87.4%). 44% of idiopathic lymphedema cases were bilateral edema, of which more than half were bilateral edema from onset. Besides, even the unilateral edema cases probably become bilateral within approximately nine years. As for secondary lymphedema, while 26% of cases were bilateral soon after surgery, approximately 69% of cases became bilateral from unilateral. On average, secondary lymphedema occurred on one side within 4.5 years post operation and also occurred on the opposite side within approximately 7 years post operation, with the result that they converted to bilateral lymphedema. This showed that 26% of cases of unilateral lymphedema had the possibility to become bilateral edemas. We also experienced a cases in which edema of the unilateral lower limb shifted to bilateral limbs and that progressed rapidly during preoperative compressive treatment[10]. It cannot be said that the unaffected lower limbs will not develop an edema in unilateral cases.

7-6. 症例提示

VI 予防的吻合術の必要性

　筆者らが過去 10 年以上にわたって提唱している浮腫発生後早期の予防的吻合術後の長期経過では、その有効性が証明されている。

　これまで 10 年以上にわたり、予防的吻合術を試みその有効性を報告してきた[2)−4)]。さらに乳癌または子宮癌の切除術と同時の予防的な吻合術を行えば浮腫発生率は激減することも報告してきた。藤原ら（前川崎医科大学婦人科）も子宮癌切除時の大網移行術を併用することによって浮腫の発生頻度を半数に減少できたと述べている。Takeishi らもその有効性を報告している[11)]。われわれは現在、浮腫発生前の集合リンパ管の還流能が残っている間に吻合術を行う予防的吻合術を導入している。

VI. Necessity of prophylactic anastomosis

　As we have advocated for more than ten years, the early prophylactic anastomosis after initial lymphedema has been proved to be effective upon long-term follow-up.

　We have attempted prophylactic anastomosis for over 10 years and reported the effectiveness[2)−4)]. Furthermore, we also reported that prophylactic anastomosis that performed simultaneously with resection of breasts or uterine cancers leaded to a dramatic decrease in the incidence of lymphedema. Fujiwara et al. (formerly the Gynecology Department, Kawasaki Medical University) also described that concomitant use of omentum transfer with resection of uterine cancer could lead to a decrease in the frequency of lymphedema by half. Takeishi et al. also reported on its effectiveness[11)]. Currently, we perform prophylactic anastomosis prior to the occurrence of lymphedema while the drainage capacity of lymphatic vessel remains.

VII 陰部リンパ浮腫（瘻）(Fig. 7-6-15)

　陰部浮腫例は、進行性であり両下肢の浮腫を合併することが多い。また、性機能や排尿障害があり、圧迫療法は不可能でその QOL は大きく障害されている。これまでに陰部の難治性浮腫またはリンパ瘻例 13 症例（14〜80 歳、男 8 例、女 5 例）に局麻下 LVA を行った。このうち 10 例で両下肢浮腫を合併していた。その内訳は、一次性浮腫 3 例、二次性 10 例であった。浮腫（漏）が発生してからの期間は 2ヵ月〜12 年（平均 4 年 4ヵ月）で、リンパ管の吻合数は 1〜5 本（平均 2.6 本）で、術後の経過観察期間は 2ヵ月〜2 年 3ヵ月（平均 13ヵ月）であった。下肢浮腫が発生している例に対しては、術前後の圧迫療法がなされた。結果として、圧迫療法は効果がなかった。下肢も含めた複数の吻合で術中の良好な還流（全吻合 34 吻合の 67.6%）が得られた。ほとんどの症例で、最低 1 本は良好な吻合が可能であった。術後の浮腫は著減し、リンパ漏（タオル 5 枚分/日例もあり）も止まるものもみられた。陰部浮腫（リンパ漏）発生後長期例でも、LVA は症状を軽減できる可能性がある。その理由として、長期例でもリンパ還流機能がかなり温存されているためと思われる。

（辛川　領、伊藤太智、水田栄樹、森下悠也、森脇裕太、光嶋　勲）

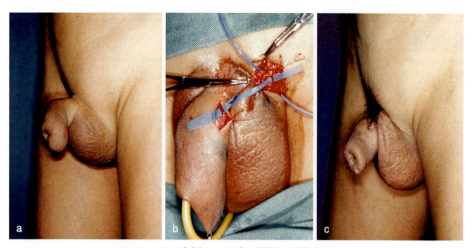

Fig. 7-6-15. 症例9：13歳、男児。陰部浮腫7年
Case 9：A 13-year-old boy. Genital lymphedema for 7 years
a：心臓手術後1ヵ月で発生した両下肢と陰部浮腫の7年目。
b：小切開にて2吻合した。
c：術後2年5ヵ月。浮腫の改善がみられる。
a：Bilateral legs and pudendal lymphedema of 7 years', duration occurred 1 month after the cardiac operation.
b：2 anastomoses were performed at small incisions.
c：2 years and 5 months post operation. Lymphedema was improved.

VII. Genital lymphedema(lymphorrhea)(Fig. 7-6-15)

Many cases of genital lymphedema are progressive and combined with edemas of the bilateral lower limbs. Moreover, as it causes disturbance in sexual function and dysuria, in which compressive treatment is impossible, it greatly affects the patients' quality of life. So far, 13 cases of refractory edema or lymphorrhea of the pubic area (14 to 80 years old, 8 male cases, 5 female cases) have undergone lymphaticovenular anastomosis under local anesthesia. 10 of these cases were associated with lymphedema in both lower limbs. 3 cases were primary lymphedema and 10 cases were secondary lymphedema. The duration of edema (lymphorrhea) was 2 months to 12 years (4 years and 4 months on average), and the number of lymphaticovenular anastomoses was 1 to 5 (2.6 on average), with a follow-up period following surgery from 2 months to 2 years and three months (13 months on average). For cases in which edema developed in the lower limbs, compressive treatment was carried out before and after surgery. The results showed that compressive treatment was ineffective. Regarding multiple anastomoses that performed at sites including the lower limbs, good drainage was obtained during surgery (67.6% of all 34 anastomoses). In most cases, at least one good anastomosis was obtained. Postoperative edemas significantly improved, and the lymphatic leakage (even including cases that needed 5 towels/day) were also cured. Even for long-term cases of genital lymphedema (lymphorrhea), lymphaticovenular anastomosis showed the potential to relieve the symptoms. The reason is probably that lymphatic drainage function is substantially preserved even in long term cases.

(Ryo Karakawa, Taichi Ito, Haruki Mizuta, Yuya Morishita, Yuta Moriwaki, Isao Koshima)

1) Koshima I, Kawada S, Moriguchi T, et al：Ultrastructural observation of lymphatic vessels in lymphedema in human extremities. Plast Reconstr Surg 97：397-405, 1996.

2) Koshima I, Inagawa K, Urushibara K, et al：Supermicrosurgical lymphaticovenularanastomosis for the treatment of lymphedema in the upper extremities. J Reconstr Microsurg 16：437-442, 2000.

3) Koshima I, Nanba U, Tsutsui T, et al：Long-term follow-up after lymphaticovenular anastomosis for lymphedema in the legs. J Reconstr Microsurg 19：209-215, 2003.

4) Koshima I, et al：Minimal invasive lymphaticovenular anastomosis under local anesthesia for leg lymphedema. Is it effective for Stage III and IV? Ann Plast Surg 53：1-6, 2004.

5) O'Brien MB, Sykes P, Threlfall GN, et al：Microlymphaticovenous anastomoses for obstructive lymphedema. Plast Reconstr Surg 60：197-211, 1977.

6) O'Brien BM, Shafiroff BB：Microlymphaticovenous and resectional surgery in obstructive lymphedema. World J Surg 3：3-15, 121-123, 1979.

7) O'Brien MB, Mellow CG, Khazanchi RK, et al：Long-term results after microlymphaticovenous anastomoses for the treatment of of obstructive lymphedema. Plast Reconstr Surg 85：562-572, 1990.

8) Földi E, Földi M, Clodius L：The lymphedema Chaos；A lancet. Ann Plast Surg 22：505-515, 1989.

9) Földi M：Discussion for Koshima's paper "Ultrastructural observations of lymphatic vessels in lymphedema in human extremities". Plast Reconstr Surg 97：406-407, 1996.

10) 光嶋　勲, ほか：下肢リンパ浮腫35症例の病因と病像；特に片側性から両側性への移行例について. 日形会誌 108：138-143, 1998.
Koshima I, et al：Etiology of 35 cases of lower limb lymphedema. Nikkeikaishi（Japanese journal） 108：138-143, 1998.

11) Takeishi M, Kojima M, Mori K, et al：Primary intrapelvic lymphaticovenular anastomosis following lymph node dissecdtion. Ann Plast Surg 57：300-304, 2006.

CHAPTER 7

外科治療
Surgical treatment

7. その他の外科治療および有用なテクニック

Other surgical treatment and valuable technique

a. IVaS 法を用いた LVA

IVaS（intravascular stenting）method for LVA

■はじめに

血管吻合技術の確立は諸説あるが、1877 年に初めてイヌの門脈を用いて吻合を Eck らが行い、1902 年には Carrel によって 3 点縫合法が行われた。微小血管吻合については、1960 年に Jacobson らはイヌの小血管を用いて成功している[1]。このときの血管径は 1.4 mm（1,400 μm）であったとされている。1968 年、玉井らによって切断指再接着の初成功が報告されると、整形・災害外科における手外科分野は飛躍的に発展を遂げることとなった[2]。さらに 1972 年に波利井らによって世界で初めて遊離皮弁の成功が報告され、今まで不可能とされてきたさまざまな難治症例を救済することが可能となった。その後、微小血管吻合の機器が開発され、現在マイクロサージャリーは一般化している。さらに 1989 年に光嶋らによって perforator flap とともにスーパーマイクロサージャリーという 0.5 mm 前後の血管を吻合することが要求される技術が報告された。世界的にみても高難度な技術であるが、低侵襲でかつ精密で微細な部位の再建まで可能となった。このスーパーマイクロサージャリーと呼ばれる微小血管吻合を一般的に行えるようにしたのが、intravascular stenting method（IVaS 法）である[3]。この方法を用いれば、またマイクロサージャリーの技術があれば、supermicrosurgery が可能となる。今回はこの方法を用いた、リンパ管静脈吻合への利用について述べる。

■Introduction

Eck et al. performed the first anastomosis of a dog portal vein in 1877. In 1902 Carrel performed vessel anastomosis with using 3 points' anastomosed procedure. Classic articles published in 1960 by Jacobson and Suarez described the microsurgical anastomosis of small vessels（1.4 mm）in dogs[1]. In 1968 Tamai et al. reported the first finger replantation, hand surgery was developed dramatically after this success[2]. Harii et al. then performed the first free flap transfer in a human patient in 1972. Throughout the 1970s, only a few plastic surgeons successfully applied microsurgical techniques. Many techniques and instruments have been developed to improve and simplify microsurgery. And in the 1989, Koshima et al. developed the supermicrosurgery technique. The intravascular stenting method greatly facilitates anastomosis of vessels less than 0.5 mm in diameter. In this article, we report the application of the intravascular stenting method to performing multiconfiguration lymphaticovenous anastomoses for the treatment of extremity lymphedema in a minimally invasive fashion.

7-7. その他の外科治療および有用なテクニック

I　IVaS 法とは

　管腔が非常に細く、内腔に攝子の先を保持しながら血管吻合ができない場合や、静脈やリンパ管のように壁が薄くすぐに管腔が潰れてしまって、内腔がはっきりしないような場合に、色付きのナイロンの糸を内腔に挿入することによって、内腔を確保しながら、確実に微小血管の吻合を行う方法のことである。

I．Intra- Vascular Stenting method(IVaS method)

　The diameter of very small vessels (about 0.5 mm or less) causes difficulties in placing forceps into the lumen and in completing anastomosis without inadvertently catching the back wall during supermicrosurgery. The insertion of nylon monofilaments into small vessels has overcome this problem. The back wall is not inadvertently caught using the intravascular stenting (IVaS) method.

II　IVaS 法の実際

1．はじめに

　IVaS を作成するために、まず挿入する脈管の径を計測する(**Fig. 7-7-1**)。測れない場合には、ナイロンの糸を用いればおおよその径を計測することが可能である。実際のところ外径が約 0.6 mm には 4-0、約 0.4 mm には 5-0、約 0.2 mm では 6-0 を選択することが多い(**Table 7-7-1**)。

　色付きナイロンは脈管の外から透見でき、吻合が容易になることや、管内に置き忘れるリスクが少ないため、青色か黒色のナイロンを使用し、透明のナイロンは避ける。

　糸の長さは、短いと抜けやすく長過ぎると抜けないため、血管吻合の場合、吻合部断端からクリップの掛かっているところまでの長さよりわずかに長くする。リンパ管静脈の場合には、静脈側にはクリップを掛けるがリンパ液は透明であり、また流れも緩やかなためクリップをとめる必要がない。このため長めに作成し余裕をもって安定性を保つことが可能である。ナイロンの糸は、剪刀で切ると IVaS 断端が潰れて尖り、内膜を傷つける危険性がある。カミソリかまたはメスにて転がすように切るときれいな断端になる(**Fig. 7-7-2**)。また断端を丸めて挿入しやすくした IVaS(crownjun 社製、4-0、5-0、6-0 スケール付)の購入も可能である。

2．挿　入

　IVaS を作成したら、血管内腔を確認し挿入する(**Fig. 7-7-1-b**)。入れる順番は、同じくらいの径であればどちらからでもよいが、径が違う場合には、細い方から挿入するとスムーズである。そのとき IVaS は一番遠位を鑷子にて把持して内腔を探るように 2～3 mm 入れる。少し入ったところで IVaS をいったん放し、IVaS の後面をトントンと叩くように挿入すると周囲に引っかかることなく挿入が容易である。両側とも挿入したら脈管の断端が内反していないか確認する。

269

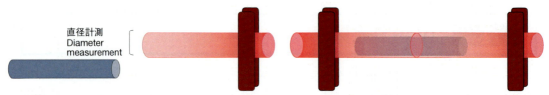

a：血管のサイズを測り、中に挿入するナイロンを選択する。
The diameter of a nylon is measured and a nylon stent is selected.

b：内腔を確認し血管内に挿入する。
A nylon stent is inserted into both vessel ends.

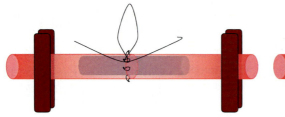
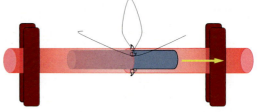

c：血管吻合を順次行っていく。最後の1針をuntieとする。
Last one or two stitches are left untied to allow stent removal.

d：Untieにした糸の間からIVaS（黄矢印）を抜去する。
IVaS is removed from lumen.

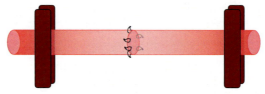

e：Untieにした糸を縫合し吻合を完了する。
Last stitch is tied.

Fig. 7-7-1. IVaS 法の順序　Process of IVaS method

Table 7-7-1. ナイロンサイズ Nylon size variations

USP	直径 diameter (mm)
0	0.35〜0.399
2-0	0.27〜0.349
3-0	0.20〜0.269
4-0	0.15〜0.199
5-0	0.10〜0.149
6-0	0.070〜0.099
7-0	0.050〜0.069
8-0	0.040〜0.049
9-0	0.030〜0.039

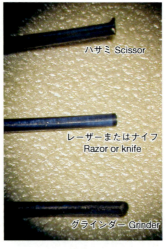

Fig. 7-7-2. IVaS 作成時のナイロン断面
IVaS cut plane of nylon monofilament

自分で作成する場合にはメスを推奨する。ほか、断端を研磨したものが販売されている。
Surgical knife is recommended for making IVaS. In addition, polished stumps are on sale.

3. 吻 合

　11-0 ナイロンまたは 12-0 ナイロンを使用して吻合する。一般的なマイクロ吻合に慣れていると、ナイロン糸を縫合する際に、血管を引っ張ってしまい、中に挿入してある IVaS が誤って抜けてしまうことがある。吻合の途中で抜けないようにするコツは、吻合部の血管の位置をずらさないことである。特に針を刺して、糸を引いてくるときに起こりやすいため、鑷子または持針器にて吻合部血管のところを軽く押さえながら糸を引くと、吻合部が安定して IVaS が抜けることはない。脈管周囲を順に縫合していく。このとき、初めの糸を縫合したら、次の糸を掛ける際、1 針目の糸を手前に軽く引く。そうすることにより IVaS が重しとなって IVaS と脈管の内腔に隙間が生じる。この生じた隙間に次の糸を掛ける（**Fig. 7-7-1-c**）。これによって、後壁を誤って掛けることなく吻合できる。最後の 1 針は untie にする（**Fig. 7-7-1-d**）。

> **ポイント**
>
> 　微小血管吻合時のリスクの 1 つに、術中糸が周囲の血餅に引っかかり、血管が裂けて治療結果にも重大な影響を及ぼすことが挙げられる。このリスクを避けるには、吻合直前に手袋を新しいものに交換することと、吻合部周囲に血の付いていない濡れガーゼを敷くだけである。非常に単純であるが、これによって糸が周囲に引っかからない。

4. IVaS の抜去

　Untie にした隙間より IVaS を抜去する（**Fig. 7-7-1-d**）。まずどちらか片方の血管内へ IVaS をズボンのゴムを引き出すときのようにしゃくりながら移動させる。次に IVaS の後方を脈管上から軽く把持し untie の隙間へ押し出すようにする。押し出された IVaS を対側の鑷子で受け取りそっと引き抜く。

5. 最終段階

　IVaS を取り除いたことを再度確認し、最後の 1 針を縫合する。吻合が終了したところで、血管に掛けたクリップを外し、完了となる（**Fig. 7-7-1-e**）。

II. How to Intra- Vascular Stenting method(IVaS method)

　1. **Background**：A nylon monofilament was specifically prepared for each vessel to be anastomosed using the IVaS method. The diameter of the nylon was two fifths that of the external diameter of the vessel. The first step of this technique begins with the measurement of the diameter of the vessel and also the width from the free end of the vessel and the clip（**Fig. 7-7-1**）. Based on these measurements, a suitable nylon monofilament was selected for the IVaS. If it is difficult to measure concisely, you can choose the 4-0, 5-0, and 6-0 nylon for 0.6 mm, 0.4 mm, and 0.2 mm of the vessels' diameter respectively（**Table 7-7-1**）. Blue or black nylon was used because it is more easily detected than clear nylon, thus reducing the risk of the monofilament's being left behind in the vessel. To ensure stable anchorage and easy ejection, the length of

the nylon monofilament was made equal to the width of the gap between the free end of the vessel and the clip.

As the end of a nylon must be smooth to avoid damage to the vessel lumen, we used a razor or surgical knife to produce a clean cut instead of using scissors (**Fig. 7-7-2**). You can buy the IVaS which edge is grained and blunt for prevention of vessels' lumen (Crownjun co.ltd Japan).

2. Insertion : Next, the nylon stent was inserted into the vessels with using forceps. The vessels were pulled closely together for anastomosis (**Fig. 7-7-1-b**). When the diameters of both ends of vessels are same, you can choose the first side to insert the nylon due to the situation. When the diameters of both ends of vessels are different, you should start inserting the nylon to the end of smaller vessels firstly. After inserting the edge of the nylon, you should hit the distal edge of the nylon gently. It is the secret of easy insertion of the nylon stent without catching on the vessels lumen.

3. Anastmosis : The vessel wall was carefully sutured using 11-0 or 12-0 nylon (**Fig. 7-7-1-c**). The last one or two stitches were left untied to allow removal of the nylon stent. You should more carefully pull the 11-0 or 12-o nylon because the vessels lumen is easy broken and IVaS is easy removed. The position of both vessels' ends need to keep on the same place when you pull the needle of nylon. So when you anastomose around the vessels and pull the needle, you should hold the vessels with using forceps or needle-folder. Holding the vessels and pulling the nylon that sutured previously allow us to anastomose easily because it makes the space of lumen for insert the needle-tip. It is the most important point to use the IVAS for preventing to catch the back wall inadvertently. The last one or two stitches were left untied to allow removal of the nylon stent.

> **Point** One of the risks that cause the failure of anastomosis is rupture of blood due to clot formation at surrounding area.
> Wet new gauze and new gloves are effective for preventing to get caught the needle and nylon strings to the surrounding tissues. To avoid this risk, we recommend you to change gloves just before starting anastomosis, and the area around anastomosis is covered by new wet gauzes. This is the simple, but very useful.

4. Removal of IVaS : The IVaS was then removed from the space between the free vessel ends (**Fig. 7-7-1-d**). First, IVaS is moved into either one side of the blood vessels. The point of moving is to push the stent like moving rubbers of trousers. Next, gently the back of the IVaS from the vessel is grasped and pushed out into the gap of untie. Last, the extruded IVaS is gently pulled out with the contralateral forceps.

5. Last stage : After reconfirming that the IVaS had securely removed from the vessel, the last one or two stitches were sutured. Finally, the clips were removed and blood flow was restarted (**Fig. 7-7-1-e**).

Ⅲ　さまざまな吻合法

　吻合方法としては、いわゆる端端吻合以外に、①Y字の静脈と吻合する flow-through、②端側吻合（end-to-side）、③端端吻合と端側吻合を組み合わせたラムダ吻合、も行われることがある（**Fig. 7-7-3～5**）。それぞれの吻合は IVaS 使用上、単純化すれば端端吻合と端側吻合の組み合わせである。そこで IVaS 端側吻合法について追記する。

1.　IVaS を用いた端側吻合法

　端側吻合の場合には 2 通りの使用方法がある。

7-7. その他の外科治療および有用なテクニック

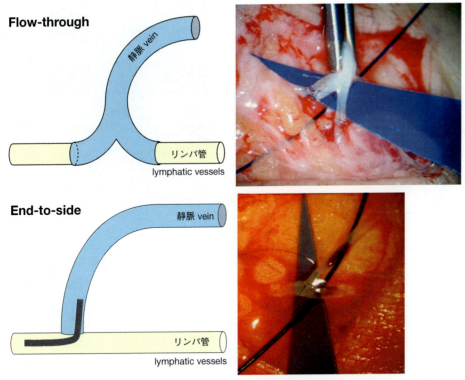

Fig. 7-7-3. Flow-through 吻合と端側吻合　Flow-through and end-to-side anastomosis

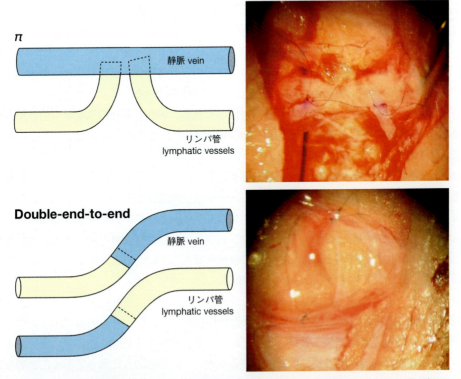

Fig. 7-7-4. π吻合と double-end-to-end　π and double-end-to-end anastomosis

273

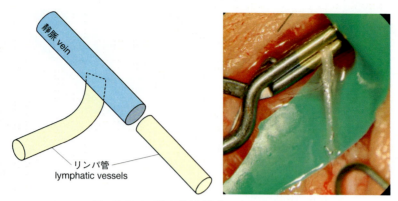

Fig. 7-7-5. ラムダ(λ)吻合　λ anastomosis

①血管の側壁に 27 G 針またはマイクロ剪刀を用いて孔を空け、IVaS を側壁よりリンパ管内に挿入して孔が IVaS の中央にくるようにセッティングする。後壁より吻合し前壁の最後の 1 針を untie として抜去する。

②IVaS を挿入する前に持針器または剥離子で IVaS の中央部を数回挟みナイロン中央部を平坦化させる。一端を血管内に挿入し対側をもう 1 本の血管内に挿入する(L 型挿入)。吻合は①と同様に行っていく。

IVaS 方法の利点と欠点についてまとめると以下のようになる。

a．IVaS 法の利点

①スーパーマイクロサージャリーの技術的特徴は、片手縫いである。内腔を針先で感じて縫合する超人的な職人技が必要となる。しかし IVaS を用いることにより内腔を容易に確保できるため、マイクロサージャリーの技術をもっていれば、吻合が可能である。

②ナイロンのサイズが多様にあるため、どのような径のリンパ管や静脈にでも対応できる。しかもナイロンはどの病院にもあるものなので、どこでも利用できる。

③径の違う場合にもアンカーとなって均等に吻合ができる。周囲の縫合の糸を軽く引き緊張をもたせると、IVaS が重しとなって違う径のものでも同じ径にすることができる。そのため縫合の位置が決めやすくなる。

④Back wall をかける危険がないため、縫い直すことがない。これが一番の目的。内腔を確実に確認できるので二度縫いがなくなり、術中のストレスが激減する。

⑤背面を吻合する際に、反転する必要がない。IVaS が挿入されている脈管はひねってもねじれず内腔を保つことが可能となる。このためクリップを反転させて後壁を吻合する必要はなく、狭い術野でも掛けた糸を持ちながら少しずつ後壁を縫合していくことが可能。

⑥IVaS はナイロンの糸を使うので、経済的である。

b．IVaS 法の欠点

①IVaS を丁寧に扱わないと血管内腔を傷つける恐れがある。しかし一般的なマイクロサージャリーの場合、幾度となく内腔に攝子を入れて縫合することを考えれば、逆に低侵襲である。

②抜き忘れる危険がある。これについては入れるときに一言周囲の人に言っておくことでリスクを回避できる。

③挿入にコツがいる。いきなり実践では難しい。ラットなどで練習する環境があれば、試してからをお勧めする。
YouTube "IVaS 2008" にて動画視聴可能である。

2. 症　例[4]

67歳、女性、悪性リンパ腫に対して放射線化学療法および両側鼠径部リンパ節郭清後のリンパ浮腫である（**Fig. 7-7-6**）。複合理学療法を行ったが、改善しないためリンパ管静脈吻合を行った。

右脚にはflow-through吻合を膝と足関節部に行い、右脚には鼠径部で端側吻合、膝部ではflow-through吻合、足関節部では端端吻合を2吻合行った。術後6ヵ月の時点で右脚18.9%、左足17%の縮小を認めた。術後ストッキングは不要となりスカートもはけるほどの改善を認めた。

III. Modified anastomosis method with using IVaS

We can use IVaS method for ①flow-through anastomosis, ②end-to-side anastomosis, ③λ anasomosis (**Fig. 7-7-3 to 5**). When end-to-side anastomoses are performed, we bend the intravascular stent using a dissector to hold the two vessel ends in the appropriate configuration.

1. End-to-Side anastomosis with IVaS：①The side wall of lymphatic channel was opened by 27G needle or surgical knife. Then IVaS is inserted to the lymphatic channel and is located at the center of hole.

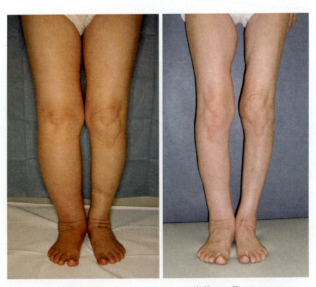

術前 Pre　　　　術後6ヵ月　Po 6M

Fig. 7-7-6.　下肢リンパ浮腫（67歳、女性）：術前術後
67-year-old female preoperative and postoperative findings of lower lymphedema

（Narushima M, Mihara M, et al：The intravascular stenting method for treatment of extremity lymphedema with multiconfiguration lymphaticovenous anastomoses. Plast Reconstr Surg 125(3)：935-943, 2010 による）

Anastomosis is performed from back wall to frontal wall. ②The central part of IVaS is bended by forceps or needle folder before insertion. One side of IVaS is inserted to the vein and the other side of IVaS is inserted to lymphatic channel like L shape.

a. Advantages of IVaS : ①It is available for an average microsurgeon to anastomosis with using IVaS without any special instruments.

②Nylon of various sizes is available, allowing the application of appropriate size of IVaS for various vessel diameters.

③To anastomose the different diameters of vessels' ends, IVaS can use as a stable anchorage.

④IVaS can be performed completing anastomosis without inadvertently catching the back wall during supermicrosurgery.

⑤IVaS procedure does not need to turn the vessel during anastomosis.

⑥IVaS has an economic aspect because of nylon stent.

b. Disadvantages of IVaS : One is that the surgeon could forget to remove the nylon from the vessel. Another is that the lumen can become injured if the IVaS is not correctly applied. However, the back wall did not invert and obstruct blood flow in any anastomosis in the present study with IVaS.

Electron microscopic observation revealed that the lumens of the vessels that were anastomosed using the IVaS method were not damaged, indicating that the lumen will remain intact if this method is correctly applied.

2. Case[4] : A 67-year-old woman had bilateral lymph node excisions and chemoradiotherapy for malignant lymphoma (**Fig. 7-7-6**). She developed bilateral lower extremity lymphedema. We performed 6 LVAs At 6-month follow-up, average girth reduction considering all five measurement sites was decreased 18.9 percent and 10.5 percent in the right leg and the left leg. The patient no longer needs to wear compression stockings and has improved leg function.

■おわりに

特にリンパ浮腫の患者のリンパ管は、正常では静脈よりも壁が薄いものが、リンパ内圧の慢性的な上昇によって壁肥厚をきたしていることが多い。この場合、外径で判断せず、リンパ管断面を確認した後、適切な IVaS を選択することが重要と考える。この IVaS 法を応用することで、最良の手術を確実に行っていける可能性がある[5]。

ちなみに IVaS 法を用いた脈管吻合の最小径は、われわれの経験では 8-0 IVaS を用いて外径 0.15 mm である。これは Jacobson の吻合血管に比べて直径で約 1/10 であり、着実に進歩を遂げている。

（成島三長）

■Conclusion

The wall of lymphatic channel is thinner than vein normally. However Lymphatic channels of lymphedema change to hypertrophic wall due to the hyper pressure of lymph. So after cutting the vessel and checking the wall thickness, you should decide to the size of IVaS.

The IVaS method can be used in procedures such as finger-tip replantation, true perforator flap transplantation[5], and lymphaticovenous anastomosis of lymphedema. The IVaS method can assure safe and accurate anastomosis and will contribute to further advances in supermicrosurgery.

By the way, the minimum diameter of the vascular anastomosis using the IVaS method is 0.15 mm in outer diameter using 8-0 IVaS in our experience. This is approximately 1/10 in diameter as compared with Jacobson's anastomotic vessel, and steadily progresses.

(*Mitsunaga Narushima*)

1) Jacobson JH, Suarez EL：Microscopy in anastomosis of small vessels. Surg Forum 45：243-495, 1960.
2) Komatsu S, Tamai S：Successful replantation of completely cut-off thumb. Plast Reconstr Surg 42：374-377, 1968.
3) Mitsunaga N, Isao K, Makoto M, et al：Intravascular stenting(IVaS) for safe and precise super-microsurgery. Ann Plast Surg 60：41-44, 2008.
4) Narushima M, Mihara M, Yamamoto Y, et al：The intravascular stenting method for treatment of extremity lymphedema with multiconfiguration lymphaticovenous anastomoses. Plast Reconstr Surg 125(3)：935-943, 2010.
5) 成島三長, ほか：IVaS法(intravascular stenting method)を用いたsuper-microsurgery. 整形・災害外科 55(4)：343-350, 2012.
  Narushima M, et al：Super-microsurgery using IVaS method(Intravascular stenting method). Orthopedics Surgery and Traumatology 55(4)：343-350, 2012.

b．LVA 小技集
Little tricks for LVA

Ⅰ　術野の展開

　リンパ管細静脈吻合術（LVA）ではなるべく小さい切開からの手術を心がけるべきであるが、手術部位に応じて術野を展開する器具を使い分けるとよい。通常の開創器は術野に入らないため、釣り針式の開創器を基本的に用いるが、釣り針式開創器も掛けにくいような数 mm の切開ではナイロン糸で創縁を皮膚に固定するとよい。釣り針式開創器の牽引糸が術中操作の邪魔になる鼠径部などではＫワイヤーを折り曲げて開創器として用いると便利である（**Fig. 7-7-7**）。

　大腿内側では術野の創面が視線に対して平行となり、剝離操作が困難なことがある。このような場合は、釣り針を内側創縁に掛けて手術用顕微鏡のドレープに固定するとよい（**Fig. 7-7-8**）。こうすることで、背面へ落ち込んでいる内側創縁が上方向へ牽引されて創面が視線に対して垂直に近づくため剝離しやすくなる。

　リンパ浮腫肢では間質液が極めて豊富で、皮切後に術野に水があふれ手術操作が困難となることがある。軽度であれば、適宜ガーゼで水分を吸い取ることで問題ないが、多量の間質液があるような症例ではガーゼで吸い取るだけでは術野をコントロールできなくなる。吸引チューブを留置することで持続的に水分を吸い取れるが、硬い吸引チューブは手術操作の妨げとなり不便である。術野の妨げにならないためには、濡れたガーゼの端を術野に差し込んで、術野外にある部位

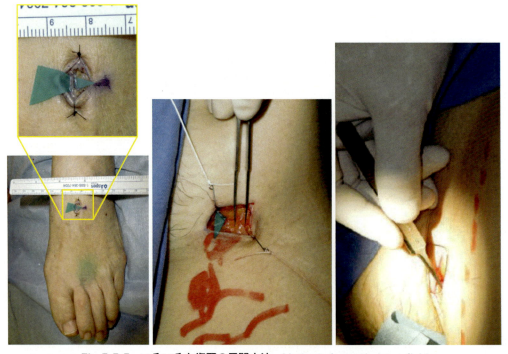

Fig. 7-7-7. いろいろな術野の展開方法　Methods for exploring a field

7-7. その他の外科治療および有用なテクニック

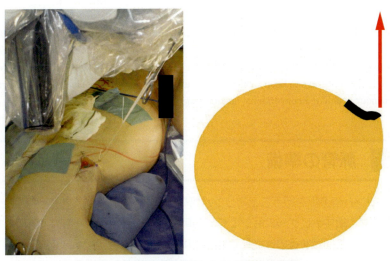

Fig. 7-7-8. 大腿内側における術野の展開
Field preparation in the medial aspect of the thigh

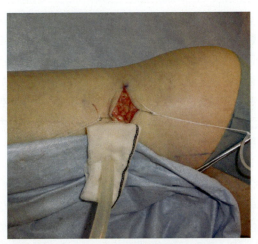

Fig. 7-7-9. 浸出が多い術野での工夫
A method for field clearance in a very-wet field

で濡れたガーゼを吸引するとよい(**Fig. 7-7-9**)。wet-to-dry dressing のようにガーゼが吸引され余分な水分を吸い取られ続けるため、術野に挿入された部位でガーゼは毛細管現象による吸引効果を持続させることができる。吸引管が術野外にあるため手術操作を妨げない。

I. A surgical field exploration

To minimize the incision length for LVA, various instruments can be used. Hooks are helpful to explore a small surgical field where a conventional retractor cannot be used. Suturing skin edges using a nylon thread is useful, when hooks cannot be used in a millimeter surgical field. In the groin region where strings of hooks can disturb a surgeon's procedure, a bent wire can be used as a retractor (**Fig. 7-7-7**).

In the medial aspect of the thigh, a surgeon usually feels difficulty to explore a surgical field because a plane of the field is horizontal to the surgeon's view. To make the plane more vertical to the surgeon's view,

279

the medial edge of the wound is retracted upward using a hook fixed to a surgical microscope (**Fig. 7-7-8**).

　Abundant interstitial fluid disturbs a surgeon's procedure especially in a severe lymphedematous limb. When interstitial fluid is too much to be absorbed by putting gauzes, continuous indirect aspiration (CIA) method is useful: an edge of a wet gauze is put into an edge of a surgical field, and a suction tube is put onto another edge of the wet gauze to keep capillary action effective (**Fig. 7-7-9**). This method does not disturb a surgeon's maneuver unlike a conventional suction tube placement.

II　脈管の準備

　術前にICGリンパ管造影を行うことでリンパ管の走行・状態を予測することができLVAに極めて有用であるが、術中ナビゲーションとしても用いることできる。黄色い脂肪の中から透明もしくは白いリンパ管を同定するのは容易ではないが、術中ナビゲーションにより初心者でも容易にリンパ管を同定することができる。近赤外線装置が内蔵された手術用顕微鏡を用いると、ICG注射を追加することなく術中に造影されたリンパ管を確認しながら手術を行える(**Fig. 7-7-10**)。Linear部位ではもちろんのこと、Stardust部位でも術中にリンパ管が造影されていることを確認できる。Diffuse部位では造影されることはあまりないため有用性が低い。

　LVAでは適切なリンパ管はもちろんこと、適切な静脈を用意することが極めて重要である。適切な静脈とは、静脈弁が正常で吻合後に静脈逆流をきたさない静脈のことである。ICGリンパ管造影で使用される近赤外線モニターは、静脈も可視化することができるため、術前の位置同定と静脈弁の機能検査として有用である。静脈を体表からミルキングテストを行うことで、静脈弁の位置を同定することができる(**Fig. 7-7-11**)。ICGリンパ管造影と合わせて術前マッピングを行い、適切なリンパ管と静脈のある部位に皮切部位を決めるとよい。

　SE吻合・SS吻合は1吻合で末梢側・中枢側両方のリンパ液をバイパスできるため、EE吻合・ES吻合に比べて効率的である(**Fig. 7-7-12**)。しかし、SE吻合・SS吻合はリンパ管に側孔を作成する必要があり、硬化の強いリンパ管では側孔作成に失敗するリスクが高い。したがって、リンパ管切開前にリンパ管硬化を評価することが重要であるが、temporary lymphatic expansion(TLE)法が有用である(**Fig. 7-7-13**)。術野に出ているリンパ管の中枢側を攝子・クランプで

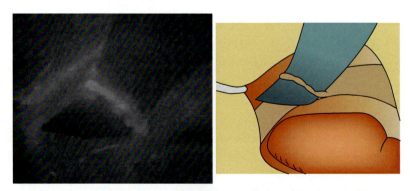

Fig. 7-7-10. ICGリンパ管造影による術中ナビゲーション
Intraoperative navigation using ICG lymphography

7-7. その他の外科治療および有用なテクニック

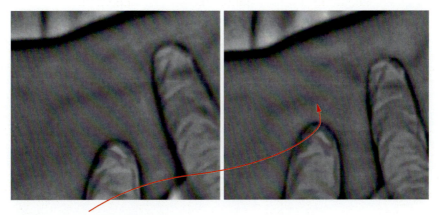

静脈逆流が止まる位置に静脈弁があることがわかる
Location of a venous valve is shown

Fig. 7-7-11. 近赤外線装置による静脈の評価
Preoperative evaluation of veins using a near-infrared device

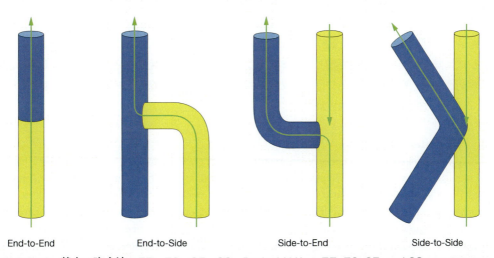

Fig. 7-7-12. 基本4吻合法：EE・ES・SE・SS　Basic 4 LVAs：EE, ES, SE, and SS anastomoses

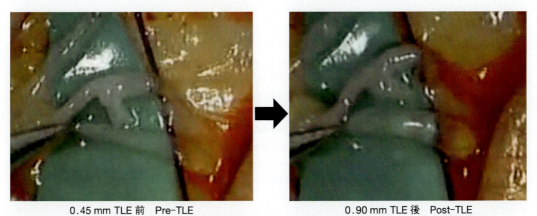

0.45 mm TLE 前　Pre-TLE　　　　　　　　　0.90 mm TLE 後　Post-TLE

Fig. 7-7-13. TLE法によるリンパ管拡張操作　TLE maneuver for dilatation of a lymphatic vessel

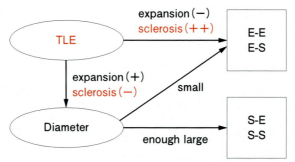

Fig. 7-7-14. TLE 法による吻合方法の選定
Selection of anastomotic configurations using TLE maneuver

一時的に遮断し、術野の末梢側をマッサージすることでリンパ管内圧を上昇させる。リンパ管硬化が軽度であればリンパ管は拡張し、硬化が高度であればリンパ管径は変わらない(**Fig. 7-7-14**)。TLE 法によりリンパ管が拡張するため、側孔作成もより正確・容易にできる。

リンパ管硬化が高度の場合はリンパ管を切断し EE 吻合・ES 吻合することになるが、リンパ管切断時には切断面を強拡大で観察する必要がある。リンパ管炎の既往がある場合では、近接するリンパ管同士が炎症により癒着し、1本のリンパ管のように見えることがあるためである。リンパ管切断面を観察し内腔を2つ以上認めた際は、隔壁を切断・切除し内腔を1つにするとよい(**Fig. 7-7-15**, mono-canalization)。

II. Preparation of vessels

ICG lymphography is useful not only for preoperative prediction of lymphatic vessels' conditions but also for intraoperative navigation of lymphatic surgery. It is difficult to identify a translucent or white lymphatic vessel in a yellow fat tissue, but a beginner LVA surgeon can easily find lymphatic vessels under ICG lymphography navigation. A near-infrared camera-integrated operating microscope facilitates navigation lymphatic surgery without additional ICG injection ; preoperative ICG injection is enough to enhance lymphatic vessels intraoperatively (**Fig. 7-7-10**). ICG lymphography navigation visualizes lymphatic vessels not only in Linear region but also in Stardust region, however, hardly visualizes in Diffuse region.

It is important to find an "appropriate" recipient vein for LVA. "Appropriate" veins are those with intact valves to prevent post-anastomotic venous backflow into the anastomosis site. A near-infrared camera visualizes also subcutaneous veins, and is useful for preoperative venous evaluation. Localization and evaluation of venous valves are possible with squeeze test (**Fig. 7-7-11**). Skin incision sites are determined based on preoperative ICG lymphography and venous mapping.

SE or SS anastomoses are more efficient than EE or ES anastomoses, because SE/SS anastomoses can bypass both normograde and retrograde lymph flows via one anastomosis (**Fig. 7-7-12**). Lymphotomy, creation of lateral window on a lymphatic vessel, is required for SE or SS anastomoses. It is difficult and of failure risk to do lymphotomy on a sclerotic lymphatic vessel. Temporary lymphatic expansion (TLE) maneuver is useful to evaluate severity of lymphosclerosis before lymphotomy (**Fig. 7-7-13**). The proximal side of a lymphatic vessel is clamped, and then skin distal to the field is massaged to increase the lymphatic pressure. When the lymphatic vessel is expanded, the vessel's sclerosis is mild and suitable for lymphotomy (**Fig. 7-7-14**). Since TLE maneuver expand a lymphatic vessel, lymphotomy becomes easier than before TLE maneuver.

When lymphosclerosis is severe, a lymphatic vessel to be anastomosed should be transected and

7-7．その他の外科治療および有用なテクニック

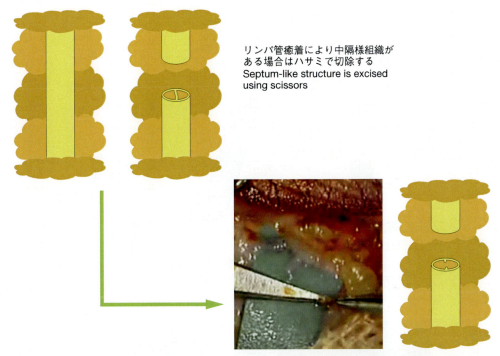

Fig. 7-7-15. Mono-canalization 法　Mono-canalization method for firmly-adhered lymphatic vessels

anastomosed in an EE or ES fashion. A surgeon should precisely observe the intraluminal structure of the lymphatic vessel under a high magnification (×20-30), because there can be multiple lymphatic vessels due to previous lymphangitis. When the lumen has a septum-like structure, the septum should be resected to make the lumen mono-canalized (**Fig. 7-7-15**).

III　吻合

　微小血管吻合で用いられる動静脈に比べると、リンパ管は細く透明で壁が薄いため内腔の視認・確保が難しいことがある。ナイロン糸を stent として用いた IVaS 法が内腔確保に有用である。初心者でも確実に吻合することができる。単純な EE 吻合のほか、ナイロン糸を分割して挿入するなど工夫することで ES 吻合・SE 吻合・SS 吻合にも用いることができる（**Fig. 7-7-16**）。
　遠く離れたリンパ管と静脈を吻合する際は、1 針目の縫合部にテンションがかかり脈管が潰れ内腔が確認しにくくなることがある。このようなときは連続縫合によるパラシュート法が有用である（**Fig. 7-7-17**）。結紮することなく後壁を連続で縫合し、後壁が縫い終わった段階で糸を引きリンパ管と静脈を引き寄せる。その後、前壁を同じ糸で連続縫合し、1 周したところで結紮する。テンションによって内腔が潰れることがなく縫合しやすく、また連続縫合なので吻合時間も短い（1 吻合に最短 3 分）。術野に間質液があふれている際は糸が絡まりやすく連続縫合しにくいので不向きである。
　静脈逆流を防ぎ吻合部に血液が触れないようにすることが吻合の長期開存に重要である。静脈

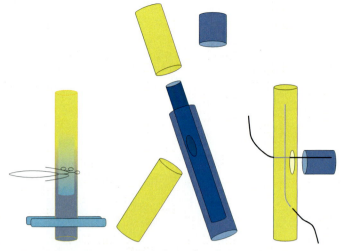

Fig. 7-7-16. ナイロン糸による stent
Intravascular stenting (IVaS) method using a nylon thread

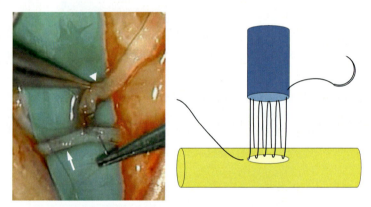

Fig. 7-7-17. パラシュート法による SE 吻合
Parachute technique for fast SE anastomosis

　弁の効いている静脈を確保することが肝要であるが、術野にそのような静脈がないことも多い。術野の静脈が静脈逆流をきたしているものの静脈弁があれば、壁外から静脈弁を縫合し締めることで弁不全を改善することもできるが、静脈弁がない場合は静脈弁を"つくる"（neo-valvuloplasty）必要がある。吻合に用いられた細静脈が中枢で太い静脈に合流する部位が術野にあれば、合流部で細静脈を全層で太い静脈内に内挿し壁外で縫合固定することで、新たな静脈弁を作成することができる（Fig. 7-7-18）。血栓形成を避けるために、neo-valvuloplasty では「血管内に内膜以外の組織が露出しない」ことを厳守しなければならない。neo-valvuloplasty ができない場合は、他の術野から静脈弁を有した静脈を移植することができる（Fig. 7-7-19）。鼠径部では多数の静脈が確保でき静脈が余ることも多い。そのような術野から静脈移植することでドナーの犠牲なく静脈移植が可能である。
　吻合の長期開存に重要なもう1つのポイントは、リンパから静脈へのリンパ流が豊富であるこ

7-7. その他の外科治療および有用なテクニック

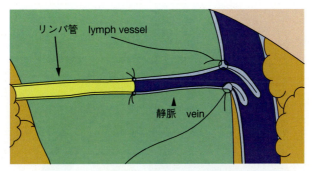

Fig. 7-7-18. Neo-valvuloplasty 法　Neo-valvuloplasty for a branched vein

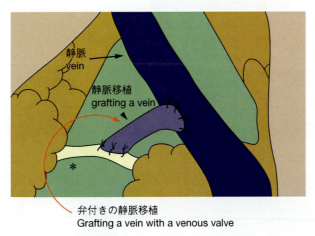

Fig. 7-7-19. 静脈移植を用いた LVA　Vein grafting for LVA

とである。恒常的で豊富なリンパ流により静脈が吻合部に逆流しにくくなる。そのためには1つの静脈になるべく多くのリンパ流をバイパスさせるべきであるが、静脈閉塞時にリンパ流が閉塞しないよう EE 吻合・ES 吻合・SE 吻合・SS 吻合を駆使して吻合形態を工夫しなければならない (**Fig. 7-7-20～23**)。

(山本　匠)

III. Anastomoses

Lymphatic vessels are smaller and thinner than blood vessels, that makes it difficult to identify the vessel lumen. Intravascular stenting (IVaS) method, in which a nylon thread is inserted into a vessel lumen as a stent, is useful to facilitate supermicrosurgical lymphatic anastomosis. The IVaS method can be applied not only in EE anastomosis, but also in ES, SE, and SS anastomoses by splitting an IVaS (**Fig. 7-7-16**).

During anastomosis of distant vessels, the second stich is usually difficult due to invisibility of the vessels' lumen that is caused by tension created on the first stich. Parachute method, untied continuous suture, addresses this challenge (**Fig. 7-7-17**). The anastomosis starts from the back wall in a continuous fashion. The suture is run loosely to make the lumen always visible. The suture is only tightened after completion of

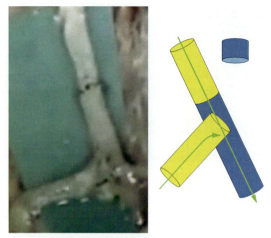

Fig. 7-7-20. λ吻合 (EE+ES)
Lambda anastomosis (EE+ES)

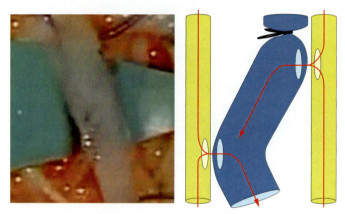

Fig. 7-7-21. Sequential 吻合 (SS+SS)
Sequential anastomosis (SS+SS)

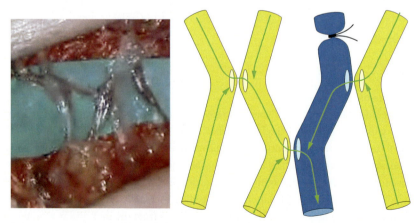

Fig. 7-7-22. Ladder 吻合 (SS+SS+SS：SS-LVA×2+SS-LLA)
Ladder anastomosis (SS+SS+SS：SS-LVA×2+SS-LLA)

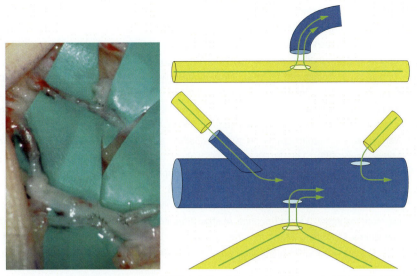

Fig. 7-7-23. All-star 吻合(EE＋ES＋SE＋SS)　All-star anastomosis(EE＋ES＋SE＋SS)

the back wall suturing. The lumens of both vessels are kept open by the traction from the tightened sutures. The same suture is used to suture the anterior wall as in the back wall suture. After anterior wall suture completion, the sutures are tightened and tied with care taken to avoid purse-stringing. Parachute technique is especially useful for distant vessels in a SE anastomosis, and shortened anastomosis time (shortest time 3 min). It would be helpless when there is abundant interstitial fluid in a field.

　It is important for long-term anastomosis patency that blood does not contact with the anastomosis site by preventing venous reflux with an intact venous valve. When a venous valve exists but is not enough functional to avoid venous reflux, external valvuloplasty is useful. When there is a small vein branched from a larger vein but no venous valve, neo-valvuloplasty is helpful to prevent venous reflux. The adventitia of the small vein is sutured to make a neo-valve at the branching site. Two vertical mattress sutures are placed at the proximal and distal sites along the larger vein axis to invert the branched small vein into the larger vein; the inverted vein makes a valve-like structure within the larger vein (**Fig. 7-7-18**). It is necessary for only the endothelium to be exposed in lumen. When both valvuloplasty and neo-valvuloplasty are not applicable, vein grafting is useful. Since there are many veins more than required there, a vein can be used as a graft without additional invasiveness (**Fig. 7-7-19**).

　Another important point for long-term anastomosis patency is abundant lymph-to-venous flow. Continuous and abundant lymph flow prevents venous reflux into an anastomosis site. To increase lymph-to-venous flow, more lymph flows should be bypassed into a vein. Care should be taken to avoid native lymph flow obstruction by combining EE, ES, SE, and SS anastomoses (**Fig. 7-7-20 to 23**).

(Takumi Yamamoto)

1) Yamamoto T, Narushima M, et al：Minimally invasive lymphatic supermicrosurgery (MILS)；indocyanine green lymphography-guided simultaneous multi-site lymphaticovenular anastomoses via millimeter skin incisions. Ann Plast Surg 72(1)：67-70, 2014.

2) Kato M, Yamamoto T：Simple wire retractor for supermicrosurgical lymphaticovenular anastomosis. Microsurgery 35(4)：335-336, 2015.

3) Yamamoto T, Koshima I : Upward retraction for lymphaticovenular anastomosis in the deep fat layer. Microsurgery 34(7) : 586-587, 2014.

4) Yamamoto T, Yoshimatsu H, Hayashi A : A method of continuous indirect aspiration (CIA) for field clearance in lymphatic supermicrosurgery. Microsurgery 36(2) : 175, 2016.

5) Yamamoto T, Yamamoto N, et al : Near-infrared illumination system-integrated microscope for supermicrosurgical lymphaticovenular anastomosis. Microsurgery 34(1) : 23-27, 2014.

6) Yamamoto T, Ishiura R, Kato M : Hands-free vein visualizer for selection of recipient vein with an intact valve in lymphatic supermicrosurgery. J Plast Reconstr Aesthet Surg 68(6) : 871-873, 2015.

7) Yamamoto T, Yoshimatsu H, et al : A modified side-to-end lymphaticovenular anastomosis. Microsurgery 33(2) : 130-133, 2013.

8) Yamamoto T, Yoshimatsu H, et al : Side-to-end lymphaticovenular anastomosis through temporary lymphatic expansion. PLoS ONE 8(3) : e59523, 2013.

9) Yamamoto T, Yamashita M, et al : Mono-canalization of adhered lymphatic vessels for lymphatic supermicrosurgery. J Plast Reconstr Aesthet Surg 67(11) : e291-e292, 2014.

10) Narushima M, Mihara M, et al : The intravascular stenting method for treatment of extremity lymphedema with multiconfiguration lymphaticovenous anastomoses. Plast Reconstr Surg 125 : 935-943, 2010.

11) Yamamoto T, Narushima M, et al : Lambda-shaped anastomosis with intravascular stenting method for safe and effective lymphaticovenular anastomosis. Plast Reconstr Surg 127(5) : 1987-1992, 2011.

12) Yamamoto T, Yoshimatsu H, et al : Split intravascular stents for side-to-end lymphaticovenular anastomosis. Ann Plast Surg 71(5) : 538-540, 2013.

13) Yamamoto T, Chen WF, Yamamoto N, et al : Technical simplification of the supermicrosurgical side-to-end lymphaticovenular anastomosis using the parachute technique. Microsurgery 35(2) : 129-134, 2015.

14) Yamamoto T, Koshima I : Neo-valvuloplasty for lympahtic supermicrosurgery. J Plast Reconstr Aesthet Surg 67(4) : 587-588, 2014.

15) Yamamoto T, Koshima I : *In situ* vein grafting for lymphatic supermicrosurgery. J Plast Reconstr Aesthet Surg 67(5) : e142-e143, 2014.

16) Yamamoto T, Mito D, Hayashi A, et al : Multiple-in-one concept for lymphatic supermicrosurgery. Microsurgery 35(7) : 588-589, 2015.

17) Yamamoto T, Kikuchi K, et al : Ladder-shaped lymphaticovenular anastomosis using multiple side-to-side lymphatic anastomoses for a leg lymphedema patient. Microsurgery 34(5) : 404-408, 2014.

18) Yamamoto T, Furuya M, Harima M, et al : Triple supermicrosurgical side-to-side lymphaticolymphatic anastomoses on a lymphatic vessel end-to-end anastomosed to a vein. Microsurgery 35(3) : 249-250, 2015.

19) Yamamoto T, Yoshimatsu H, et al : Sequential anastomosis for lymphatic supermicrosurgery ; multiple lymphaticovenular anastomoses on one venule. Ann Plast Surg 73(1) : 46-49, 2014.

c. The Superior-Edge-of-the-Knee Incision method
― Effective LVA for lower extremity lymphedema ―

■はじめに

　リンパ管細静脈吻合術（lymphaticovenular anastomosis；LVA）の治療技術により、上肢・下肢リンパ浮腫患者への外科治療は飛躍的に向上した。多施設からのLVAの治療報告から、施設ごとの方法論によりLVAの治療効果も異なることが示唆されるが、それ以上に同じ術者が同一方法でLVAを行っても、治療効果が症例により大きく異なることが、この術式の普及を妨げる一因であると考えられる。

　LVAの治療効果は、硬化した皮膚変化の改善や周径減少を含め、吻合部周囲に限局して認めることが多いため、一肢においても基本的にmultiple LVAを行うことが推奨される。また、苦労して作成したリンパ管細静脈吻合自体が術後の中・長期経過で閉塞してしまい、効果を認めなくなるケースも少なからず経験することから、保険的な意味合いでmultiple LVAを行うといった意義も大きい。

　しかし、multiple LVAを行うには複数術者による同時進行手術が必須要件となる。そもそも、手術用顕微鏡を用いた比較的高度な吻合技術が求められるLVAを、同一症例に対して複数の手術用顕微鏡を用い、複数の術者が同時に行うことが可能な施設は限られてしまい、現実的にmultiple LVAを世界に広く普及させることは困難と考えられる。

　ここで求められる理想的なLVAは、①少数の術者でも患者の治療効果を最大限に引き出せる、②中・長期的に閉塞することのない、③すべての患者において一定の治療効果を認めるもの、である。

　われわれはmultiple LVAをこれまで多くの患者に施行してきたが、筆者の経験ではおよそ50〜70皮切に1度の頻度で、豊富なリンパ流を伴い、かつ0.65 mmから時として1.2 mm以上の径をもつリンパ管を同定する。これらのリンパ管を静脈と吻合すると、そのリンパ管から静脈への持続的リンパ流は、patency testにおいて血管吻合時の流量に匹敵する。理論的には流量は半径の4乗に比例することからも、当然これらリンパ管を同定し得た症例では、上肢リンパ浮腫・下肢リンパ浮腫患者共に、通常のLVAでは考えられないほどの劇的な治療効果を認めることが多い（**Fig. 7-7-24**）。

　下肢リンパ浮腫患者において、その豊富なリンパ流を伴う太いリンパ管は、大腿部に多く認め、下腿部や足背には稀に認める。特にうっ滞したリンパ液によるリンパ管拡張期の患者において認められることが多く、リンパ管硬化の進んだ症例で認めることは稀である。

　豊富なリンパ流を伴う太いリンパ管の同定例では、治療効果は長期持続する。しかし、1年以上続いた劇的な周径減少を伴う治療効果が、蜂窩織炎の発症もなく、ある瞬間に突然消失し、リンパ浮腫が再燃した症例を数例経験した。その原因としては、長期合併症であることから、吻合自体に問題があったというよりは、その劇的周径減少とリンパ灌流の改善により、リンパ管の拡張がなくなり、結果的に細くなった吻合リンパ管と静脈との口径差が拡大し、LVAが自壊してしまったと推察される。これら症例から、浮腫の程度にかかわらず、一定量のリンパ流が常に存在する部位でLVAを行うことが重要であると考える。

　そこで筆者らは、症例にかかわらず、常に豊富なリンパ流を伴う太いリンパ管が存在している

Hagen-Poiseuille equation

$$Q = \frac{\Delta P \pi}{8\mu L} r^4$$

Q : volumetric flow rate L : length of pipe
μ : dynamic viscosity ΔP : pressure loss

流量は管の半径 α の 4 乗に比例！

The flow rate is theoretically proportional to 4th power of the radius (r) of the pipe.

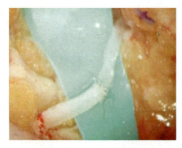

Lymphatic vessel of 0.75 mm

21.1 本分！

← 21.1 Flow

Equivalent to 21.1 0.35 mm LVAs

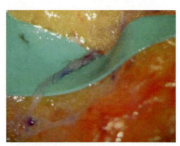

Lymphatic vessel of 0.35 mm

Fig. 7-7-24. Hagen-Poiseuille 式とリンパ流量 Lymph flow and Hagen-Poiseuille equation
一般的に管径が一定の円管を粘性流体が層流で流れる場合、管腔の流量は半径の 4 乗に比例する（Hagen-Poiseuille 式）。リンパ流量が Hagen-Poiseuille 式に従うと仮定した場合、0.75 mm のリンパ管のリンパ流量は、0.35 mm のリンパ管 21.1 本分に相当するため、LVA においてもより太く、流量の多いリンパ管を吻合することが重要と考えられる。
Based on Hagen-Poiseuille equation, flow rate of incompressible and Newtonian fluid in a constant circular and long pipe is theoretically proportional to forth power of the radius of the pipe. On the assumption that flow of lymph follows Hagen-Poiseuille equation, LVA with lymphatic vessel of 0.75 mm diameter is equivalent to 21.1 LVAs with lymphatic vessel of 0.35 mm diameter. LVA using large and high flow lymphatic vessels is important for good clinical results.

部位をさまざまな方法で探し続けた。そして最終的に、患者間で大きく異なるさまざまなリンパ管走行の中から、全患者で走行が一致している部位が膝上内側に存在していることを突き止め、かつ同部位での効果的な吻合法を開発し、膝上切開法（The Superior-Edge-of-the-Knee Incision method；SEKI 法）として報告した。本章では、SEKI 法の理論と方法について解説する。

■**Introduction**

Surgical treatment for lymphedema is greatly advanced recently by technical improvements of lymphaticovenular anastomosis (LVA). In spite of its' high therapeutic effect for lymphedema, LVA is not performed in many institutions yet. The difficulty in spreading LVA worldwide might be originated from not only the difficulty of procedure itself but also the complex pathology of lymphedema ; surgical improvements in lymphedema differ from patient to patient even when LVA was performed by experts.

Improvement in the edema, including reduction in the stiffness and size of the affected limb, is often seen only around the site of lymphaticovenular anastomosis. This is why multiple sites LVAs are recommended as a strategy of LVA operations. Moreover, LVAs are at risk of occlusion in mid- or late postoperative course. Especially, small-diameter lymphatic vessels with low flow might be easily occluded in mid- or late postoperative course. Then multiple sites LVAs are also effective as insurance implications for risk of future occlusion of LVA.

However, multiple sites LVAs require two or three microsurgeons performing LVA simultaneously in the limited operation time. It is almost impossible for many institutions to keep many LVA surgeons and operating microscopes for each case.

Therefore, we think that ideal LVA should fulfil the following requirement : ideal LVA is performed by only one microsurgeon with one operating microscope ; ideal LVA is not occluded in mid- or late postoperative course ; ideal LVA is effective for all lymphedema patients.

In our multiple LVAs experiences, we occasionally found one large lymphatic vessel in 50-70 vessels at non-specific area which had over 0.65 mm diameter with abundant lymph. LVA using these high flow lymphatic vessels has continuous lymph-to-venous flow as strong as blood flow with optimum postoperative improvements in lymphedema.

Based on Hagen-Poiseuille equation, flow rate is theoretically proportional to a forth power of the radius of the pipe. In clinical cases, LVA using these high flow lymphatic vessels actually had incredible high therapeutic effect for upper and lower extremity lymphedema (**Fig. 7-7-24**).

In lower extremity lymphedema patients, these high flow lymphatic vessels were mainly detected in the thigh and occasionally detected in the lower leg and the dorsal foot. Patients with progressive lymphedema with sclerosis of lymphatic vessels rarely have these high flow lymphatic vessels.

High clinical effects of LVA were gained when LVAs were performed using these high flow lymphatic vessels. However, we had some cases of lower extremity lymphedema patients who revealed sudden recurrence of lymphedema even though their lymphedema was dramatically improved with high volume reduction in mid- to late postoperative course. We think the reason of sudden recurrences was the spontaneous collapse of LVAs, which might happen by improvements of lymphedema. Lymphatic vessels in LVA which had been dilated by lymphedema were considered to be shrunk in many areas in the extremities especially in the distal area when the lymphedema was improved with no accumulation of lymph. Then shrunk diameter of lymphatic vessel does not match to the diameter of the vein in the LVA. As the result of tremendous improvement of lymphedema using high flow lymphatic vessels, LVAs might be at risk of spontaneous collapse in the late postoperative course. Therefore large lymphatic vessels for LVA with abundant lymph flow should be selected from the area, where the continuous flow of lymph will be maintained in each stage of lymphedema.

The authors continued to search the area, in which large diameter of lymphatic vessels with abundant lymph flow are always detected in any patients. Finally, we found the best location for LVA at the thigh using high flow lymphatic vessels. In this section, we introduce the superior-edge-of-the-knee incision (SEKI) method.

I　SEKI 法に必要な基本吻合技術

　一般的に大腿部の LVA は、他部位と比較して困難である。その理由は、大腿部の比較的太く吻合可能なリンパ管は脂肪層の深層に多く存在し、やせ形の症例でも皮膚から 1.5 cm 以上の深さでの多方向からの吻合操作が必要になることがほとんどで、豊富な脂肪組織に阻まれながらのリンパ管同定と吻合を要求されるからである。本法は切開部が決定していることから、繰り返して同じ部位で手術を行うことが困難なため、初回手術は大腿の他部位での LVA に精通した術者が行うことが望ましい。

I. Skills for the SEKI method

Lymphaticovenular anastomosis at the thigh is one of the most difficult procedures for microsurgeons to perform because lymphatic vessels in the thigh region reside in rich fatty tissue in the deep layer. In performing the SEKI method, the microsurgeon should anastomose lymphatic vessels and veins with multidirectional sutures in the deep layer in fatty tissue. Because reoperation of the SEKI method might be difficult to perform from the same incision point, the procedure should be performed only by experts in LVA at the thigh region.

Ⅱ　SEKI 法の手術方法

　SEKI 法の位置決定は、患者が仰臥位で下肢をまっすぐに伸ばした状態で行う。最初に、①膝蓋骨上縁の高さで、大腿外側から大腿内側への横方向の直線 a を引く、②大腿下方の最内側を走行する縦方向の直線 b を想定する、③直線 a と直線 b の交点から、後方に向かって大腿の皺に沿った 2.5 cm の直線が、本法の皮膚切開線である（**Fig. 7-7-25**）。

　手術は基本的に局所麻酔下に行い、近年われわれは局所麻酔薬の総量を減らす目的で 0.5%のキシロカイン® E を好んで用いている。切開線に沿って、真皮内に 27 G 針で 2.0 mL の局所麻酔を行った後、切開線の両端で、27 G 針を根本まで押しつけながら、深さ 3 cm 程度の脂肪層深層（浅筋膜と筋膜の間の層）に各々 1.5 mL ずつ局注し、1ヵ所あたり合計 5 mL の局注を行う。浅筋膜と筋膜の間の層に十分な鎮痛効果を得ることが可能で、また切開部の両端の皮下に十分な圧をかけることで、本法の特徴である浅筋膜と筋膜の間のリンパ管が容易に脂肪浅層に引き出されるため、本法の重要なポイントである。

　皮膚を切開し、東大式釣り針（単鉤式、クラウンジュン社）4 本で術野を展開し、最初に吻合に適した静脈を同定する。本法の切開線は、大伏在静脈の second branch または third branch 上にあるため、容易に静脈を同定できる。また皮下静脈も同定した場合は確保しておく。大伏在静脈そのものを同定してしまった場合は、剥離範囲が内側後方に行き過ぎているため、より外側前方を剥離しないと本法で使用するリンパ管は同定できない。

　次に吻合するリンパ管の同定であるが、本法の切開線からは、浅筋膜上でも他部位より比較的太いリンパ管を 3〜5 本は同定できる。しかし、本法ではこれらのリンパ管は吻合には用いない。浅筋膜を鈍的に貫通した後、皮膚から 1.5〜3.0 cm の深さで、豊富なリンパ流を伴う太いリンパ管を探索する。本法の特徴は、この切開部位で、浅筋膜と筋膜に挟まれて存在するリンパ管を利用して LVA を行うことである。筆者はアドソン有鉤攝子で縦方向に脂肪をよけ、血管剥離子でさらに脂肪をかき分けながら、脂肪の隙間から一瞬覗いたリンパ管を血管剥離子ですくいあげ、3-0 ナイロン糸を通してリンパ管を確保している（**Fig. 7-7-26**）。リンパ管を 3-0 ナイロン糸で確保した後は、ピオクタニンでリンパ管を marking すると切断後のリンパ管を見失い難い。3-0 ナイロンで注意深くリンパ管を牽引しながら、血管剥離子でリンパ管を近位方向に 1.5 cm 程度全周性に剥離する。この際、リンパ管を損傷しないように細心の注意が必要である。剥離した近位端でリンパ管を切断し、遠位のリンパ管を浅筋膜上の脂肪浅層に引き出して、このリンパ管と同定した複数の静脈から最も位置と口径が適切な静脈を 11-0 ナイロンで端々吻合する。

　本法を行うにあたって重要なことは、浅筋膜下のリンパ管を同定するために作成する浅筋膜の穴を大きくし過ぎないことであると考えている。吻合リンパ管の通り道である浅筋膜に作成した穴が大き過ぎれば、歩行時の関節運動時に吻合リンパ管にかかる圧力が減弱してしまい、十分な治療効果が得られない可能性があるためである。そのために筆者は、浅筋膜下のリンパ管の同定の難易度が高くなったとしても、切開長を 2.5 cm に限局している。

　なお、切断したリンパ管の近位端はそのまま放置して差し支えない。この部位では探索すれば

7-7. その他の外科治療および有用なテクニック

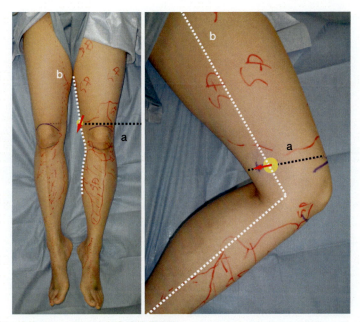

Fig. 7-7-25. SEKI 法の皮膚切開部位　Incision point of the SEKI method

リンパ管の走行は患者間で大きく異なるため、切開部の決定は LVA において最も重要である。特に深部にリンパ管が存在する大腿部では、リンパ管が複数存在している部分を切開した場合でさえ、脂肪をかき分けてリンパ管を同定することの難易度は高い。切開部によっては、吻合可能なリンパ管が存在していない場合もあるため、大腿部でリンパ管を探索することは常にチャレンジ要素のある手技となる。その点においても、常に太いリンパ管が存在している膝上切開法の切開部位は、術者に多くの余裕を与えてくれる。本法の切開位置は、仰臥位で膝蓋骨中央が時計の 0 時方向となった体位で決定する。膝蓋骨上縁に平行に引いた直線 a と、大腿内側縁に想定した直線 b の交点を起点とし、皮膚の皺に沿って後方に 2.5 cm の切開を design することで得られる。

Determination of incision site is one of the most important points for LVA, because the locations of the lymphatic vessels differ from patient to patient anatomically. Detection of lymphatic vessels itself is a difficult procedure for microsurgeons especially at the thigh region where lymphatic vessels are residing in rich fatty tissue. Moreover, it is possible that there is no lymphatic vessel at the incision site in traditional LVA because lymphatic vessels at the thigh region are difficult to be detected by ICG lymphography which has depth limit of 2.0 cm from the body surface. The SEKI method relieves microsurgeons to undertake LVA at the thigh with constant presence of effective lymphatic vessels there. The incision site is defined as the intersection of a transverse *line a* drawn at the superior edge of the patella and a longitudinal *line b* drawn along the medial axis of the distal thigh with the patient in the supine position in which the center of the patella is in the 0 o'clock direction of the clock. From the point of intersection, a 2.5-cm-long transverse incision was made posteriorly.

豊富なリンパ流を伴う太いリンパ管を 3 本以上は同定でき、大腿にうっ滞を伴う進行例ではこれらが互いに吻合し合っているために（ICG lymphography での Splash パターンに該当）、近位断端からリンパ漏が生じることは極めて稀であると考えられる。本法で作成した LVA では、その豊富なリンパ流により、静脈からリンパ管への血液の逆流を認めることはごく稀であり、patency test で静脈への豊富なリンパ流を確認できることも多い。

293

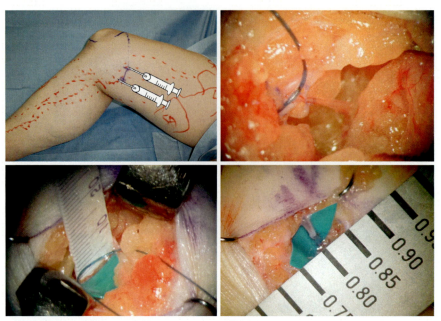

Fig. 7-7-26. SEKI 法で吻合に用いるリンパ管を深部から引き出すためのテクニック
Techniques to pull out lymphatic vessels under the superficial fascia in the SEKI method

浅筋膜下の深い部位に存在するリンパ管を表面に引き出すため、切開部の両端で、浅筋膜下に 1.5 mL ずつ局所麻酔を注射し、浅筋膜下の内圧を高めておく。SEKI 法の切開部では、浅筋膜上にも比較的太いリンパ管を複数同定できるが、通常これは吻合に利用しない。吻合に利用するリンパ管は、浅筋膜下に存在するリンパ管で、これは深さ 1.5〜3.0 cm に存在する（本例では体表から 2 cm の深さで同定した）。脂肪を分けながらようやくリンパ管を同定しても、すぐに深い脂肪の中に埋もれて見失ってしまうため、いったん血管剥離子ですくいあげたリンパ管を 3-0 ナイロン糸で確保している。ピオクタニンでリンパ管を marking し、3-0 ナイロン糸を丁寧に牽引しながら、リンパ管を近位方向に向かって全周性に十分剥離する。近位端でリンパ管を切断してナイロン糸を引っ張ると、リンパ管は浅筋膜下の圧により、表面に自然と出てくる。
After an intradermal injection along the 2.5 cm incision, 1.5 mL injections under the superficial fascia at both edges of the incision were done for efficient anesthesia and pressure control under the superficial fascia to pull out the lymphatic vessel. Lymphatic vessels over the superficial fascia were not selected for LVA. Only lymphatic vessels which located under the superficial fascia at a depth of 1.5 to 3.0 cm (2.0 cm in this case) from the cutis were selected for LVA in the SEKI method. Once the lymphatic vessel was detected under the superficial fascia from rich fatty tissue, the 3-0 nylon suture was used to catch the vessel. After pigmentation of the lymphatic vessel using surgical marker, the lymphatic vessel was dissected proximally with careful traction of the vessel with the 3-0 nylon suture helps. After a careful cut of the lymphatic vessel at the most proximal point of dissection, the lymphatic vessels were easily pulled out for LVA.

II. Procedure of the SEKI method

The area of the SEKI method incision point is defined as the intersection of a transverse **line a** drawn at the superior edge of the patella and a longitudinal **line b** drawn along the medial axis of the distal thigh with the patient in the supine position. From the point of intersection, a 2.5-cm-long transverse incision was made posteriorly (**Fig. 7-7-25**).

All surgical procedure can be carried out under local anesthesia. We recently prefer to use 0.5% lidocaine with epinephrine to reduce total amount of local anesthesia. After a 2.0 mL intradermal injection along the 2.5 cm incision, 1.5 mL injections under the superficial fascia at both edges of the incision were done for efficient anesthesia in the deep layer of subcutaneous tissue. Because lymphatic vessels under the superficial fascia are compressed bilaterally by the local anesthesia, the lymphatic vessels are easily pulled out for LVA.

At the SEKI point, second to third branch of the great saphenous vein can be detected. If the great saphenous vein itself is appeared in the incision point, then the dissection should be done more anteriorly to detect the large and high-flow lymphatic vessels under the superficial fascia. The great saphenous vein itself should not be apparent in procedures of the SEKI method.

Traction of the incision point is important for the long time searching (around 20 to 30 minutes) of the lymphatic vessels under the superficial fascia. We prefer to use four hooks named the University of Tokyo fishhook to fix the surgical site.

Many lymphatic vessels can be identified over the superficial fascia layer in subcutaneous tissue at the SEKI point. But these lymphatic vessels over the superficial fascia layer are not usable for effective LVA. Only lymphatic vessels under the superficial fascia layer are selected for LVA in the SEKI method. Once the lymphatic vessel is detected under the superficial fascia layer from rich fatty tissue, careful traction of the vessel with the 3-0 nylon suture helps proximal dissection of the vessel (**Fig. 7-7-26**). After pigmentation of the lymphatic vessel using a surgical marker, the lymphatic vessel is carefully cut with microscissors at the most proximal point of dissection and pulled out over the superficial fascia for LVA. Large lymphatic vessels can be anastomosed to veins with 11-0 nylon suture.

We think dissection of the superficial fascia should be limited within narrow area (2.5 cm or less) for the clinical efficacy of the SEKI method. Although a large incision at the SEKI point makes the detection of the lymphatic vessels easy under the superficial fascia, it also makes a big hole at the superficial fascia. Because upward propulsion of lymphatic fluid to the site of LVA is derived from compression of the lymphatic vessels between the deep and superficial fascia layers, the big hole in the superficial fascia layer might diminish the power of compression to the lymphatic vessel during walking. That is why the authors limit the incision within 2.5 cm in the SEKI method.

At least three large lymphatic vessels were detected under the superficial fascia at the SEKI point whenever we tried to detect several. Each lymphatic vessel has connections in patients with lower extremity lymphedema at the thigh as the splash patterns in ICG lymphography, and that is why we can cut the lymphatic vessels proximally in the SEKI method without any postsurgical complications. Prevalence of dynamic lymphatic flow to veins without venous reflux is usually obtained with the SEKI method.

Ⅲ　SEKI 法の治療効果とメカニズム

LVA の治療効果が患者間で異なる最大の理由として、リンパ管変性の程度の違いが考えられる。リンパ管変性が進行しリンパ管硬化をきたすと、壁肥厚により内腔が狭小化したリンパ管の平滑筋細胞は、その自動収縮能を果たせず、それによるリンパのうっ滞がさらなるリンパ管の硬化を生じ、浮腫はなお増悪するという悪循環に陥る。そのため、リンパ管変性が進行した患者では、LVA の部位までリンパ液を輸送することが困難なことから治療効果が乏しくなり、またリンパ流量の少ない LVA が中・長期的に閉塞することで治療効果が限定されると考えられる (**Fig. 7-7-27**)。

これら進行例では、リンパ管平滑筋に代わる新しいリンパ輸送の力源が必要である。本法で吻合に用いる膝上内側の、浅筋膜と筋膜に挟まれたリンパ管は、歩行時の膝関節運動が直接ポンプとしてリンパ液を駆出し続けることで、リンパ管の平滑筋機能が低下した進行例の患者でも治療効果を発揮すると考えられる (**Fig. 7-7-28**)。それは、歩行開始とともに術後早期から局所のリン

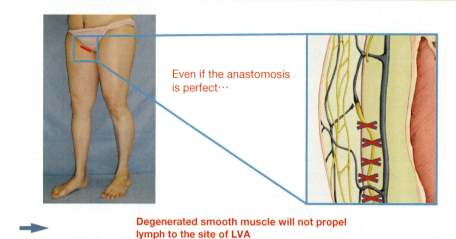

Fig. 7-7-27. Less effective LVA using lymphatic vessel with sclerosis

リンパ浮腫の進行とともに、リンパ管硬化は進行する。硬化して内腔が狭小化すると、リンパ管平滑筋機能の低下により、リンパ液の自動輸送能はさらに低下し、浮腫はさらに進行する。硬化が進んだ状態でLVAを行ったとしても、LVA吻合部までリンパを駆出することが困難なため、従来のLVAでは治療効果は限定されると考えられる。

Lymphedema develops sclerosis of lymphatic vessels. Once lymph perfusion is decreased by dysfunction of lymphatic vessels due to sclerosis with narrowed lumen, congestion of lymph itself also exacerbates lymphedema more. LVA using lymphatic vessel with sclerosis has the limitation of clinical effect because degenerated smooth muscle is not enough as a power source to propel lymph to the site of LVA. The original source of this figure is partially from Ref. 1.

（Seki Y, Yamamoto T, Yoshimatsu H, et al：The Superior-Edge-of-the-Knee-Incision Method in Lymphaticovenular Anastomosis for Lower Extremity Lymphedema. Plast Reconstr Surg 136：665e-675e, 2015 による）

パ灌流の改善を示し、リンパうっ滞による皮膚の発赤が徐々に改善してくる現象や、吻合部へのリンパドレナージで発赤が消失するという、従来のLVAでは得られない早期治療効果からも確認できる。また、その持続的リンパ流は、浮腫の程度にかかわらず一定量をもつことから、中・長期的なLVAの閉塞も予防すると考えられる。これからの長期的な経過観察が必要であるが、本法をLVAに取り入れて3年が経過した現在までに、効果の減退や浮腫の増悪を認めた症例はない。

Ⅲ．Therapeutic effect and mechanism of the SEKI method

One of the main hindrances to resolution of progressive lower extremity lymphedema by traditional LVA is sclerosis of lymphatic vessels. Once lymph perfusion is decreased, congestion of lymph itself develops degenerations of lymphatic vessels, in which sclerosis of lymphatic vessels will occur. Sclerosis of lymphatic vessels leaves the vessels too weak to propel lymph to the site of LVA (**Fig. 7-7-27**). Then LVA with a small amount of lymph flow is at risk of occlusion in the mid- or late postoperative course. This is why the effectiveness of traditional LVAs tends to be limited in severe lymphedema patients.

At the SEKI point, one of the most superior lymphatic vessels for LVA can be found；lymphatic vessels at

7-7. その他の外科治療および有用なテクニック

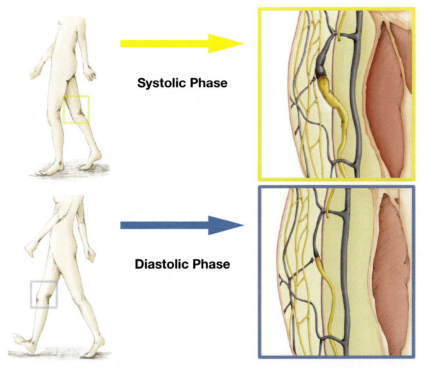

Fig. 7-7-28. The theory of the SEKI method using normal walking as the power source to propel lymph to the site of the SEKI-LVA

膝周囲の大腿内側部では、通常歩行における筋収縮が膝関節運動と連動し、浅筋膜と筋膜の間で加圧と減圧が繰り返され、筋ポンプ作用が生じる。リンパ浮腫の患者ではリンパ管平滑筋機能が低下しているため、従来型のLVAを行ってもその吻合部まで有効にリンパ液を駆出できていないケースが多いと考えられる。SEKI法では、大腿内側の筋ポンプ作用を新たなリンパ輸送の力源とし利用することで、歩行によりLVAの吻合部までリンパ液を有効に駆出している。なお、浅筋膜が広範囲で剥離された場合、歩行時に浅筋膜の穴を通過するリンパ管にかかる圧力が減じるため、2.5 cm以上の切開は推奨されない。

At the medial thigh around the knee, the knee joint movement works as a pumping system to propel lymph proximally especially at the lymphatic vessels between the superficial and deep fascia layers. Traditional LVA in which only the smooth muscle of lymphatic vessels with sclerosis works as a power source to propel lymph to the site of LVA has limitation on its' therapeutic effect. In the SEKI method, not only the smooth muscle of lymphatic vessels but also the knee joint movement during normal walking works as power sources to propel lymph to the site of SEKI-LVA. Length of the incision should be limited within 2.5 cm or less, because a big hole at the superficial fascia might decrease the pressure to the lymphatic vessels through the hole of the superficial fascia. The original source of this figure is from Ref. 1.

(Seki Y, Yamamoto T, Yoshimatsu H, et al：The Superior-Edge-of-the-Knee-Incision Method in Lymphaticovenular Anastomosis for Lower Extremity Lymphedema. Plast Reconstr Surg 136：665e-675e, 2015による)

the SEKI point are strongly compressed between the superficial fascia and the deep fascia, and the normal movement of the knee joint during walking is employed as a power source that can effectively propel lymph to the site of LVA instead of the degenerated smooth muscle in severe lower extremity lymphedema patients (**Fig. 7-7-28**).

　Clinical effectiveness of the SEKI method can be confirmed just after the surgery with signs of improvement including the early lightening phenomenon, manual lymphatic drainage to the site of the SEKI-LVA, and volume reduction of the affected limb. Continuous and strong flow of lymph through the SEKI-LVA reduces risk of occlusion of LVA. No mid- or late occlusion of lymphaticovenular anastomosis has occurred for three years after the SEKI method was applied in the treatment of lower extremity lymphedema as far.

■おわりに

本法は、これまで難易度が高く実践が困難であった大腿部でのLVAを容易にし、かつ高い治療効果をもつことから、今後の下肢リンパ浮腫治療に対する標準的な手法の1つになると考えられる。本法が1人でも多くの患者QOLの改善に結びつくことを願う。

（関　征央）

■Conclusion

The SEKI method facilitates the LVA in the thigh with high therapeutic effect. The method has a possibility to be a first-line surgical treatment for patients with lower extremity lymphedema.

(*Yukio Seki*)

1) Seki Y, Yamamoto T, Yoshimatsu H, et al : The Superior-Edge-of-the-Knee-Incision Method in Lymphaticovenular Anastomosis for Lower Extremity Lymphedema. Plast Reconstr Surg 136 : 665e-675e, 2015.

CHAPTER 8

Future prospects
今後の展望

Ⅰ 世界におけるリンパ浮腫外科治療の現況

　最近は、リンパ浮腫外科治療の普及を目的として手術手技の講習会が頻繁に開催されている。2007、2009 年にはアジア・太平洋スーパーマイクロサージャリー講習会（国立シンガポール大学）が開催された。また、2010 年 3 月に第 1 回ヨーロッパ・リンパ浮腫外科治療学会＆ヨーロッパ・スーパーマイクロ講習会（バルセロナ）が開催され、約 600 名のコメディカルと 200 名の専門医が参加した（**Fig. 8-1**）。次いで、2010 年 7 月、北フランス穿通枝皮弁・スーパーマイクロ講習会（アミアン）には約 100 名の形成外科医が参加した。さらに、2010 年 10 月、アメリカ形成外科学会（トロント）でリンパ浮腫外科治療に関するパネルが組まれ、アメリカから 3 名（スレイバン、チャン、須網）、日本から 1 名（光嶋）、台湾から 1 名（ミンティン・チェン）が招待発表した（**Fig. 8-2**）。

　2000 年以後、光嶋は国際講習会でライブデモ（18ヵ国 28 施設）と講演（350 演題以上）を行ってきた。これらの講習会には毎回 100～600 名が参加し、参加者の一部がさらに東京大学形成外科に研修に来ている。これによって海外にも吻合術が広まっていった。これまでリンパ浮腫外科治療のライブデモを行った主な施設は以下のとおりである。

　　2001 年　ベルギー・ゲント大学
　　2002、2014、2016 年　台北・チャンカン記念病院
　　2005、2008 年　バルセロナ・サンパウ大学病院
　　2007 年　北京・日中友好病院
　　2007、2009 年　国立シンガポール大学
　　　　　　　　　アジア太平洋超微小外科講習会においてリンパ管 LVA を供覧した。
　　2009 年　ロシア・シベリア・トムスク大学病院
　　2009 年　オランダ・ズウォール市民病院
　　2010 年　バンコク・国立シルラジ大学病院
　　　　　　　インド・チェンナイ市・ライト病院
　　　　　　　フィラリア症下肢重症リンパ浮腫に対する世界初の足背リンパ管移植法をライブデモで行った。
　　　　　　　クウェート国立大学病院
　　2015 年　北京・北京大学天壇病院
　　　　　　　台北・三軍大学病院
　　　　　　　ソウル・アザン大学病院

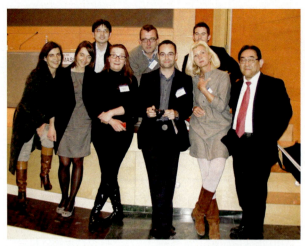

Fig. 8-1. 2010年3月、第1回ヨーロッパ・リンパ浮腫外科治療学会＆ヨーロッパ・スーパーマイクロ講習会（バルセロナ）でのライブデモ
In March 2010, live demonstration was performed at the 1st European Lymphedema Surgical Treatment Society & Europe Super-microsurgery Seminar (Barcelona)
同講習会開催メンバー。前列右から光嶋、ベッカー、マシア、ポンス、後列中：ランデュイト、左：成島らが集まった。
Members of seminar. From right in the front row：Koshima, Becker, Masià, Pons, Middle in the back row：Landuyt, left in the back row：Narushima.

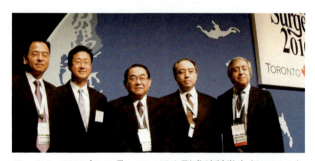

Fig. 8-2. 2010年10月、アメリカ形成外科学会（トロント）
In October 2010, Annual Meeting of the American Society of Plastic Surgeons (Toronto)
リンパ浮腫外科治療に関するパネルが組まれた（左からチェン、チャン、光嶋、須網、スレイバン）。
The Panel on lymphedema surgical treatment was organized (from left Cheng, Chang, Koshima, Suami, Slavan).

I. Current situation of lymphedema surgical treatment in the world

Nowadays, workshops of surgical procedure for the purpose of disseminating lymphedema surgical treatment are being held frequently. In 2007 and 2009, the Asia-Pacific Ocean Super microsurgery Seminars (National University of Singapore) were held. In addition, the 1st European Lymphedema Surgical Treatment Society & Europe Super microsurgery Seminar was held in March 2010 (Barcelona), with approximately 600 co-medical and 200 specialists participated (**Fig. 8-1**). Then, in July 2010, about 100

8. 今後の展望

plastic surgeons took part in the Northern France Perforator Flaps & Super microsurgery Seminar in Amiens. In addition, in October 2010 the American Society of Plastic Surgeons organized the panel on lymphedema surgical treatment at Toronto. 3 surgeons from the United States (Slavin, Chang, Suami), 1 from Japan (Koshima), and 1 from Taiwan (Cheng) were invited for presentations (Fig. 8-2).

Since 2000, the author has performed live demonstrations (18 countries, 28 facilities) and lectures (more than 350 subjects) at the international seminars. There were 100-600 participants in each seminar, and some of them came to the department of Plastic Surgery, University of Tokyo for training. By this way, the anastomosis technique is spread abroad. So far, the facilities where the author has presented live demonstrations on surgical treatment of lymphedema are as follows :

2001 Ghent University, Belgium

2002, 2014, 2016 Chang Gung Memorial Hospital, Taipei

2005, 2008 Hospital de la Santa Creu i Sant Pau, Barcelona, Spain

2007 China-Japan Friendship Hospital, Beijing, China

2007, 2009 National University of Singapore, Singapore
    Lymphaticovenular anastomosis (LVA) was performed in Asia Pacific Ocean Super microsurgery Seminar.

2009 Siberian State Medical University, Tomsk, Russia

2009 Hospital Zwolle, Netherland

2010 Siriraj Hospital, Bangkok, Thailand

2010 Lite hospital, Chennai, India
    The first live demonstration of Lymphatic tissue transfer from dorsal foot for severe lymphedema of lower extremity caused by filariasis was performed.

2010 Kuwait National University Hospital, Kuwait

2015 Beijing Tian Tan Hospital, Capital Medical University, Beijing, China

2015 Tri-Service General Hospital, Taipei

2015 Asan Medical Center, Seoul, Korea

■Ⅱ リンパ浮腫外科治療の世界のパイオニアたち (Fig. 8-3～11)

　現在、何人かの海外の形成外科医がリンパ管細静脈吻合法（LVA）を行っている。彼らは、最近頻繁に国際学会で良好な結果を報告している。以下に海外の拠点病院とリンパ浮腫外科治療を行っている代表的な外科医を挙げる。

・オルゼオスキー教授（ワルシャワ大学）：リンパ節静脈吻合を 1960 年台に報告された最高齢のリンパ外科医である。既に 80 歳を超えているが今なお精力的に患者の治療にあたっている。時々日本に来られ意見交換している。

・バウ・マイスター教授（ミュンヘン大学）：下肢からの血行のない遊離リンパ管移植による上肢浮腫の治療を報告した。現在でもミュンヘンでは彼の後継者によってこの方法による治療が継続されている。

・ブローソン医師（スウェーデン・ウプサラ大学）：脂肪吸引法によるリンパ浮腫の治療を一貫して行っている。LVA に対しては肯定的であり微小外科手技をもたない外科医の治療法として脂肪吸引法があると主張されている。

・キャンピシ教授（イタリア）：リンパ管静脈移植による上下肢の治療法を報告した。

301

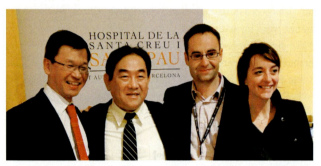

Fig. 8-3. (右より)テオ教授(ロンドン)、光嶋、マシア教授＆ポンス(バルセロナ)
From right side：Prof. Teo (London), Koshima, Prof. Masià & Pons (Barcelona)

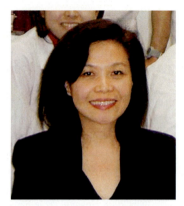

Fig. 8-4. リン准教授(国立シンガポール大学)
Associate Prof. Lim (National University of Singapore)

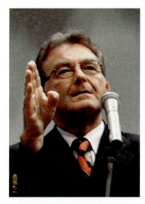

Fig. 8-5. バウ・マイスター教授(ミュンヘン大学)[1]
Prof. Baumeister (University of Munich, Germany)[1]
上肢リンパ浮腫に対する下肢からのリンパ管移植の提唱者
Advocate of lymphatic transplantation from the lower extremities for the upper extremity lymphedema

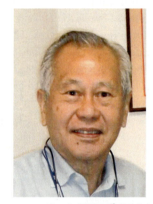

Fig. 8-6. ポー名誉教授[2] (国立シンガポール大学手の外科)
Honorary Prof. Pho[2] (Hand surgeon, National University of Singapore)

・コーリン・ベッカー医師(パリ・形成外科女医)：血管柄付きリンパ節移植による上肢浮腫の治療を行っている。
・ハンチー・チェン教授(台湾、形成外科医)：血管柄付きリンパ節移植による上肢浮腫の治療
・ミン・フェイ・チェン教授(台北・チャンカン記念大学病院)：血管柄付きリンパ節移植による上肢浮腫の治療を行っている。
・マシア教授＆ポンス准教授(女医)(バルセロナ・サンパウ病院形成外科)：リンパ管細静脈吻合、深下腹壁穿通枝皮弁と下腹部からのリンパ節移植による乳房再建と上肢浮腫の同時再建法を提唱した。東京大学形成外科で研修した後そのテクニックをヨーロッパで最初に広めた。
・アウバ医師(スペイン・パンプローナ大学形成外科女医)：リンパ管細静脈吻合。東京大学形成外科で研修した後スペインで治療を開始した。

8. 今後の展望

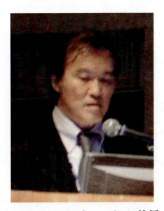

Fig. 8-7. ハンチー・チェン教授（中国医科大学、台湾）
Prof. Hung-chi Chen (China Medical University Hospital, Taiwan)

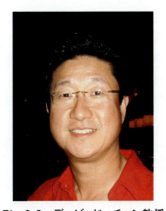

Fig. 8-8. デービッド・チャン教授（アンダーソン癌センター、ヒューストン）
Prof. David W. Chang (University of Chicago, USA)

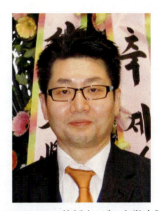

Fig. 8-9. ホン教授（アザン大学病院、ソウル）
Prof. Hong (Asan University Hospital, Seoul)

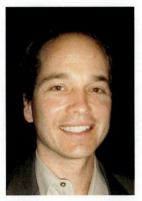

Fig. 8-10. グランツォウ准教授（UCLA、アメリカ）
Associate Prof. Granzow (UCLA, USA)

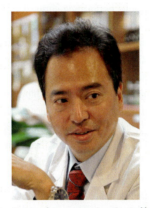

Fig. 8-11. ミン・フェイ・チェン教授（チャンカン記念大学病院、台湾）
Prof. Ming-Huei Cheng (Chang Gung Memorial Hospital, Taiwan)

・テオ教授（ロンドン・形成外科医）：リンパ管細静脈吻合、血管柄付きリンパ節移植。東京大学形成外科で研修した後イギリスで初めて外科的治療を開始した。

・リン准教授（女医）＆ウェイ・チェン講師（国立シンガポール大学形成外科女医）：リンパ管細静脈吻合。東京大学形成外科で研修した後シンガポールで外科治療を開始した。

・デービッド・チャン教授（アメリカ・シカゴ大学形成外科）：リンパ管細静脈吻合。東京大学形成外科で研修した後アメリカで初めてアンダーソン癌センターで外科治療を開始した。その後シカゴ大学に移りコメディカルを対象としたリンパ浮腫の外科的治療に関する講習会を開催している。毎回約300人のコメディカルが外科的治療に必要な複合的理学療法の最先端を学んでいる。

・ホン教授（ソウル・アザン大学病院形成外科）：リンパ管細静脈吻合。東京大学形成外科で研修した後韓国で初めて外科治療を開始した。
・グランツォウ准教授（アメリカ・UCLA 形成外科）：リンパ管細静脈吻合。東京大学形成外科で研修した後アメリカで外科治療を開始した。
・デミルカン医師（アンカラ・トルコ）：リンパ管細静脈吻合。ヨーロッパで行われたリンパ浮腫外科治療の講習会で学んだ後にトルコで外科治療を開始した。
・ランデュイト教授（ベルギー・ゲント大学）：リンパ管細静脈吻合、リンパ節移植。東京大学で研修した後ゲント大学で外科治療を行っている。
・グイドー・ジアカローネ医師（ベルギー・ブリュッセル）：リンパ管細静脈吻合。東京大学で毎年２回来日して研修しながらベルギーで外科治療を行っている。
このように、若手外科医が精力的に外科治療を進めている。

II. The pioneers of lymphedema surgical treatment in the world (Fig. 8-3 to 11)

Currently, some plastic surgeons outside Japan are performing the lymphaticovenular anastomosis. They are reporting good results frequently at international conferences. The following lists the representative surgeons and hospitals performing surgical treatment of lymphedema outside Japan.

・Professor Olszewski (University of Warsaw)：He is the oldest lymph surgeon who reported Lymphnode-venous anastomosis in 1960s. He has been more than 80 years old, but is still energetic in the treatment of patients. Sometimes he comes to Japan to exchange academic opinions with other physicians.

・Professor Baumeister (University of Munich)：He reported treatment of lymphedema of upper extremity by free lymphatic grafting without blood supply transferred from lower extremity. In Munich, this treatment is still continued by his successor.

・Doctor Broson (Uppsala University, Sweden)：He consistently performs liposuction for lymphedema. He agrees with LVA, and recommends that a surgeon who does not have the micro-surgical technique could choose liposuction as one of the treatment methods.

・Professor Campisi (Italy)：Treatment for lymphedema of upper and lower extremities with autologous venous grafts and lympho-venous anastomosis.

・Doctor Corinnel Becker (female plastic surgeon, Paris)：Treatment of lymphedema of upper extremity with vascularized lymph node transfer.

・Professor Hung-chi Chen (Department of Plastic and Reconstructive Surgery, China Medical University Hospital, Taiwan)：Treatment of lymphedema of upper extremity with vascularized lymph node transfer.

・Professor Ming-Huei Cheng (Chang Gung Memorial Hospital, Taipei)：Treatment of lymphedema of upper extremity with vascularized lymph node transfer.

・Professor Masià and Associate Professor Pons (female plastic surgeons, Hospital de la Santa Creu i Sant Pau, Barcelona)：They proposed the simultaneous breast reconstruction and upper limb lymphedema treatment by using lymph node transfer from lower abdomen, LVA and the deep inferior epigastric perforator (DIEP) flap. After receiving training at the department of Plastic Surgery, University of Tokyo, they spread the technique in Europe.

・Doctor Aubá (female plastic surgeon, University of Navarra, Spain)：LVA. After training at the department of Plastic Surgery, University of Tokyo, she began to treat patients in Spain.

・Professor Teo (plastic surgeon, London)：LVA and vascularized lymph node transfer. He practiced at the department of Plastic Surgery, University of Tokyo, and began to perform surgical treatment of lymphedema for the first time in England.

・Associate Professor Lim and Senior Consultant Ong Wei Chen (female plastic surgeons, National University of Singapore)：LVA. After receiving training at the department of Plastic Surgery, University of

Tokyo, they began to treat patients in Singapore.

· Professor David W. Chang (University of Chicago, USA) : LVA. He practiced at the department of Plastic Surgery, University of Tokyo, and began to perform surgical treatment of lymphedema for the first time in MD. Anderson Cancer Center, USA. In 2013, he transferred to University of Chicago. Since then, he has held seminars on surgical treatment of lymphedema for co-medicals. Each time, about 300 co-medicals staffs learned complex physiotherapy methods necessary for the updated surgical treatment.

· Professor Hong (Department of Plastic Surgery, Asan University Hospital, Seoul) : LVA. He practiced at the department of Plastic Surgery, University of Tokyo, and began to perform surgical treatment of lymphedema for the first time in Korea.

· Associate Professor Granzow (Division of Plastic Surgery, University of California, Los Angeles, USA) : LVA. After receiving training at the department of Plastic Surgery, University of Tokyo, he began to treat patients in USA.

· Doctor Demirkan (Ankara, Turkey) : LVA. He began to perform surgical treatment of lymphedema after joining to the seminar of lymphedema surgical treatment in Europe.

· Professor Landuyt (Ghent University, Belgium) : LVA and lymph node transfer. He started to perform surgical treatment of lymphedema after learning at the University of Tokyo.

· Doctor Guido Giacalone (Brussels, Belgium) : LVA. He is doing surgical treatment in Belgium, while he comes to the University of Tokyo twice a year.

Young surgeons are vigorously promoting surgical treatment of lymphedema.

Ⅲ　今後の治療戦略：より効果的な外科的治療法の必要性

　最近は、長期経過した重症のリンパ浮腫例に対しては、健側から、正常な平滑筋収縮機能をもつ血管柄付きリンパ管移植を行い、リンパ液を静脈系に誘導するという方法を行っている。今後は、形成外科と乳腺外科、産婦人科、泌尿器科などと合同のチーム・アプローチによる集学的治療によってリンパ浮腫の発生率が激減する日がくるものと確信している。また、筆者らの経験では、浮腫発生前や直後に予防的吻合術を行えば、浮腫は発生しにくいことがわかっている[3)-7)]。子宮癌手術時に大網移行術を併用することによって浮腫の発生頻度を減少できたという報告もある。同様に、リンパ節摘除と同時に吻合術を行うと有効であることが判明しつつある。

Ⅲ. Treatment strategies for the future : necessity of more effective surgical treatment

Nowadays, for severe cases of lymphedema with long duration, vascularized lymphatic vessels from the healthy side, of which the smooth muscle cells have normal function, have been transferred to the affected limb to lead the lymph flow drainage into veins. In the future, the incidence of lymphedema will be dramatically reduced because of the multimodal therapy on which surgeons of plastic surgery, breast surgery, obstetrics and gynecology, and urology collaborate with each other. In addition, in authors' experience, if prophylactic anastomosis is performed before or immediately after the occurrence of lymphedema, the incidence of edema will be significantly reduced[3)-7)]. It has been reported that the combination of the uterine cancer resection with the omentum transfer could reduce the incidence of lymphedema. Similarly, it is being revealed that LVA at the same time of lymph nodes resection is effective.

Ⅳ 今後の治療の進め方：チーム医療を含めて

　チーム医療では、理学療法の専門家、特に医師（婦人科、乳腺外科、骨盤外科、泌尿器科など）、コメディカルとの協調体制が重要であろう。また、ICG 造影法による浮腫の早期診断も重要である。この造影法によってリンパ流の異常が早期に診断できるようになった。Stage 0 の四肢のリンパ浮腫、骨盤内リンパ嚢胞や下腹部の初期の浮腫、大腿部の軽度浮腫の時点で ICG 検査を行うと重度のリンパ流の障害があることが判明した。

　今後は重症例に対する合併外科治療法や予防のための術式の開発がさらに進むであろう。またリンパ浮腫の改善から完治、血管肉腫をはじめとした他の進行癌に対する免疫外科治療、致死性免疫不全疾患に対する外科治療法の確立が進むであろう。難治肉腫などを含めたリンパ系疾患治療を目的とするリンパ外科学が発生し、その専門医が新しい外科的治療法を開発していくであろう。同時に免疫学を含む基礎リンパ学の導入による複雑なリンパ系疾患の機序解明や治療法の開発、さらにこの領域に関する最新の専門知識をもったコメディカルの育成も重要となるであろう。

（辛川　領、伊藤太智、水田栄樹、森下悠也、森脇裕太、光嶋　勲）

Ⅳ. How to proceed treatment for the future : including team medical care

　Team medical care : cooperative system among professionals of physical therapy, special doctors (gynecology, breast surgery, pelvic surgery, urology, etc.), co-medical would be important. In addition, early diagnosis of lymphedema by using ICG lymphography is also important. Abnormality of the lymph flow can be diagnosed at an early stage by this lymphography. Even if the patients have Stage 0 lymphedema of extremities, pelvic lymph cyst, initial lymphedema of abdomen or mild lymphedema of thigh, severe disorder of lymph flow can be revealed by ICG lymphography.

　In the future, the combined surgical treatment for severe cases and the operation method for prevention will be developed further. Improvement from lymphedema to complete cure, immunosurgical treatment for other advanced cancers including angiosarcoma and surgical treatment for lethal immunodeficiency diseases will be advanced. Lymphatic surgery aimed at treating lymphatic system diseases including intractable sarcoma, and the specialist will be raised. They will develop new surgical treatments for the entire lymphatic disorders. At the same time, mechanisms of complicated lymphatic diseases and treatments are developed by introduction of basic lymphology including immunology. It will also be important to develop co-medicals with the latest expertise on this area.

(Ryo Karakawa, Taichi Ito, Haruki Mizuta, Yuya Morishita, Yuta Moriwaki, Isao Koshima)

1) Baumeister RG, Siuda S：Treatment of lymphedema by microsurgical lymphatic grafting ; What is proved? Plast Reconstr Surg 85：64-74, 1990.
2) Pho RWH, Bayon P, Tan L：Adipose veno-lymphatic transfer for management of post-radiation lymphedema. J Reconstr Microsurg 5：45-52, 1989.
3) Koshima I, Kawada S, Moriguchi T, et al：Ultrastructural observation of lymphatic vessels in lymphedema in human extremities. Plast Reconstr Surg 97：397-405, 1996.
4) Koshima I, Inagawa K, Urushibara K, et al：Supermicrosurgical lymphaticovenularanastomosis for

8. 今後の展望

the treatment of lymphedema in the upper extremities. J Reconstr Microsurg 16 : 437-442, 2000.
5) Koshima I, Nanba U, Tsutsui T, et al : Long-term follow-up after lymphaticovenular anastomosis for lymphedema in the legs. J Reconstr Microsurg 19 : 209-215, 2003.
6) Koshima I, et al : Minimal invasive lymphaticovenular anastomosis under local anesthesia for leg lymphedema. Is it effective for Stage III and IV? Ann Plast Surg 53 : 1-6, 2004.
7) Takeishi M, Kojima M, Mori K, et al : Primary intrapelvic lymphaticovenular anastomosis following lymph node dissecdtion. Ann Plast Surg 57 : 300-304, 2006.

和文索引

足立文太郎　1
杉田玄白　1
前野良沢　1
舟岡省吾　1,3
山田行男　12

あ

アキレス腱　38
アディポサイトカイン　235
アディポネクチン　235
悪性腫瘍　57
圧迫療法　230,251

い

インドシアニングリーン　5
　──(蛍光)リンパ管造影　67,70,112,119,135,137,148,157,158,168,280
　──検査　128,214
　──所見　183
　──の感度・特異度　168
　──分類　81,82,83,84
　──,ダイナミック　71,72
陰嚢水腫　49
陰部のリンパ流評価　158
陰部リンパ浮腫　123,265

う

内深頸リンパ節　29

え

エコー　194
エストロジェン　224
腋窩リンパ節　37
炎症性サイトカイン　235
　──,抗　235

お

オトガイ下リンパ節　27
黄金顆粒　91,102

か

下肢リンパ浮腫　113,119,251
　──,家族性先天性　49
下腹壁リンパ管移植法　18
加齢退縮　222
可逆性リンパ浮腫　62
家族性先天性下肢リンパ浮腫　49
外側胸動脈深枝　237
外側胸動脈浅枝　237
外側胸リンパ管移植　18
外側胸リンパ節移植　203,208
獲得免疫　235
顎下リンパ節　27,211

き

基本吻合　281
機能的外側胸リンパ節挙上　203
機能的リンパ脂肪弁移植　201
逆行性リンパ流　64,70,157
胸腺の退縮　223
胸背動静脈　237
筋皮弁移行術　10
筋膜弁筋内挿入術　8
筋膜有窓術　8

け

血管吻合技術　268
血管柄付きリンパ管移植　17,258,305
血管柄付きリンパ節移植　16,140,141,145,156,160,170,258
血管柄付きリンパ脂肪弁　237
顕微鏡下リンパ管静脈吻合術　14,243
顕微鏡下リンパ管細静脈吻合術　244
原発性リンパ浮腫　81,82,115,116,167

　──の治療戦略　169

こ

コロイド　119
古典的リンパ管静脈吻合術　14,160
広背筋　237
抗炎症性サイトカイン　235
抗原提示　235
後頭リンパ節　27
後腹膜腫瘍　57
国際リンパ学会　70
骨盤内リンパ嚢胞　113,260
骨盤リンパ嚢胞　172

さ

鎖骨上リンパ節　29,211
細網組織　220
最小侵襲リンパ超微小外科　139,164
三角胸筋リンパ節　37

し

指動脈神経　36
脂肪　222
　──吸引　7,160,170,229,232,233,239
　──減量術　140,141,145,235
　──塞栓　161
　──沈着　70,141,145,156
　──浮腫　219
脂肪組織　220
　──切除　239
　──増生　229
耳後リンパ節　27
耳前リンパ節　27
自己免疫病　224
膝関節内側　39
膝上切開法　290,291,292
島状鼠径皮弁・広背筋(皮)弁(脂肪筋膜弁)移行術　10

i

写真撮影　194
手術のナビゲーション　158
樹状細胞　235
周径の測定　194
集学的治療　305
集合リンパ管　35,36,167
　——，浅　34
　——，前　167
重症度評価　70,157
術前マッピング　280
術中所見予測　137
小伏在静脈　39
上肢リンパ浮腫　211,249
静脈移植　284
静脈血栓　161
真皮弁埋没法　8,9
深リンパシステム　34
進行リンパ浮腫　142

す

スーパーマイクロサージャ
　リー　160,180,208,268
ステロイドホルモン　223

せ

センチネルリンパ節再建　217
センチネルリンパ節生検　57
性差　224
性染色体異常　47
性ホルモン　223
切断指再接着　268
先天性リンパ浮腫　41,47,
　56,81,84,167
浅筋膜下　160
浅頸リンパ節　29
浅集合リンパ管　34
浅鼠径リンパ節　39
浅腸骨回旋動静脈　203,211
線維性中隔　88
潜在性リンパ浮腫　62
遷移相　72,75
全身性リンパ浮腫　51
前集合リンパ管　167

そ

早期リンパ浮腫　142
早発性リンパ浮腫　41,56,
　81,84,167
造影剤　114
　——アレルギー　115
象皮症　62,219
側胸動静脈　237
続発性リンパ浮腫　41,44,
　45,58,156

た

ターナー症候群　47,48
ターニケット　232
ダイナミックICGリンパ管
　造影　71,72
胎児浮腫　103
大胸筋　237
大伏在静脈　39,120
大網移行術　8,9
第1趾間リンパ管移植法　18
端側吻合　272
弾性着衣　230,233

ち

チーム医療　306
治癒　145
治療戦略　142
遅発性リンパ浮腫　41,81,84,
　167
中皮細胞　221
中皮腫　221
超音波式脂肪吸引器　231
腸管弁移行術　8

つ

釣り針式開創器　278

て

テストステロン　224
デスモゾーム　65
定常相　72,75

と

特発性リンパ浮腫　41,43

な

内皮間接着　65
内皮細胞間隙　101
内皮小孔　94

に

二次性リンパ浮腫　64,156,
　157
二重睫毛　51
乳癌　216
乳腺切除術　216
乳び腹胸水　261
乳房再建　216

ぬ

ヌーナン症候群　48

ね

ネクスト分類　215

の

囊胞性リンパ管腫　48

は

バンクロフト糸状虫　57
パラシュート法　283,284
白色線維　88
腫れ　54
反復性蜂窩織炎　91,94

ひ

皮切　237
皮膚壊死　161
非可逆性リンパ浮腫　62
微小血管吻合　268

ふ

フィラリア感染　57
プロスタグランディン E₁
　247
不顕性リンパ浮腫　62,142,
　163,165
伏在静脈　240
副神経リンパ節　29
腹膜硬化症　221
複合的理学療法　6,215,258
吻合　272
　——, λ　192,286
　——, π　191
　——, all-star　287
　——, EE　280,281,282
　——, ES　272,280,281,
　282
　——, Ladder　286
　——, multiple　192
　——, SE　191,280,281,
　282
　——, SS　280,281,282
　——, 基本　282
　——, 端側　272
　——, 微小血管　268
　——, 輸出リンパ管静脈
　164
　——, 予防的　21,153,265
　——, ラムダ　272

へ

ヘルパー T 細胞 2　235
平滑筋細胞　243,258
閉鎖血管系　54
閉所恐怖症　115
閉塞性リンパ浮腫　156,169
扁平線維芽細胞　102

ほ

母児相関　225
放射線被曝　127
蜂窩織炎　60,156
　——, 反復性　91,94

ま

マイクロ剪刀　274
マクロファージ　229
　——, 2 型　235
マッピング　72
マレー糸状虫　57
前川分類　120
　——タイプ I　121
　——タイプ II　121
　——タイプ III　122
　——タイプ IV　122
　——タイプ V　123
慢性リンパ浮腫　221,224

み

ミルキングテスト　280
ミルロイ病　49,56
脈管外通液路　220

む

むくみ　54

め

メージュ病　51
免疫不全状態　235

も

毛細リンパ管　34,55,167

ゆ

輸出リンパ管　2,160
　——静脈吻合　164
遊離皮弁　268
遊離リンパ管移植法　15

よ

予防的吻合　21,153,265

ら

ラムダ吻合　272

り

リンパ液　54,59
　——還流障害　114
リンパ管　25,104
　——拡張　64
　——奇形　116,167
　——機能　232
　——系統発生　25
　——個体発生　25
　——硬化　141,157,160
　——内圧　64,70
　——の電顕像　22
　——の同定　130
　——のポンプ作用　35
　——変性・硬化　64
　——, 集合　35,36,167
　——, 浅集合　34
　——, 前集合　167
　——, 毛細　34,55,167
リンパ管炎　57
リンパ管細静脈吻合術　34,
　160,180,181,243,252,258,
　289,301
　——, 顕微鏡下　244
　——, 超微小的　16
リンパ管腫　221
　——, 嚢胞性　48
リンパ管静脈吻合術　12,14,
　60,180,181
　——, 顕微鏡下　14,243
　——, 古典的　14,160
リンパシンチグラフィ　70,
　112,119,126,137,157,158,
　168,195
リンパ脂肪弁　202
　——挙上　202
　——(第 1 趾間)　202,204
　——, 血管柄付き　237
リンパ循環動態　64,71,142,
　157
リンパ静脈シャント　160
リンパ節　25

――，郭清　25
――，系統発生　25
――，個体発生　25
――，の再生　25
――，内深頸　29
――，腋窩　37
――，オトガイ下　27
――，顎下　27,211
――，後頭　27
――，鎖骨上　29,211
――，三角胸筋　37
――，耳後　27
――，耳前　27
――，浅頸　29
――，浅鼠径　39
――，副神経　29
リンパ節移植　6,170,211,
　213,215,216
　　――，血管柄付き　16,140,
　　141,145,156,160,170,258
リンパ節炎　57

リンパ組織　25
　　――，系統発生　25
　　――，個体発生　25
リンパ側副路　64,70,143
リンパ道の回復　25
リンパ嚢胞　113,167
　　――，骨盤内　113,260
　　――，骨盤　172
リンパ浮腫　48,55,59,219
　　――病期分類　70
　　――，陰部　123,265
　　――，下肢　113,119,251
　　――，可逆性　62
　　――，家族性先天性下肢　49
　　――，原発性　81,82,114,
　　116,167
　　――，上肢　211,249
　　――，進行　142
　　――，先天性　41,47,56,
　　81,84,167
　　――，潜在性　62

――，全身性　51
――，早期　142
――，早発性　41,56,81,
84,167
――，続発性　41,44,45,
48,156
――，遅発性　41,81,84,
167
――，特発性　41,43
――，二次性　64,156,157
――，非可逆性　62
――，不顕性　62,142,163,
165
――，閉塞性　156,169
――，慢性　221,224
リンパ流閉塞　156
リンパ漏出　70

レーザードプラ　232

欧文索引

2型マクロファージ　235
λ吻合　192,286
π吻合　191

Brorson H　7,229,231
Kinmonth JB　1,8,9,41,47
O'Brien MB　14,243

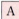

ADB(arm DB) stage　75,
　183
adipose tissue　220
aging regression　223
all-star anastomosis　287
anastomosis
　　――，all-star　287
　　――，classical lymphatico-
　　venous　160
　　――，double end-to-end
　　191
　　――，EE(end-to-end)　280,
　　281,282
　　――，ES(end-to-side)　272,

280,281,282
　　――，flow-through　191
　　――，Ladder　286
　　――，Lambda　286
　　――，multiple　192
　　――，SE(side-to-end)　191,
　　280,281,282
　　――，SS(side-to-side)　280,
　　281,282
angiosarcoma　156
aplasia　41
autoimmune diseases　225

CCT(controlled compression
　therapy)　230
CDT(combined physical thera-
　py)　6,215,258
CEBPファミリー　235
Charles法　7
chronic lymphedema　222,225
classical lymphaticovenous
　anastomosis　160

compression therapy　230
congenital　47
　　――lymphedema　41,56,
　　81,84,167

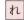

DB(Dermal Backflow)　57,
　72,77,149
DB stage　75,142
　　――Ⅰ　143,163
　　――Ⅱ　144,163
　　――Ⅲ　145
　　――Ⅳ　145
　　――Ⅴ　145
DDB(distal DB) pattern　81,
　82,84,168,169,170
degeneration　66
Degni法　14
Diffuse　67,68,77,135,136,
　137,139,141,157,280
dry technique　230

索引

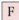

early diagnosis　148
early lymphedema　142
early transient phase　74
EE(end-to-end) anastomosis　280,281,282
elastography　129
elephantiasis　63,219
ELVA(efferent lymphatic vessel-to-venous anastomosis)　144,164,165
embryonic edema　104
estrogen　225
ES(end-to-side) anastomosis　272,280,281,282
extravascular fluid pathways　220

fat deposition　223
FDB(facial DB) stage　76
feto-maternal relationship　225
flow-through　272
Földi 法　6,215,258

GDB(genital DB) stage　75
Gillies & Fraser 法　8

Hennekam syndrome　51
Homan 法　7
hyperplasia　41
hypoplasia　41

I

ICG(indocyanine green)　5
ICG classification　81,82,83,84
ICG lymphography　67,70,112,119,135,137,148,157,158,168,280
──検査　128,215
──所見　182
──の感度・特異度　168
──, ダイナミック　71,72
ICGv(ICG velocity)　72,74,145
irreversible lymphedema　63
ISL(International Society of Lymphology)　70
──stage　163
IVaS(intra-vascular stenting)　269,283,285
──端側吻合法　272
──の欠点　274
──の実際　269
──の抜去　271
──の利点　274

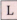

Kinmonth 法　8,9
Kondoleon 法　7,8

L

Ladder anastomosis　286
Lambda anastomosis　286
late plateau phase　74
LDB(leg DB) stage　75,183
LDI(laser Doppler imaging)　232
LE(less enhancement) pattern　81,83,84,168,170
Linear　67,68,77,135,137,139,140,157,280
lipedema　219
liposuction　232
LNT(lymph node transfer)　16,140,141,145,156,160,170,258
LS(liposuction)　7,160,170,229,232,233,239
LVA(lymphaticovenular anastomosis)　140,141,144,156,165,170,175,180,243,278,289
lymph extravasation　70
lymphangiomas　222

lymphatic vessel　25,104
lymphedema　219
Lymphedema distichiasis syndrome　51
lymphedema precox　41,56,81,84,167
lymphedema tarda　41,81,84,167
lymphodynamics　64,70,71,142,157
lymphoscintigraphy　70,112,119,126,137,157,158,168
lymphosclerosis　68,139,156

M

MCLMR syndrome　50
MCP-1(monocyte chemoattractant protein-1)　235
Meige disease　51
mesothelial cells　222
mesothelioma　222
midaxial line　38
Milroy disease　50
Milroy-like lymphedema　50
MILS(minimally invasive lymphatic supermicrosurgery)　139,140,143,164,165
mono-canalization　282
MR/CT lymphography　158
MRCP(magnetic resonance thoracic ductography)　116
MRL(magnetic resonance lymphography)　114,119
MR 胆膵管撮影　115
MR リンパ管造影法　114,119
MSKCC(Memorial Sloan-Kettering Cancer Center) 分類　31
multiple anastomosis　192

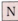

NECST 分類　215
NE(no enhancement) pattern　81,83,84,168,169,170
neo-valvuloplasty　284,287
non-pitting edema　62,70

v

Noonan syndrome 48

O'Brien 法 14, 243
obstructive lymphedema 156
on-pitting edema 141

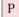

Parachute technique 283, 284
Patency test 245
PDB (proximal DB) pattern 81, 82, 84, 168, 169, 170
perforator flap 268
peritoneal sclerosis 222
pitting edema 70
PLC (pelvic lymphocele) 172, 173
PLC (prelymphatic channel) 101
PPARγ 235
Praecox 47
primary lymphedema 43, 58, 84, 167, 168
progressed lymphedema 142

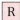

real-time elastography 132
Reticular 74, 75

reticular tissue 220
reverse lymphatic mapping 216, 217
reversible lymphedema 63

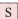

sclerosis 66
secondary lymphedema 41, 44, 45, 58, 156
SEKI (superior-edge-of-the-knee incision) method 290, 291, 296
sensitivity/specificity 169
sequential anastomosis 286
sex difference 225
sex hormones 224
SE (side-to-end) anastomosis 191, 280, 281, 282
Sistrunk 法 7
ski-jump 爪変形 49
SPECT/CT 126, 157, 158
Splash 67, 68, 77, 135, 136, 137, 139, 143, 157, 163, 165
SS (side-to-side) anastomosis 280, 281, 282
Stardust 67, 68, 77, 135, 136, 137, 139, 140, 141, 144, 157, 163, 165, 280
steroid hormones 223
Stewart-Treves syndrome 156

subclinical lymphedema 62, 142, 163, 165
supermicrosurgery 160, 180, 208, 268
supermicrosurgical lymphaticovenular anastomosis 160

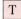

tarda 47
testosterone 225
therapeutic strategy 170
Thompson 法 8
thymic involution 224
thymus 223
TLE (temporary lymphatic expansion) 法 280, 281, 282
TNF-α (tumor necrosisfactor-α) 235
Turner syndrome 47, 48

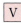

valvuloplasty 287

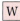

wet-to-dry dressing 279
WILD syndrome 52

vi

略歴 Curriculum Vitae

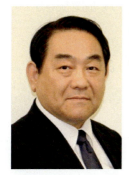

光嶋　勲 (こうしま　いさお)
Isao KOSHIMA
広島大学病院国際リンパ浮腫治療センター　特任教授
Professor and Chief of the International Center for Lymphedema, Hiroshima University Hospital

1976	鳥取大学医学部卒業	Graduated from Tottori University School of Medicine
1983-90	筑波大学臨床医学系形成外科　講師	Assistant Professor, Department of Plastic and Reconstructive Surgery of Tsukuba University
1990-2000	川崎医科大学形成外科　助教授	Associate Professor, Department of Plastic and Reconstructive Surgery of Kawasaki Medical School
2000-04	岡山大学医学部形成再建外科　教授	Professor and Chief, Department of Plastic and Reconstructive Surgery, Okayama University Medical School
2004-17	東京大学医学部形成外科・美容外科　教授	Professor and Chief, Department of Plastic and Reconstructive Surgery, Graduate School of Medicine, University of Tokyo
2011-13	東京大学付属病院　副院長	Vice Director of Tokyo University Hospital
2017	広島大学病院国際リンパ浮腫治療センター　特任教授	Professor and Chief, International Center of Lymphedema, Hiroshima University Hospital
2017	東京大学　名誉教授	Emeritus Professor, University of Tokyo

【主な所属学会】　　　　　　　　　　　　　　　Societies：
世界再建マイクロサージャリー学会(理事長)　　　World Society of Reconstructive Microsurgery
世界リンパ浮腫外科シンポジウム(理事長)　　　　World Symposium on Lymphedema Surgery
国際リンパ学会(バルセロナ名誉会長)　　　　　　International Society of Lymphology
国際形成外科学会　　　　　　　　　　　　　　　International Society of Plastic, Reconstructive and Aesthetic Surgery

日本マイクロサージャリー学会　　　　　　　　　Japanese Society for Reconstructive Microsurgery
日本形成外科学会(特別会員)　　　　　　　　　　Japan Society of Plastic and Reconstructive Surgery
日本手外科学会(特別会員)　　　　　　　　　　　Japanese Society for Surgery of the Hand
日本リンパ学会(常任理事)　　　　　　　　　　　Japanese Society of Lymphology

【近年の国際活動】
2011　シンガポール大学にてリンパ浮腫症例の招聘ライブ手術執刀・講演(2011.2)
　　　バルセロナ大学・サンパウ病院講習会にてリンパ浮腫症例の招聘ライブ手術執刀・講演、見学者300名(2011.3)
　　　ヘルシンキ・世界再建マイクロサージャリー学会ディベートシンポジウム演者(リンパ浮腫)(2011.6)
　　　マドリード・ヨーロッパ頭頸部外科講習会にて招待講演(キメラ型合併移植による顔面広範再建)(2011.9)
　　　ソウル・アサン大学病院講習会にてリンパ浮腫症例の招聘ライブ手術執刀・講演、見学者200名(2011.10)
　　　台北・チャンカン・メイヨー大学カンファランスにて招待講演(超微小外科、リンパ浮腫、穿通枝皮弁など)(2011.10)
　　　チューリッヒ・スイス形成外科学会総会招待講演＆ディベート(リンパ浮腫外科治療を巡って)(2011.11)
　　　スタンフォード大学講習会・超微小外科手術の招聘ライブデモ・講演、見学者50名(2011.11)
　　　北京・日中友好病院にてリンパ浮腫2例招聘手術デモ(2011.12)

2012	ラスベガス・アメリカ微小外科学会にて講演、インストラクショナルコース（リンパ浮腫）（2012.1）
	インド・チェンナイ・ライト病院講習会にてリンパ浮腫3例、顔面神経麻痺例2例の招聘ライブ手術執刀と講演、見学者200名（2012.2）
	バルセロナ大学・サンパウ病院講習会にてリンパ浮腫症例の招聘ライブ手術執刀・講演、見学者300名（2012.3）
	中国無錫（ウーシー）・手外科講習会にて招待講演、参加者150名（2012.4）
	海外向け動画・講演Web-Site開始（http//nmed.jp/koshima/）（2012.5）
	ヘルシンキ大学講習会にてリンパ浮腫症例の招聘ライブ手術執刀、参加者200名（2012.6）
	フランス・アミアン大学講習会にて超微小外科招聘ライブデモ・講演、参加者100名（2012.6）
2013	台北三軍大学病院ライブオペ（2013.3）
	台北・チャンカン記念医科大学にてリンパ浮腫国際シンポジウムライブオペ、参加者200名（2013.4）
	アメリカ手外科学会インストラクショナルコース（サンフランシスコ・2013.10）
	中国手外科招待講演（青島・2013.10）
	ペルー穿通枝皮弁講習会にて招待講演（リマ・2013.10）
	ハーバード大学招聘講演（グランドレクチャー）（ボストン・2013.11）
	ニューヨーク州立大学ライブオペ＆講演（2013.11）
	ペンシルバニア大学屍体解剖デモ＆講演（フィラデルフィア・2013.11）
2014	バンキ教授記念講演（ハワイ・カウアイ島・2014.1：アメリカ再建外科学会でノーベル賞に相当する講演）
	バルセロナ大学にて欧州超微小外科講習会ライブオペ（2014.3）
	国際形成再建美容外科学会にて招待keynote lecture（シンガポール・2014.8）
	トムスク大学にて招待ライブオペ＆講演（シベリア・2014.9）
2015	世界再建マイクロサージャリー学会keynote lecture（ムンバイ・2015.6）

リンパ浮腫の外科的治療

ISBN978-4-907095-40-6 C3047

平成 29 年 9 月 1 日　第 1 版発行

編　集─────光　嶋　　　勲
発 行 者─────山　本　美　惠　子
印 刷 所─────三　報　社　印　刷 株式会社
発 行 所─────株式会社 ぱーそん書房
　　　　　〒101-0062 東京都千代田区神田駿河台 2-4-4 (5 F)
　　　　　電話 (03) 5283-7009 (代表) /Fax (03) 5283-7010

Printed in Japan　　　　　　　　　　　　Ⓒ KOSHIMA Isao, 2017

・本書の複製権・翻訳権・上映権・譲渡権・公衆送信権（送信可能化権を含む）は
　株式会社ぱーそん書房が保有します.
・ JCOPY ＜出版者著作権管理機構 委託出版物＞
　本書の無断複写は著作権法上での例外を除き禁じられています. 複写される場合
　には, その都度事前に出版者著作権管理機構（電話 03-3513-6969, FAX 03-3513-
　6979, e-mail：info@jcopy.or.jp）の許諾を得て下さい.